Advances in Ginsenosides

Advances in Ginsenosides

Editor

Jen-Tsung Chen

MDPI • Basel • Beijing • Wuhan • Barcelona • Belgrade • Manchester • Tokyo • Cluj • Tianjin

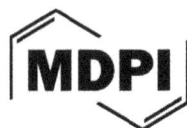

Editor
Jen-Tsung Chen
National University of
Kaohsiung
Taiwan

Editorial Office
MDPI
St. Alban-Anlage 66
4052 Basel, Switzerland

This is a reprint of articles from the Special Issue published online in the open access journal *Biomolecules* (ISSN 2218-273X) (available at: https://www.mdpi.com/journal/biomolecules/special_issues/ginsenosides).

For citation purposes, cite each article independently as indicated on the article page online and as indicated below:

LastName, A.A.; LastName, B.B.; LastName, C.C. Article Title. *Journal Name* **Year**, *Volume Number*, Page Range.

ISBN 978-3-0365-1953-1 (Hbk)
ISBN 978-3-0365-1952-4 (PDF)

© 2021 by the authors. Articles in this book are Open Access and distributed under the Creative Commons Attribution (CC BY) license, which allows users to download, copy and build upon published articles, as long as the author and publisher are properly credited, which ensures maximum dissemination and a wider impact of our publications.

The book as a whole is distributed by MDPI under the terms and conditions of the Creative Commons license CC BY-NC-ND.

Contents

About the Editor .... **vii**

Jen-Tsung Chen
Advances in Ginsenosides
Reprinted from: *Biomolecules* **2020**, *10*, 681, doi:10.3390/biom10050681 .... **1**

Anshul Sharma and Hae-Jeung Lee
Ginsenoside Compound K: Insights into Recent Studies on Pharmacokinetics and
Health-Promoting Activities
Reprinted from: *Biomolecules* **2020**, *10*, 1028, doi:10.3390/biom10071028 .... **5**

Myung Joo Han and Dong-Hyun Kim
Effects of Red and Fermented Ginseng and Ginsenosides on Allergic Disorders
Reprinted from: *Biomolecules* **2020**, *10*, 634, doi:10.3390/biom10040634 .... **47**

Saikat Gantait, Monisha Mitra and Jen-Tsung Chen
Biotechnological Interventions for Ginsenosides Production
Reprinted from: *Biomolecules* **2020**, *10*, 538, doi:10.3390/biom10040538 .... **65**

Byeong-Min Jeon, Jong-In Baek, Min-Sung Kim, Sun-Chang Kim and Chang-hao Cui
Characterization of a Novel Ginsenoside MT1 Produced by an Enzymatic Transrhamnosylation
of Protopanaxatriol-Type Ginsenosides Re
Reprinted from: *Biomolecules* **2020**, *10*, 525, doi:10.3390/biom10040525 .... **83**

Yu-Shi Wang, He Li, Yang Li, Shiyin Zhang and Ying-Hua Jin
(20S)G-Rh2 Inhibits NF-κB Regulated Epithelial-Mesenchymal Transition by Targeting
Annexin A2
Reprinted from: *Biomolecules* **2020**, *10*, 528, doi:10.3390/biom10040528 .... **95**

Jung-Mi Oh, Jae Hoon Jeong, Sun Young Park and Sungkun Chun
Ginsenoside Compound K Induces Adult Hippocampal Proliferation and Survival of Newly
Generated Cells in Young and Elderly Mice
Reprinted from: *Biomolecules* **2020**, *10*, 484, doi:10.3390/biom10030484 .... **111**

Dong-Soon Im
Pro-Resolving Effect of Ginsenosides as an Anti-Inflammatory Mechanism of *Panax ginseng*
Reprinted from: *Biomolecules* **2020**, *10*, 444, doi:10.3390/biom10030444 .... **125**

Wei Chen, Prabhu Balan and David G Popovich
Comparison of Ginsenoside Components of Various Tissues of New Zealand Forest-Grown
Asian Ginseng (*Panax Ginseng*) and American Ginseng (*Panax Quinquefolium* L.)
Reprinted from: *Biomolecules* **2020**, *10*, 372, doi:10.3390/biom10030372 .... **137**

Muhammad Zubair Siddiqi, Sathiyaraj Srinivasan, Hye Yoon Park and Wan-Taek Im
Exploration and Characterization of Novel Glycoside Hydrolases from the Whole Genome
of *Lactobacillus ginsenosidimutans* and Enriched Production of Minor Ginsenoside Rg3(S) by a
Recombinant Enzymatic Process
Reprinted from: *Biomolecules* **2020**, *10*, 288, doi:10.3390/biom10020288 .... **153**

Young-Jun Park, Minkyoung Cho, Garam Choi, Hyeongjin Na and Yeonseok Chung
A Critical Regulation of Th17 Cell Responses and Autoimmune Neuro-Inflammation by Ginsenoside Rg3
Reprinted from: *Biomolecules* **2020**, *10*, 122, doi:10.3390/biom10010122 173

Wenna Guo, Zhiyong Li, Meng Yuan, Geng Chen, Qiao Li, Hui Xu and Xin Yang
Molecular Insight into Stereoselective ADME Characteristics of C20-24 Epimeric Epoxides of Protopanaxadiol by Docking Analysis
Reprinted from: *Biomolecules* **2020**, *10*, 112, doi:10.3390/biom10010112 185

In-Seon Lee, Ki Sung Kang and Song-Yi Kim
Panax ginseng Pharmacopuncture: Current Status of the Research and Future Challenges
Reprinted from: *Biomolecules* **2020**, *10*, 33, doi:10.3390/biom10010033 197

Weijie Xie, Ting Zhu, Xi Dong, Fengwei Nan, Xiangbao Meng, Ping Zhou, Guibo Sun and Xiaobo Sun
HMGB1-triggered inflammation inhibition of notoginseng leaf triterpenes against cerebral ischemia and reperfusion injury via MAPK and NF-κB signaling pathways
Reprinted from: *Biomolecules* **2019**, *9*, 512, doi:10.3390/biom9100512 217

Dahye Yoon, Bo-Ram Choi, Young-Chang Kim, Seon Min Oh, Hyoung-Geun Kim, Jang-Uk Kim, Nam-In Baek, Suhkmann Kim and Dae Young Lee
Comparative Analysis of *Panax ginseng* Berries from Seven Cultivars Using UPLC-QTOF/MS and NMR-Based Metabolic Profiling
Reprinted from: *Biomolecules* **2019**, *9*, 424, doi:10.3390/biom9090424 239

About the Editor

Jen-Tsung Chen is currently a professor at the National University of Kaohsiung in Taiwan. He teaches cell biology, genomics, proteomics, medicinal plant biotechnology, and plant tissue culture. Dr. Chen's research interests include bioactive compounds, chromatography techniques, plant tissue culture, phytochemicals, and plant biotechnology. He serves as an editorial board member of Plant Methods, Biomolecules, International Journal of Molecular Sciences, and a guest editor in Frontiers in Plant Science, Frontiers in Pharmacology, and Journal of Fungi.

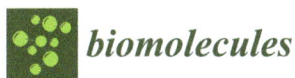

Editorial

Advances in Ginsenosides

Jen-Tsung Chen

Department of Life Sciences, National University of Kaohsiung, Kaohsiung 811, Taiwan; jentsung@nuk.edu.tw

Received: 24 April 2020; Accepted: 27 April 2020; Published: 28 April 2020

Ginsenosides are unique to plants that belong to the *Panax* genus. The genus name *Panax* means "all-curing" in Greek, and one of the representative plants, Asian ginseng (*Panax ginseng* Meyer), has been classified as a top-grade herb in traditional Chinese medicine according to the Divine Husbandman's Herbal Foundation Canon. It has been used as medicine as well as a tonic for over two thousand years and is still popular with increasing demand in oriental countries nowadays. It has long been recognized that ginseng remedies possess a wide range of benefits for human health. However, their bioactivities are diverse, interconnective, and complicated that need to be clarified. Hence, this special issue attempts to explore new insights into characterization, quantitation, production, biotechnology as well as bioactivities of ginsenosides.

1. Characterization and Quantitation

Up to date, there are more than one hundred ginsenosides have been identified. Jeon et al. reported a new protopanaxatriol-type ginsenoside, namely ginsenoside MT1, that occasionally obtained from enzymatic converted products derived from ginsenoside Re [1]. They suggested potential commercial applications of MT1 with nutraceutical, pharmaceutical or cosmeceutical values, and further tests for the pharmacological effects are ongoing. Chen et al. profiled ginsenoside components from various parts of Asian ginseng (*P. ginseng* Meyer) and American ginseng (*P. quinquefolium* L.) that grown in the North Island of New Zealand mainly using liquid chromatography-tandem mass spectrometry (LC-MS/MS) analysis [2]. They found these two species of ginseng have a similar number and total amounts of ginsenosides. Yoon et al. profiled primary metabolites and ginsenoside constituents of *P. ginseng* berries from seven cultivars using high-resolution magic-angle-spinning nuclear magnetic resonance (HR-MAS NMR) spectroscopy and ultra-performance liquid chromatography-quadrupole-time-of-flight mass spectrometry (UPLC-QTOF/MS), respectively [3]. They confirmed that a characteristic metabolic pattern presented in the cultivar Gopoong, and a differential content of 20(S)-protopanaxatriol (PPT)-type ginsenosides was found in the cultivars Kumpoong and Sunwon.

2. Production and Biotechnology

In the ginseng extract, ginsenoside Rg3(S) only presents a limited amount and its production could be enhanced conventionally by the steaming method and heat acid treatment but some inevitable by-products were also produced in the meantime. Siddiqi et al. established an alternative way using a novel glycoside hydrolase for the enzymatic conversion of ginsenoside Rg3(S) from ginsenosides Rb1 and Rd [4]. The enzyme originated from *Lactobacillus ginsenosidimutans* EMML 3041^T that exited in Korean fermented pickle (kimchi), and subsequent has been modified into a recombinant enzyme, namely BglL.gin-952. According to the results, the authors proposed that BglL.gin-952 has a high ability of biotransformation that could be applied in the industrial level production of ginsenoside Rg3(S) in the future. Gantait et al. summarized the approaches of in vitro plant biotechnology for ginsenosides production [5]. It is an intensive topic that many tools that have been reported for this purpose, including bioreactor, genetic transformation, in vitro mutagenesis, hairy root culture, polyploidy induction, as well as conventional tissue-culture protocols such as adventitious root culture, callus culture, cell suspension, direct organogenesis, liquid culture, protoplast culture, and somatic embryogenesis, together with the utilization of additives, elicitors, and precursors.

3. Bioactivities

Epithelial–mesenchymal transition (EMT) is crucial for differentiation and development, and it is also a key step in cancer metastasis. Wang et al. studied the effect of the (20S)ginsenoside Rh2 (G-Rh2) on EMT, and they concluded that in a human breast cancer cell line, G-Rh2 could inhibit the NF-κB activation as well as the related EMT by targeting an NF-κB p50 subunit binding protein annexin A2 [6].

It has been recognized that adult neurogenesis in the hippocampus is the main contributor to prevent age-related cognitive impairments as well as neurodegenerative diseases. Oh et al. investigated the effect of compound K (CK), a product from ginsenosides Rb1, Rb2, and Rc through intestinal microbial conversion, on hippocampal neurogenesis in mice [7]. They found CK promoted cell proliferation in the dentate gyrus of both young and elderly mice. Hence, the authors proposed that CK has the potential benefit against neurodegenerative disorders such as Alzheimer's disease.

Ischemic stroke is a serious cerebrovascular disease and it is one of the leading causes of death worldwide. Xie et al. studied the bioactivity of notoginseng leaf triterpenes (PNGL) on cerebral ischemia and reperfusion injury of ischemic stroke [8]. The results showed that PNGL decreased the expression of the high mobility group box-1 protein (HMGB1) and consequently inhibited HMGB1-triggered inflammation. In addition, a reduction of several pro-inflammatory mediators, as well as a suppression of the activation of MAPKs and NF-κB signaling pathways, were found in the presence of PNGL.

In autoimmune diseases, IL-17A-producing CD4$^+$ T cells (Th17) were recognized as critically pathogenic immune cells that mediate tissue inflammation. Park et al. demonstrated that ginsenoside Rg3 inhibited Th17 differentiation as well as Th17-mediated neuro-inflammation in a dendritic cell-T co-culture system [9]. The authors suggested that Rg3 could be a potential agent for treating certain autoimmune disorders driven by Th17 cells.

Allergies including allergic rhinitis, anaphylaxis, asthma, atopic conjunctivitis, atopic dermatitis, pruritus, and so on, are common disorders worldwide with prevalence ranges from 10% to 40% population. Han and Kim summarized the effects of white ginseng (WG, dried root of *Panax* sp.), red ginseng (RG, steamed and dried root of *Panax* sp.), and fermented WG and RG (fWG and fRG) on allergic disorders [10]. Overall, the extract of fRG and ginsenosides CK, Rh1, and Rh2 have better potential than other ginseng remedies to alleviate allergic disorders.

Inflammation is part of immunity associated with diseases and physiological conditions. Im refined the knowledge of ginsenosides for anti-inflammation and summarized the action mechanism [11]. It was proposed that ginsenosides exert their anti-inflammation actions through retarding expressions of pro-inflammatory cytokines, TNF-α, IL-1β, and IL-6, and enzymes, iNOS, and COX-2, in M1-polarized macrophages. Besides, it was mentioned that a new focusing on the pro-resolving effect of ginsenosides in M2-polarized macrophages is emerging.

Theoretically, the understanding of molecular mechanisms involved in ligand–protein interactions is crucial for drug design. Guo et al. investigated the chirality of C20-24 epimeric epoxides that transformed from protopanaxadiol-type ginsenosides [12]. Through the analysis of molecular docking, the authors confirmed consistency in some previous cell/animal-based experimental findings and gain insights into the stereo-selectivity of ginsenosides. Their findings could support the rational development of ginseng products in the future.

An overview of the *P. ginseng* pharmacopuncture was reported by Lee et al. to systematically refine safety, physiological responses, and clinical effects regarding the manufacturing processes [13]. The authors concluded that the process should be standardized including a comprehensive comparison of the quantity and quality of ginsenoside components of injections for improving clinical outcomes in the future.

4. Conclusions and Perspectives

This special issue collected recent innovative research and review articles on analytical techniques, production protocols, biotechnological tools, and new insights into bioactivities of ginsenosides including the effects on epithelial–mesenchymal transition, hippocampal neurogenesis and inflammation as well as on diseases such as ischemic stroke, autoimmune diseases, and allergic disorders. In addition, the analysis through molecular docking and an overview of the *P. ginseng* pharmacopuncture were also included. With the rapid development of molecular tools such as high-throughput technologies and integrative multi-omics, there are more opportunities for scientists to clarify the efficacy of ginseng products and the ginsenoside components in the future.

Conflicts of Interest: The author declares no conflicts of interest.

References

1. Jeon, B.-M.; Baek, J.-I.; Kim, M.-S.; Kim, S.-C.; Cui, C.-H. Characterization of a Novel Ginsenoside MT1 Produced by an Enzymatic Transrhamnosylation of Protopanaxatriol-Type Ginsenosides Re. *Biomolecules* **2020**, *10*, 525. [CrossRef] [PubMed]
2. Chen, W.; Balan, P.; Popovich, D.G. Comparison of Ginsenoside Components of Various Tissues of New Zealand Forest-Grown Asian Ginseng (*Panax ginseng*) and American Ginseng (*Panax quinquefolium* L.). *Biomolecules* **2020**, *10*, 372. [CrossRef] [PubMed]
3. Yoon, D.; Choi, B.-R.; Kim, Y.-C.; Oh, S.M.; Kim, H.-G.; Kim, J.-U.; Baek, N.-I.; Kim, S.; Lee, D.Y. Comparative Analysis of *Panax ginseng* Berries from Seven Cultivars Using UPLC-QTOF/MS and NMR-Based Metabolic Profiling. *Biomolecules* **2019**, *9*, 424. [CrossRef] [PubMed]
4. Siddiqi, M.Z.; Srinivasan, S.; Park, H.Y.; Im, W.-T. Exploration and Characterization of Novel Glycoside Hydrolases from the Whole Genome of *Lactobacillus ginsenosidimutans* and Enriched Production of Minor Ginsenoside Rg3(S) by a Recombinant Enzymatic Process. *Biomolecules* **2020**, *10*, 288. [CrossRef] [PubMed]
5. Gantait, S.; Mitra, M.; Chen, J.-T. Biotechnological Interventions for Ginsenosides Production. *Biomolecules* **2020**, *10*, 538. [CrossRef] [PubMed]
6. Wang, Y.-S.; Li, H.; Li, Y.; Zhang, S.; Jin, Y.-H. (20S)G-Rh2 Inhibits NF-κB Regulated Epithelial-Mesenchymal Transition by Targeting Annexin A2. *Biomolecules* **2020**, *10*, 528. [CrossRef] [PubMed]
7. Oh, J.-M.; Jeong, J.H.; Park, S.Y.; Chun, S. Ginsenoside Compound K Induces Adult Hippocampal Proliferation and Survival of Newly Generated Cells in Young and Elderly Mice. *Biomolecules* **2020**, *10*, 484. [CrossRef] [PubMed]
8. Xie, W.; Zhu, T.; Dong, X.; Nan, F.; Meng, X.; Zhou, P.; Sun, G.; Sun, X. HMGB1-triggered inflammation inhibition of notoginseng leaf triterpenes against cerebral ischemia and reperfusion injury via MAPK and NF-κB signaling pathways. *Biomolecules* **2019**, *9*, 512. [CrossRef] [PubMed]
9. Park, Y.-J.; Cho, M.; Choi, G.; Na, H.; Chung, Y. A Critical Regulation of Th17 Cell Responses and Autoimmune Neuro-Inflammation by Ginsenoside Rg3. *Biomolecules* **2020**, *10*, 122. [CrossRef] [PubMed]
10. Han, M.J.; Kim, D.-H. Effects of Red and Fermented Ginseng and Ginsenosides on Allergic Disorders. *Biomolecules* **2020**, *10*, 634. [CrossRef] [PubMed]
11. Im, D.-S. Pro-Resolving Effect of Ginsenosides as an Anti-Inflammatory Mechanism of *Panax ginseng*. *Biomolecules* **2020**, *10*, 444. [CrossRef]
12. Guo, W.; Li, Z.; Yuan, M.; Chen, G.; Li, Q.; Xu, H.; Yang, X. Molecular Insight into Stereoselective ADME Characteristics of C20-24 Epimeric Epoxides of Protopanaxadiol by Docking Analysis. *Biomolecules* **2020**, *10*, 112. [CrossRef]
13. Lee, I.-S.; Kang, K.S.; Kim, S.-Y. Panax ginseng Pharmacopuncture: Current Status of the Research and Future Challenges. *Biomolecules* **2020**, *10*, 33. [CrossRef] [PubMed]

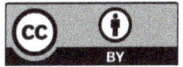

© 2020 by the author. Licensee MDPI, Basel, Switzerland. This article is an open access article distributed under the terms and conditions of the Creative Commons Attribution (CC BY) license (http://creativecommons.org/licenses/by/4.0/).

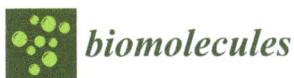

Review

Ginsenoside Compound K: Insights into Recent Studies on Pharmacokinetics and Health-Promoting Activities

Anshul Sharma [1] and Hae-Jeung Lee [1,2,*]

1 Department of Food and Nutrition, College of Bionanotechnology, Gachon University, Gyeonggi-do 13120, Korea; anshul.silb18@gmail.com
2 Institute for Aging and Clinical Nutrition Research, Gachon University, Gyeonggi-do 13120, Korea
* Correspondence: skysea1010@gmail.com; Tel.: +82-31-750-5968; Fax: +82-31-724-4411

Received: 11 June 2020; Accepted: 7 July 2020; Published: 10 July 2020

Abstract: Ginseng (*Panax ginseng*) is an herb popular for its medicinal and health properties. Compound K (CK) is a secondary ginsenoside biotransformed from major ginsenosides. Compound K is more bioavailable and soluble than its parent ginsenosides and hence of immense importance. The review summarizes health-promoting in vitro and in vivo studies of CK between 2015 and 2020, including hepatoprotective, anti-inflammatory, anti-atherosclerosis, anti-diabetic, anti-cancer, neuroprotective, anti-aging/skin protective, and others. Clinical trial data are minimal and are primarily based on CK-rich fermented ginseng. Besides, numerous preclinical and clinical studies indicating the pharmacokinetic behavior of CK, its parent compound (Rb1), and processed ginseng extracts are also summarized. With the limited evidence available from animal and clinical studies, it can be stated that CK is safe and well-tolerated. However, lower water solubility, membrane permeability, and efflux significantly diminish the efficacy of CK and restrict its clinical application. We found that the use of nanocarriers and cyclodextrin for CK delivery could overcome these limitations as well as improve the health benefits associated with them. However, these derivatives have not been clinically evaluated, thus requiring a safety assessment for human therapy application. Future studies should be aimed at investigating clinical evidence of CK.

Keywords: ginseng; compound M1; hepatoprotective; anti-cancer; anti-inflammation; anti-diabetic; safety

1. Introduction

Ginseng (*Panax ginseng*) of the Araliaceae family is a perennial plant which has been conventionally used as a functional food. It is commonly consumed as a health supplement in Korea, Japan, China, the United Kingdom, Canada, Germany, France, and Austria [1]. Ginseng's bioactive constituents, including ginsenosides, phenolic compounds, and polysaccharides, have several medical uses [2]. Ginsenosides (or panaxosides) are the key pharmacologically significant bioactive constituents of ginseng. Nearly 150 ginsenosides isolated from roots, fruits, leaves, flower buds, processed items of ginseng, and other species have been identified [3]. A category of triterpene and saponin ginsenosides are divided into two forms: tetracyclic triterpenoids (four-ring dammarane type) and pentacyclic triterpenoids (five-ring oleanolic type) [4]. The dammarane type saponins are further categorized into protopanaxadiol (PPD) and protopanaxatriol (PPT) saponins [5]. The ginsenosides of PPD group constitute Compound K (CK), Rg3, Ra1, Ra3, Ra2, Rh2, Rb1, Rb3, Rb2, F2, Rc, and Rd, while PPT group constitutes of F1, Rg1, Rg2, Rf, Re, and Rh1 [3,6]. The oleanolic type saponins, such as Ro, are very low in concentration and thus rarely detected [4,5]. Examples of rare ginsenosides are CK, Rg3, F2, and Rh2, which are either absent in unprocessed ginseng or available at low concentrations [7]. It is well-known that compared to ginsenosides, their metabolite CK is absorbed well by the body and in lieu of this property, CK is becoming the fast focus of research [8].

Ginsenoside CK (G-CK; 20-O-β-D-glucopyranosyl-20(S)-protopanaxadiol) is a minor tetracyclic triterpenoid, also known as IH901, CK, and M1 [9]. Compound K is absent from natural ginseng and was isolated by researchers from Japan in 1972 by several biotransformation approaches from saponins such as Rc, Rb1, and Rb2 [10]. The various processes used for the CK synthesis include enzymatic use [11], microbial conversion [3,4,12], heating [13], mycelial fermentation [14] and metabolic engineering [15]. The detailed procedure of biotransformation has been described in detail elsewhere [3]. Compound K is a major deglycosylated metabolite found in organs or blood after oral ingestion of PPD ginsenosides in the human gastrointestinal (GI) tract (Figure 1) [11]. The molecular weight and chemical formula of CK are 622.86 g/mol and $C_{36}H_{62}O_8$, respectively [16].

A review by Yang et al. [11] described in detail the biotransformation of CK and recorded its pharmacological activities until 2014. Another review [3] compiled information on the biotransformation and pharmacokinetics of CK, including the positive effects on neuroprotection and cognitive improvement by 2016. Like the previously published reviews, this paper documents recent papers targeting hepatoprotective, anti-inflammatory, anti-atherosclerosis, anti-diabetic, anti-cancer, neuroprotective, anti-aging/skin protective effects published from 2015 to 2020. This review, however, differs significantly from previous works, including detailed information on preclinical and clinical pharmacokinetic studies and the inclusion of anti-asthmatic and kidney-protective effects among others in vitro and in vivo activities of CK. Additionally, data are also integrated on several CK derivatives with improved solubility and health-promoting activities. Finally, recently published clinical studies are also summarized. Herein, we briefly discuss the recent reports on the pharmacokinetics and health effects of CK and elucidate on how the modification of CK improves metabolic properties, pharmacokinetics, and bioactivities of CK.

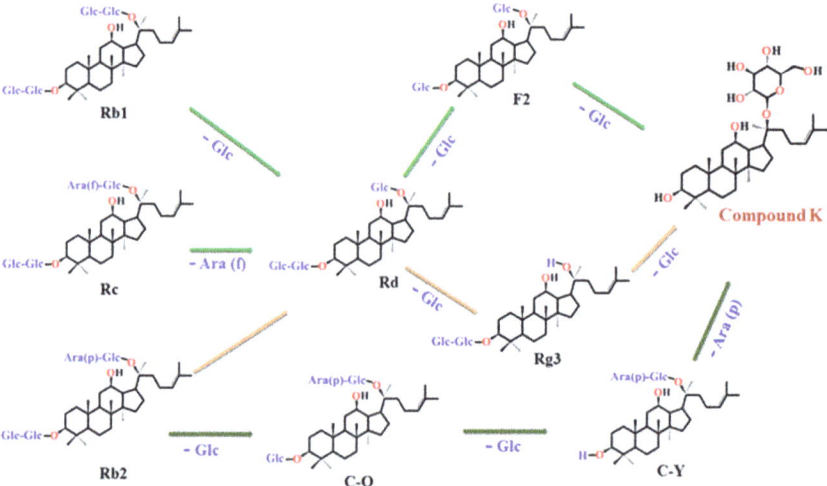

Figure 1. Schematic illustration of plausible biotransformation of major ginsenosides Rb1, Rb2 and Rc to compound K.

2. Literature Search

A precise literature search was carried out with Google Scholar, PubMed, and the Science Direct repositories for related findings between January 2015 and May 2020. The following keywords: "Ginsenoside compound K" or "Compound K" or "20-O-D-glucopyranosyl-20(S)-protopanaxadiol" or "IH901" or "M1" or "health-promoting activities of compound K," or "Ginsenoside Compound K and pharmacokinetics," "Compound M1," and "fermented ginseng," were used to find all the relevant literature published on CK, its pharmacological activities, and modifications conferred on its structure so as to augment solubility and bio permeability.

3. Pharmacokinetics, Metabolism and Safety of Compound K

Compound K has recently been the focus of research for its bioactivities; however, little is known about its pharmacokinetic behavior, solubility, bioavailability and safety.

3.1. Preclinical Perspective (Pharmacokinetic)

It is important to have an in-depth knowledge of how pro-and prebiotics affect adsorption, distribution, metabolism, and excretion (ADME) of drugs. In this line, the effect of prebiotic fiber (NUTRIOSE®) on the pharmacokinetic behavior of CK was investigated using Sprague-Dawley (SD) rats. NUTRIOSE® treatment displayed a dose-dependent rise in plasma concentration (C_{max}), area under the plasma concentration-time curve (AUC), and a decrease in time of maximum concentration (T_{max}) values compared to control. Moreover, the increased glycosidase activity led to the synthesis of CK in the internal intestinal constituents. In addition, NUTRIOSE® has substantially triggered the biotransformation of CK by in vitro grown gut microbiota [17]. This study was in par with earlier findings wherein gut microbiome and diet were reported for possible effects on the concentration of CK in plasma [8,18].

In a study, fermented and non-fermented red ginseng extracts were administered to SD rats. Based on the pharmacokinetics parameters, CK absorption was found to be more in the fermented group than non-fermented group (Table 1) [19]. In another study, the pharmacokinetics of the oral administration of *P. ginseng* extract was evaluated in plasma, urine, and fecal samples using SD rats. The study used liquid chromatography (LC)-mass spectrometry (MS)/MS for identifying and quantifying major saponins and their metabolites present in *P. ginseng* extract. The C_{max}, T_{max}, and AUC, were significantly higher for CK (in rat plasma) compared to other ginsenosides, including Re, Rg1, Rc, Rf, Rb1, Rg2, Rb2, Rd, F1, and F2. The study for the first time documented the comprehensive pharmacokinetics of ginsenosides and their metabolites following oral intake of *P. ginseng*. Earlier studies documented the pharmacokinetic properties of several individual ginsenosides only [20].

In another study from Japan, the oral pharmacokinetic behavior of CK/gamma-cyclodextrin (K/γ-CyD, 1:1) in SD rats has been described. The strong dissolution behavior of CK (K/γ-CyD) was attributed to a higher significant change in C_{max}, AUC values and a lower T_{max} compared with CK and K/β-CyD (Table 1). The stability constant for (K/γ-CyD, 1:1) complex was 18 times (1.5×10^5 M^{-1}) than that of the β-CyD complex (8.2×10^3 M^{-1}). The compound-complex (K/γ-CyD, 1:1) displayed a faster dissolution rate compared to K/γ-CyD complex at 1:3 ratios. The study concluded that partial inclusion complexes are more advantageous for improving the solubility of CK compared to complete inclusion [21].

3.2. Clinical Perspective (Pharmacokinetic)

Previously, the pharmacokinetics of CK was studied as part of the ingestion of whole ginseng extract. In one study, the intake of fermented red ginseng extract showed a higher concentration (more than 10 times) of CK in plasma compared to its unfermented counterpart in a study of healthy Korean volunteers. In the fermented group, AUC was 15.5-fold higher than the non-fermented group, and the mean C_{max} was 27-fold higher compared to the unfermented group. A lower T_{max} was observed in the fermented group than non-fermented group (Table 1). Compared to a previous study [22] where subjects were administered with 5 g of Korean red ginseng, this study showed larger AUC, higher C_{max}, and longer T_{max} values with lower (3 g) amount of fermented red ginseng. The authors described the differences in the pharmacokinetic parameters plausibly due to different methods used for fermentation of red ginseng. Of note, the study also confirmed these effects in vivo and found absorption of CK was more in humans compared to rats. The study also highlighted that absorption of CK depends upon the interspecies variability between humans and rats [19]. It has also been reported that the fermentation of white ginseng had less effect on CK absorption compared with red ginseng fermentation [23].

Likewise, another study compared the pharmacokinetics of CK after oral administering fermented ginseng (FG, by *Lactobacillus (L.) paracasei* A221) and non-fermented ginseng (NFG) in healthy Japanese adults. A higher C_{max} and a lower T_{max} value of CK was observed for FG compared to NFG (Table 1). The mean AUC value from 0 to 12 h was 58.3-times, and AUC value from 0 to 24 h was 17.5-times higher than the NFG. Furthermore, following 24 h supplementation, the mean concentration of testosterone was increased significantly in the male subjects treated with FG [24]. The findings concluded that the transformation of ginseng extract by *L. paracasei* A221 resulted in improved health in Japanese subjects. This is the first research on Japanese subjects which evaluates the health properties of *P. ginseng*. The positive bio transforming role of *L. paracasei* A221 modulating bioavailability and functional aspects has also been described [25]. In recent research, LC-MS was used to spot 13 ginsenosides in the human plasma following two-week recurrent supplementation of red ginseng extract. Among 13 ginsenosides, CK, Rh2, PPD, and PPT were detected in the subject's plasma, although initially not presented in red ginseng extract, suggesting the formation of these ginsenosides after bioconversion in the GI tract. The C_{max}, T_{max}, and AUC values were found to be higher for CK among 13 ginsenosides. The authors further identified a large variation in the concentration of CK among subjects owing to their metabolic differences associated with microorganisms of the GI tract (Table 1) [26].

In a recent randomized, open-label, single-sequence study, the participants were administered with the red ginseng product of a single dose and two-week repeated dose. The quantities of CK, Rc, Rb1, Rd, and Rb2 ginsenosides in plasma of the human subjects were measured. Of the 15 participants, three subjects revealed higher plasma levels of CK and Rd, suggesting higher bioconversion of Rb1, Rb2, and Rc to Rd and then to CK. The study showed that the multiple-dose of red ginseng extract did not boost the AUC and C_{max} values, leading to low accumulation of CK (compared to other ginsenosides) in plasma, due to the comparatively short half-life of CK (Table 1). Furthermore, the AUC values of CK and Rd were significantly correlated irrespective of the dose amount. These results suggest the upstream biotransformation of saponins and have found that the repeated dose of CK is healthy for human consumption [27].

Apart from ginseng extracts or a mixture of ginsenosides, the pharmacokinetics of monomer CK has also been described [28,29]. In one study, LC-MS/MS (positive ion mode) with lithium adducts, was used to measure CK concentration in plasma of healthy Chinese subjects. Adducts were intended to boost the MS functionality. The method used was found to be perfect, reproducible and precise compared to the LC-MS/MS (negative ion mode) study reported earlier [22] for CK determination in human plasma. In addition, the lower limit of quantification was achieved by using smaller concentrations (50 µL) compared to higher human plasma levels (100 µL) [29]. An open-label, single-center, randomized, two-period crossover trial found that high-fat food consumption with CK decreased its T_{max} value and increased its values for C_{max} and AUC relative to the overnight fasting community (Table 1). Moreover, in females, the CK consumption was higher than in males. These results suggest that both food (high-fat diet) and sex affect the pharmacokinetics of CK and its metabolite, 20(*S*)-PPD. Such findings revealed preliminary pharmacokinetics of pure CK and its metabolite. To make a stronger conclusion, further research through large population size and daily diet record should be implemented [28]. Another recent, randomized, single-center, open-label, two-period crossover trial study first applied and validated LC-MS/MS to govern the pharmacokinetics of CK and its 20 (*S*)-PPD metabolites present in plasma and urine samples of healthy Chinese volunteers (Table 1) [30].

Table 1. Pharmacokinetics of CK and its derivatives.

Subject	Compound	Dose	C$_{max}$ (ng/mL)	T$_{max}$ (h)	AUC (ng·h/mL)	V/F (L)	MRT (h)	CL/F (L·h^{-1})	T$_{1/2}$ (h)	Ref.
Preclinical Studies										
SD rats	GE (N0-G)	2000 mg/kg	24.1 ± 5.5	15.2 ± 1.8	153.1 ± 30.6					[17]
	GE ± 2.5% N		24.0 ± 9.3	12.8 ± 3.3	187.2 ± 24.0					
	GE ± 5% N		38.8 ± 21.8	12.0 ± 0.0	218.5 ± 60.7					
	GE ± 10% N		54.4 ± 26.2	12.0 ± 0.0	429.9 ± 160.8					
SD rats	HYFRG™ ***	500 mg/kg	15.19 ± 10.69	3.3 ± 0.5	58.0 ± 32.5					[19]
	CK from RG	500 mg/kg	2.55 ± 0.99	6.7 ± 3.9	9.2 ± 7.5					
SD rats	CK from PG #	100 mg/kg	1888.9 ± 403.0	8.2 ± 1.7	24.0 ± 6.0		13.9 ± 5.2		10.2 ± 8.1	[20]
SD rats	CK	30 mg/kg	192.3 ± 40.7	2.2 ± 0.5	622.3 ± 240.7		3.8 ± 0.8			[21]
	CK/γ-CyD (1:1)		366.7 ± 102.5	1.8 ± 0.1	907.3 ± 111.1		2.5 ± 0.2			
	CK/γ-CyD (1:3)		476.0 ± 81.5	1.5 ± 0.2	1074.8 ± 32.9		2.2 ± 0.0			
	CK/β-CyD (1:1)		204.0 ± 30.8	2.0 ± 0.4	867.0 ± 69.6		3.3 ± 0.5			
Clinical Studies										
24 M	HYFRG™	3 g	254.4 ± 51.2	2.5 ± 0.9	1466.83 ± 295.89					[19]
	RG	3 g	3.1 ± 1.7	9.1 ± 1.4	12.73 ± 7.83					
12 M/F	FG	1.65 g	41.5 ± 21.8	2.2 ± 0.6	204 ± 94 (0–12 h), 238 ± 105 (0–24 h), 264 ± 113 $^{\$\$}$		9.9 ± 5.5		10 ± 5	[24]
	NFG		1.1 ± 0.7	16 ± 7.0	3.5 ± 3.1 (0–12 h), 13.6 ± 9.3 (0–24 h), NC		NC		NC	
11 M	RG extract ##	Multiple	81.6 ± 112.5	9.5 ± 1.6	873.0 ± 1236.0		10.6 ± 1.2		5.2 ± 1.1	[26]
15 M	RG extract ###	Single	24.8 ± 23.2	7.8 ± 2.0	247.50 ± 269.49		13.3 ± 3.7		9.9 ± 4.9	[27]
		Multiple	18.2 ± 27.1	6.9 ± 2.4	210.88 ± 400.44		10.5 ± 3.1		7.6 ± 4.1	

Table 1. Cont.

Subject	Compound	Dose	C_{max} (ng/mL)	T_{max} (h)	AUC (ng·h/mL)	V/F (L)	MRT (h)	CL/F (L·h^{-1})	$T_{1/2}$ (h)	Ref.
24 M/F	CK + HF diet	200 mg	1,570.3 ± 587.3	2.5 (1.5–5.0)	12,599.2 ± 4098.3 $; 12,836.7 ± 4166.2 $$	652 ± 381	12.3 ± 1.2 $; 14.6 ± 1.7 $$	18.2 ± 9.8	24.8 ± 3.0	[28]
	CK + FO diet		796.8 ± 406.0	3.6 (2.0–6.0)	5748.7 ± 2830.2 $; 5879.3 ± 2871.0 $$	1875 ± 1899	11.7 ± 1.2 $; 15.1 ± 4.3 $$	43.4 ± 24.2	27.7 ± 7.9	
12 M/F	GCK	50 mg	652 ± 180	2.6 ± 1.1	3650 ± 850 $; 3810 ± 890 $$				5.9 ± 0.6	[29]
10 adults	CK	200 mg	733.9 ± 408.4	3.3 (2.5–5.0)	5960.8 ± 3524.4 $; 6094.2 ± 3598.4 $$		11.5 ± 1.4 $; 13.8 ± 1.6 $$		21.6 ± 5.5	[30]

*** The study was conducted on both rats and humans. # analysis was compared with other ginsenosides, including Rb1, Rb2, Rc, Rd, Re, Rg1, Rg2, Rf, F1 and F2. ## RG extract dose protopanaxadiol (PPD):50.2–64.7 mg/day and protopanaxatriol (PPT), 11.2–14.9 mg/day. Multiple (3 Pouches). CK was compared with Rb1, Rb2, Rc, Rd, Rg3, Rh2, PPD, and PPT. ### RG extract consisted of a pouch with > 60% of dried ginseng extract. Multiple (3 Pouches). CK was compared with Rb1, Rb2, Rc and Rd. $ AUC$_{(0-t)}$, $$ AUC$_{(0-\infty h)}$. CK, compound K; C_{max}, maximum drug concentration; T_{max}, time of maximum concentration; AUC, area under the plasma concentration-time curve; V/F, apparent volume of distribution after extravascular administration MRT, mean residence time; CL/F, oral clearance; $T_{1/2}$, half-life. Each value represents the mean ± SE of three samples. SD, Sprague Dawley; GE, ginseng extract; N, NUTRIOSE; HYFRG™, CK from fermented RG extract; RG, red ginseng; PG, *Panax ginseng*; M., Male; F, female; FG, fermented ginseng (fermented using *Lactobacillus paracasei* A221); NFG, non-fermented ginseng; NC, not-calculated; GCK, ginsenoside CK; AUC$_{(0-t)}$, AUC from zero to the time of the last quantifiable concentration; AUC$_{(0-\infty h)}$, AUC from zero to infinity; HF, high fat; FO, fasting overnight.

Furthermore, a study on healthy Chinese participants has established the relationship between ABCB1 gene polymorphisms and CK pharmacokinetics. The results indicated that the gene NR1I2 (rs1464602 and rs2472682) allied primarily to the pharmacokinetics of CK. While ABCC4 (rs1751034 and rs1189437) influenced the pharmacokinetic behavior of both CK and its metabolite 20(S)-PPD. Such hereditary variations could thus partially describe the inter-individual variances in the pharmacokinetic behavior of CK [31].

3.3. Solubility, Permeability, and Efflux

Many health-promoting activities of CK have been reported. However, low water solubility, low membrane permeability, and efflux phenomenon critically weaken its efficacy and restrict its clinical application. The use of cyclodextrin (CyD) and nanocarriers have been implemented to improve the bioavailability of CK. Table 2 summarizes various modifications of CK with their outcomes.

The use of CyD has been duly recognized to improve the pharmacological behavior of drugs. In this line, an inclusion complex, K/γ-CyD, with improved oral bioavailability and solubility [21], compared to an earlier finding (in β-CyD only solubility was improved) has been described [32]. In another study, the use of ginsenoside CK with TPGS (D-alpha-tocopheryl polyethylene glycol (PEG) 1000 succinate) (GCKT)-liposomes has been described to improve solubility, targeting tumor cells, and minimizing efflux. The D-alpha-tocopheryl polyethylene glycol (PEG) 1000 succinate and phospholipid could increase the solubility of CK in the form of GCKT-liposome, leading to significant repression of tumor growth [33]. Phospholipid use improves biocompatibility, which could restore permeability and increase the process of ADME [34]. The D-alpha-tocopheryl polyethylene glycol (PEG) 1000 succinate has widely been documented as an inhibitor of P-glycoprotein (P-gp)-mediated efflux in drug delivery systems [35], and P-gp-mediated efflux was reported to be a significant limiting factor for the efficacy of CK [36].

In another study, CK-micelles (CK-M) from TPGS, PEG, and PCL (polycaprolactone) showed enhanced solubility and improved bioactivities. After 48 h, the CK was released slowly from CK-M with a drug release percentage of more than 42.1 ± 3.2% and without bursting. In the first eight hours, the rate of in vitro drug release for free CK with bursting was 84.4 ± 4.2%. Additionally, the P-gp-mediated efflux in the CK-M group was substantially inhibited compared to free CK, suggesting drug uptake by the target cells [36]. Likewise, CK ascorbyl palmitate (AP)/TPGS micelles enhanced solubility of CK and significantly inhibited P-gp-mediated efflux [37]. Similarly, the micellar system based on phosphatidylcholine (PC) and 1,2-distearoyl-sn-glycero-3-phosphoethanolamine polyethylene glycol 2000 (DP) showed improved solubility and continued release of CK [38]. The water solubility of the CK nanoparticles (NPs)/bovine serum albumin (BSA) and CK, was compared, and BSA was found to augment the water solubility of CK. The high biocompatibility, dispersive nature, and conjugative ability to several target molecules make BSA a useful carrier molecule [39].

In another study, CK was loaded onto gold(G)NPs synthesized using probiotic bacteria (*Lactobacillus kimchicus* DCY51^T) and evaluated for the effectiveness of drug loading [40]. Furthermore, the use of deoxycholic acid (DA)-O-carboxymethyl chitosan (OCMC) has been advocated to increase solubility and ability for CK. For example, CK-NPs conjugated with DA-OCMC showed increased solubility and improved drug entrapping and drug loading efficiencies. The release pattern of CK was pH-dependent and faster at lower pH. The collective release of CK at pH 7.4 and 5.8 was 10.7 ± 0.71%, and 16.3 ± 1.4%, respectively, after the first 48 h, without bursting. Notably, over 120 h of the study, a significant increase in the release of CK was observed. These findings indicate that CK was released slowly (the pH of blood), thus the system could be used for target delivery of CK [41].

Table 2. Solubility, permeability, and efflux of CK and its derivatives.

Modified CK	Model	Major Findings	Ref.
K/γ-CyD and K/β-CyD	K/γ-CyD at different ratios 1:1 and 1:3 and K/β-CyD at 1:1	Improved solubility at lower concentrations (<0.03 M) compared to higher (<0.06 M) ↑bioavailability ↑dissolution rate compared to CK and K/β-CyD Higher dissolution rate in 1:1 ratio compared to 1:3	[21]
GCKT-liposomes	Phospholipid and TPGS (7:3 ratio)	↑High CK loading capacity and solubility GCK EE% was of above 98.4 ± 2.3% Sustained discharge of GCK from GCKT-liposomes compared to GCK solution (in PBS)	[33]
CK-M	PEG-PCL/TPGS mixed micelles at different ratios of 3:0. 3:1, 3:2, 3:3	↑drug EE% in CK-M (94.6 ± 1.4) than CK-P (62.5 ± 1.6; PEG-PCL micelles) ↑CK concentration (107.3-times) in micelles (CK-M) than free CK ↑solubility of CK with higher TPGS	[36]
CK-AP/TPGS micelles	AP/TPGS mixed micelles	↑solubility from 35.2 ± 4.3 to 1,463.2 ± 153.3 μg/mL of CK EE% = 91.3 ± 5.2% Inhibited P-gp mediated efflux	[37]
CK PC/DP micellar system	CK, DP, and PC at ratios of 5:12:18	↑water solubility (~66-fold) and long drug retention time	[38]
BSA-CK NPs	BSA	↑water solubility	[39]
DCY51T-AuCKNps	AuNPs synthesized using *Lactobacillus kimchicus*	Drug loading efficiency-11.03%	[40]
CK:DA-OCMC NPs	CK:DA-OCMC at different ratios 1:10, 2:10, 3:10	↑water solubility ↑EE% from 20.2 ± 1.4 to 42.6 ± 1.2% ↑drug loading capacity from 3.0 ± 0.2 to 10.6 ± 1.4% by ↑drug: carrier ratio Enhanced cellular uptake and increased cytotoxicity than CK	[41]
GK-OCMC NPs	GK: OCMC at different ratios of 1:10, 2:10, 3:10	↑water solubility and permeability ↑EE% from 5.9 ± 1.2 to 20.8 ± 2.5% ↑drug loading capacity from 1.9 ± 1.8 to 4.2 ± 0.7 % by ↑ drug: carrier ratio Enhanced cellular uptake and increased cytotoxicity than CK	[42]
APD-CK micelles	CK: A54-PEG-DA-OCMC at different ratios of 1: 20, 2:20, 4:20	↑EE% increased from 61.7 ± 1.4 to 76.5 ± 1.2 % ↑drug loading capacity from 1.6 ± 0.1 to 3.1 ± 1.4 % by ↑drug: carrier ratio	[43]

CK, compound K; CyD, cyclodextrin; GCKT, ginsenoside CK with TPGS; TPGS, D-α-tocopheryl polyethylene glycol 1000 succinate; EE, encapsulation efficiency; PEG, polyethylene glycol; PCL, polycaprolactone; AP, ascorbyl palmitate; P-gp, P-glycoprotein; PC, phosphatidylcholine; DP, 1,2-distearoyl-sn-glycero-3-phosphoethanolamine polyethylene glycol 2000; BSA, bovine serum albumin; NPs, nanoparticles; OCMC, O-carboxymethyl chitosan; DA, deoxycholic acid.

In a recent comparative study on CK and CK within OCMC NPs showed that the later had higher water solubility and membrane permeability [42]. Similarly, a recent study found that CK-loaded with A54-PEG-DA-OCMC, known as APD-CK micelles, enhanced the delivery of CK. A54 is a long peptide of 12 amino acids which binds explicitly to hepatic cancer cells. Drug release was pH-dependent, and its release at pH 7.4 was slow (32.69%) compared to a fast release (73.49%) at pH 5. 8 [43].

3.4. Safety

As per the new clinical guidelines, drug safety tests should be screened with two animal types, inclusive of non-rodents (usually dogs) and rodents (mice or rats) [44]. For preclinical safety evaluation, rats and mice were assessed for acute and 26-week recurrent-dose toxicity of CK.

Single oral supplementation of CK for rats (8 g/kg) and mice (10 g/kg) did not induce toxicity or mortality in the same. On the other hand, for 26-week toxicity (e.g., clinical symptoms, biochemical and hematological parameters, urine analysis, the body weights, food consumption, and histopathology of rats) were evaluated at 13, 40, or 120 mg/kg doses of CK. The NOAEL (no observed adverse effect levels) doses were 40 mg/kg and 120 mg/kg for females and males, respectively. However, a decrease in body weight, fur-loss, reduced activity, and lack of energy were transiently observed in the 120 mg/kg male test group [45]. Oral preclinical safety of CK was evaluated on Beagle dogs (4, 12, or 36 mg/kg) for 26-weeks. The NOAEL dose for dogs was 12 mg/kg [46].

Considering clinical perspective, in a randomized, double-blind trial on healthy Chinese subjects, compared to placebo, the treatment group were orally administered CK at 100, 200, or 400 mg doses for up to nine times a week. The results of this documented study showed the safety of CK during the intervention period [47]. However, it has been suggested that further evaluations are necessary to affirm the safety of CK administration in humans.

4. Health-Promoting Activities

Compound K, in terms of its bioactivity, has gained much interest as a rarely known ginsenoside [48]. Investigation on the CK metabolism is beneficial to gain better insights into the pharmacological activities of CK. Concerning this, a recent study used an ultra-performance LC quadrupole time-of-flight tandem MS to characterize CK (oral dose 50 mg/kg) in feces and urine of SD rats, resulting in the detection of tentative twelve (M1–M12) metabolites. The authors suggested sequential oxidation, deglycosylation and conjugation as the key metabolic pathways for CK metabolic profile characterization [49]. This section summarizes recent studies on various health-promoting activities of CK (Tables 3 and 4 and Figure 2).

4.1. Hepatoprotective

The hepatoprotective effects of CK were observed against the injury caused by carbon tetrachloride [50], tert-butyl hydroperoxide [51], paracetamol (acetaminophen) [52], or as in recent studies by sodium valproate (SVP) [9]. Compound K exhibited protective effects against hepatotoxicity caused by SVP via minimizing oxidative stress through triggering the hepatic antioxidant system and inhibiting lipid peroxidation [9]. Among other protecting effects, CK significantly improved liver fibrosis in a high-fat diet (HFD)-induced rats [53]. Another study evaluated the effect of CK on hepatosteatosis using a mouse model with diabetes and obesity. The beneficial effects against hepatosteatosis were described by reducing expressions of lipogenesis genes and upregulating expressions of genes involved in fatty acid oxidation through adenosine monophosphate-activated protein kinase (AMPK) phosphorylation [54].

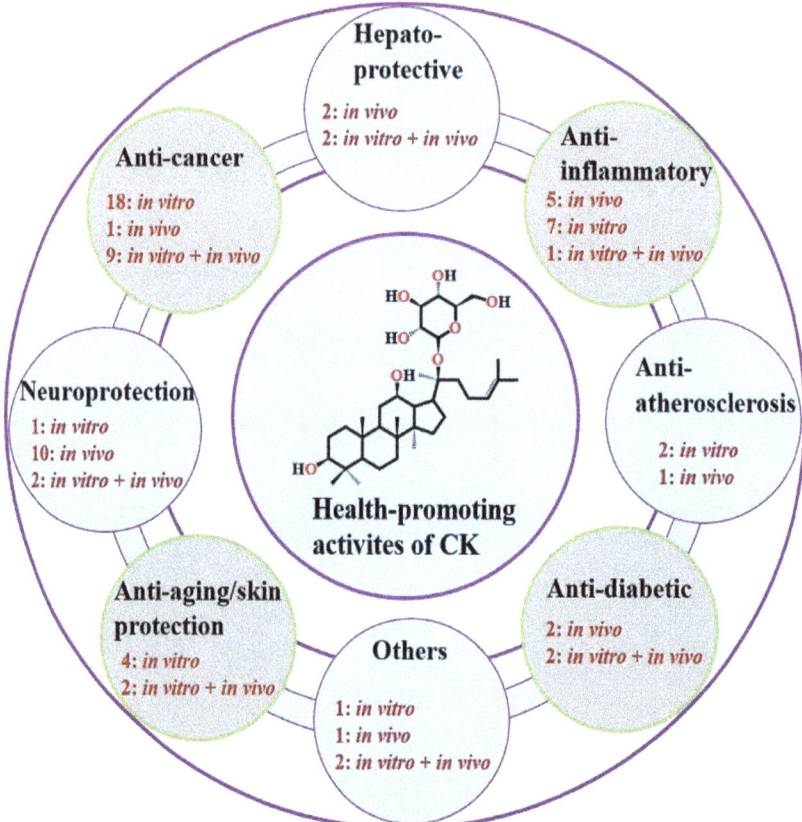

Figure 2. Schematic illustration of health-promoting activities of Compound K (CK). The numbers in the figure represent the total number of studies assessed for evaluating in vitro and in vivo, health-promoting activities of CK.

Table 3. Hepatoprotective, anti-inflammatory, anti-atherosclerosis, and anti-diabetic activities of CK and its derivatives.

Material Type	ST	Model	Treatments	Major Findings	Ref.
Hepatoprotective					
CK	In vivo	SVP-induced SD rats	LCK-80 mg/kg GCK + SVP MCK-160 mg/kg GCK + SVP HCK-320 mg/kg GCK + SVP once daily for 15 days	↓ hepatic index-LCK (7.6%), MCK (8.7%), and HCK (9.4%) ↓ AST, ALT, ALP, TG and ↑ALB ↑CAT, GPx, and SOD activities and GSH level ↓ MDA level and soluble epoxide hydrolase (better with LCK) ↑ hepcidin level	[9]
CK and Rh1	In vivo	HFD-treated SD rats	CK + phospholipid; phospholipid + Rh1; phospholipid + CK+ Rh1 (3 mg/kg/day), 1 week	Treatment either alone or in combined form (CK or Rh1) ↓ γ-GT, AST, ALT, ALP, TG, CHOL, FCHOL, LDL ↑HDL levels Anti-fibrotic effects by ↓ expressions of TIMP-1, PC-I, and PC-III Improved insulin resistance by normalizing glucose levels	[53]
	In vitro	Rat liver stellate cell line (HSC-T6)	CK, Rh1, CK+Rh1 for 6 h	↑anti-proliferative effect ↑ apoptosis in HSC-T6 CK (20.63%), Rh1(12.43%), CK+Rh1 (18%)	
CK	In vivo	HFD-treated OLETF rats	CK (25 and 10 mg/kg), 12 weeks	↓ plasma glucose level and improved morphology of liver cells ↓ FAS and SREBP-1c expressions ↑ CPT-1 and PPAR-α expressions ↑ phosphorylation of AMPK	[54]
CK from GBCK25	In vivo	C57BL/6 mice	GBCK 25 with CK (400, 200, 100, 20, and 10 mg/kg) once daily, 12 weeks	↓ liver weight ↓inflammation, degree of steatosis, and ballooning degeneration ↓ ALT, TC and TG levels ↓ TNF-α, IL-1β, IL-6 levels ↓ expressions of α-SMA and TIMP-1 Reduction in hepatic lipid accumulation and ↓ MDA levels ↓ FAS, ACCα and CYP2E1 levels ↓ levels of p-JNK (reduced JNK activation)	[55]

Table 3. Cont.

Material Type	ST	Model	Treatments	Major Findings	Ref.
	In vitro	Palmitic acid-treated AML12 cells LPS-treated RAW264.7 cells Kupffer cells (KCs)*	GBCK25 (4, 2, and 1 μg/mL), 24 h GBCK25 (0.5, 0.4, or 0.3 μg/mL), 24 h	↓ cellular toxicity ↓ TG, FAS, ACCα and CYP2E1 levels ↓ TNF-α, IL-1β, IL-6 in RAW264.7 and KC cells	[2]
Anti-inflammatory					
CK	In vitro	LPS-stimulated RAW264.7 cells and HEK293 cells transfected with HA-AKT1, HA-Src, or HA-AKT2 for 48 h	CK (10, 5, and 2.5 μM), 24 h	No effect on the viability ↓ expressions of TNF-α, IL-1β, iNOS, and AOX1 ↓ phosphorylation of Akt1, not Akt2	
BIOGF1K	In vitro	Pretreated RAW264.7 cells	BIOGF1K (200, 100, and 50 μg/mL), 1 h + LPS (1 μg/mL), 24 h	↓ NO production (67%) with BIOGF1K (200 μg/mL) Significant scavenging of DPPH ↓ expressions of iNOS and IFN-β ↓ NF-kB activity (72%), IRF3 pathway (63%) Inhibited IKK and TBK1 phosphorylation	[56]
BIOGF1K	In vitro	Pretreated RAW264.7 cells	BIOGF1K (30, 20, and 10 μg/mL), 30 min + LPS (1 μg/mL), 24 h	Dose-dependent ↓ of NO and iNOS and COX-2 expressions AP-1 signaling pathway inhibited by blocking MAPKs and MAPKKs	[57]
BSA-CK NPs	In vitro	Pretreated RAW 264.7 cells	BSA-CK NPs and CK (20,15, 10, 5, and 1 μM), 1 h + LPS (1 mg/mL)	↓ NO production by BSA-CK NPs (10 μM) compared with CK	[39]
SPIONs-CK	In vitro	Pretreated RAW 264.7 cells	SPIONs-CK and CK (100, 10, and 1 μg/mL), 24 h + LPS (1 μg/mL) Antioxidant-1 to 250 μg/mL	↓ NO production by CK and SPION-CK and inhibited iNOS production by 47.9% (CK) and 45.8% (SPION-CK) (at 10 μg/mL) ↓ ROS production by SPIONs-CK and CK Inhibition of DPPH was higher for SPIONs-CK (72%) compared to CK (21.1%) at (250 μg/mL)	[58]

Table 3. Cont.

Material Type	ST	Model	Treatments	Major Findings	Ref.
CK	In vivo	C57BL/6 mice	CK (20 mg/kg), 30 h	↑expression of SGLT1 gene and glucose uptake mediated by SGLT1	[59]
CK	In vitro	Caco-2 cells	CK (1, 0.1, 0.01, and 0.001 µM), 12, 24, 36, and 48 h	↑ SGLT1 protein level dose-dependent ↑ SGLT1 protein level time-dependent 1.70 times (24 h) to 2.01 times (48 h) ↑ glucose uptake activity by ↑ SGLT1 expressions	[60]
CK	In vivo	Xylene-induced Kunming mice with ear swelling Carrageenan-induced paw oedema SD rats	CK (224, 112, 56, 28, 14, and 7 mg/kg) every day, 5 days CK (160, 80, 40, 20, 10, and 5 mg/kg), orally every day, 5 days	CK displayed a dose-dependent inhibitory effect At 224 mg/kg- maximum (93.9%) inhibition Pain threshold induced by heat not effected ↑ rat inflammatory pain threshold significantly ↓ PGE2 level in the paw tissue, not in the gastric mucosa. ↓ COX-2 level in the gastric mucosa and paw tissue Activities COX-1 and -2 not effected	[61]
CK	In vivo	CIA-induced DBA/1 mice	CK (224, 56, and 14 mg/kg) per day, 21 days	Significant ↓ in arthritis global assessment and swollen joint count ↑ number of naïve T-cells and ↓ activated T-cells and DCs percentage Inhibited migration and priming of DCs ↓ expressions of CD80, CD86, MHC II, and CCL 21 levels (lymph nodes)	[61]
CK	In vivo	CIA-induced DBA/1 OlaHsd mice	CK (100 µl) once a day (20, 10, and 5 mg/kg/day), 6 weeks (Preventive effect), 4 weeks (Therapeutic effect)	↓ arthritis scores, ↓ serum anti-CII IgG, IFN-γ, and IL-2 ↑ IL-4 levels Non-significant ↓ TNF-α and IL-17 levels ↓ RANKL/OPG and MMP-3/TIMP-1 ratios	[62]
CK	In vivo	Adjuvant-induced arthritis	CK (160, 40, and 10 mg/kg), once daily, 15 days	Significant ↓ in global assessment scores and swollen joint counts ↓ spleen index and hyperplasia of lymph nodes ↓ memory B cells in the spleen ↓ expressions of CD40L (T cells) and CD40 (B cells)	[63]

Table 3. Cont.

Material Type	ST	Model	Treatments	Major Findings	Ref.
CK	In vivo	CIA-induced DBA/1 mice	CK (112 mg/kg/day), 24 days	Recovered body weight and ↓ arthritis symptoms, spleen index Inhibited viability and proliferation of lymphocytes ↓ IL-1β, IL-17 and TNF-α and ↑ IL-10 ↓ M1 macrophages and ↑ M2 macrophages; prevented phagocytosis ↑ Gαs expression and inhibited β-arrestin2, NF-κB, TLR4, and Gαi	[64]
CK	In vitro	H_2O_2-stimulated MC3T3-E1 cells	CK (0.01-10 μM) with or without H_2O_2, 48 h	CK formed hydrogen bonds with IKK ↑ ALP activity, Col-I expressions, and mineralization ↓ ROS and NO production, IL-1β expression	[65]
GNP-CK-CopA3	In vitro	LPS-activated RAW264.7	GNP-CK-CopA3 (10-100 μg/mL), 1 h + LPS (1 μg/mL), 24 h	NO production was inhibited (at 20 and 40 μg/mL) ROS production inhibited 40.4% (20 μg/mL) and 65.05% (40 μg/mL) ↓ levels of TNF-α, iNOS, COX-2, IL-6, and IL-1β Inhibited NF-κB and MAPK signaling pathways	[66]

Anti-atherosclerosis

Material Type	ST	Model	Treatments	Major Findings	Ref.
CK	In vivo	ApoE-/- C57BL/6 Peritoneal macrophages from apoE-/- C57BL/6	CK (9, 3, and 1 mg/kg) one dose per day, 8 weeks. ox-LDL (100 μg/mL) + CK (30, 10, and 3.3 μM)	↓ atherosclerotic plaques (55%) by activating RCT pathway ↓ IL-6, IL-1β, and TNF-α levels ↓ cleaved IL-1β, caspase-1, NLRP3, and NF-kB P65 ↓ inflammasome activity in mice and macrophages ↓ cholesterol ester (10 μM 46.21% and 30 μM 60.24%)	[67]
CK and its derivatives	In vitro	RAW264.7 cells	CK and CK derivatives (30, 10 μM)	Structure 1 ↓ cholesteryl ester contents in foam cells compared to CK ↑ ABCA1 mRNA expression Structure 1 (319%) compared to CK (151%) Structure 1 significantly activated LXRα compared to CK No effect on LXRβ activation	[68]

Table 3. Cont.

Material Type	ST	Model	Treatments	Major Findings	Ref.
CK	In vitro	HUVECs	Pretreated with CK (2.5, 1.25, and 0.625 mM), 12 h + ox-LDL (80 mg/mL), 24 h	↓ expressions of IL-6, MCP-1, TNF-α, VCAM1, and ICAM-1 ↓ expression of caspase3, cleaved caspase-3 and cytochrome c and LDH release Reversed mitochondrial membrane depolarization ↑ Bcl2/Bax	[69]
Anti-diabetic					
CK	In vivo	HFD fed ICR mice	Injected with STZ (100 mg/kg BW) after 4 weeks + CK (30 mg/kg), 4 weeks	↓ blood glucose levels, improve glucose tolerance ↓ PGC-1α expressions and inhibited PEPCK, G6Pase expressions Improved AMPK phosphorylation	[70]
	In vitro	HepG2 cells	CK (8, 4, and 2 µM), 24 h	Dose-dependent inhibition of hepatic glucose production ↓ PEPCK protein level and ↑ AMPK phosphorylation	
CK and Rb1	In vivo	Epididymal adipose tissue from ICR mice	Glucose treatment (high concentration), 24 h + CK (10 µM) and Rb1 (10 µM)	↓ROS production and ERS ↓ phosphorylation of PERK and IRE1α ↓ activation of NLRP3 inflammasome and ↓ IL-1β, IL-6 production ↓ IRS-1 phosphorylation at a serine residue ↑ IRS-1 phosphorylation at tyrosine residue ↑ PI3K activity and Akt phosphorylation	[71]
CD-CK conjugate	In vivo	Alloxan-induced diabetic zebrafish model	CK and CD-CK (15, 10, 7.5, 5, 2.5, 1, 0.5, 0.1, and 0.05 µM), 2 days	Good recovery of pancreatic islets by CD-CK compared to CK CD-CK showed less toxic (LC$_{50}$ = 20.68 µM) than CK (LC$_{50}$ = 14.24 µM)	[72]

Table 3. Cont.

Material Type	ST	Model	Treatments	Major Findings	Ref.
CK conjugate with beta-cyclodextrin	In vivo	HFD-induced C57BL/6 mice	CK (40, 20, and 10 mg/kg/day), 8 weeks	↑ body weight (6th week) ↓ fasting glucose, BUN, creatinine, and urine protein ↓ ROS production and Nox1, Nox4 expressions↓ expressions of NLRP3, Caspase-1, ASC, IL-1β, TNF-α, and IL-18 CK treatment reduced the activation of the p38 MAPK signaling pathway	[73]
	In vitro	High glucose-treated HBZY-1 cells	CK (50, 40, 20, and 10 µM), 48 h	↓ proliferation of HBZY-1 cells ↓ NLRP3, Caspase-1, and ASC levels	

* ex vivo, ST, study type; CK, compound K; SVP, sodium valproate; SD, Sprague–Dawley; LCK, low CK; GCK, ginsenoside CK; MCK, middle CK; HCK, high CK; AST, aspartate transaminase; ALT, alanine aminotransferase; ALP, alkaline phosphatase; TG, triglyceride; ALB, albumin; CAT, catalase; SOD, superoxide dismutase; GPx, glutathione peroxidase; GSH, glutathione; MDA, malondialdehyde; HFD, High fat diet; γ-GT, gamma-glutamyl trans peptidase; CHOL, total cholesterol; FCHOL, free cholesterol; LDL, low density lipoprotein; HDL, high density lipoprotein; TIMP-1, tissue inhibitors of metalloproteinase-1; OLETF, otsuka long-evans tokushima fatty; FAS, fatty acid synthase; SREBP-1c, sterol regulatory element-binding protein-1c; CPT-1, carnitine palmitoyltransferase-1; PPAR-α, peroxisome proliferator-activated receptor-alpha; AMPK, 5′ AMP-activated protein kinase; TC, total cholesterol; TNF-α, tumor necrosis factor alpha; IL, interleukin; α-SMA, alpha smooth muscle actin; ACCα acetyl CoA carboxylase alpha; CYP2E1, cytochrome P450 2E1; p-JNK, phospho c-Jun N-terminal kinase; LPS, lipopolysaccharide; iNOS, inducible nitric oxide synthase; AOX1, aldehyde oxidase 1; Akt, protein kinase B; BIOGF1K, CK and F1; NO, nitric oxide; DPPH, 2,2-diphenyl-1-picrylhydrazyl; IFN-β, interferon-beta; NF-kB, nuclear factor-kB; IRF3, interferon regulatory factor 3; IKK, inhibitor of kB kinase; TBK1, TANK-binding kinase 1; COX-2, cyclooxygenase-2; AP-1 (also known as c-jun), activator protein-1; MAPKs, mitogen-activated protein kinases; MAPKKs, MAPK kinases; BSA, bovine serum albumin; NP, nanoparticles; SPIONs, superparamagnetic iron oxide nanoparticles; ROS, reactive oxygen species; SGLT, sodium-glucose linked transporter or sodium-dependent glucose cotransporters; PGE2, prostaglandin E2; CIA, collagen-induced arthritis; DCs, dendritic cells; CD, cluster of differentiation; MHC, major histocompatibility complex; CCL21, chemokine (C-C motif) ligand 21; CII IgG, type II collagen immunoglobulin G; RANKL, receptor activator of nuclear factor-κB ligand; OPG, osteoprotegerin; MMP, matrix metalloproteinase; TLR4, Toll-Like receptor 4; Gαis, G(i,s) protein subunit alpha; Col-I, type I collagen; GNPs, gold nanoparticles; apoE, apolipoprotein E; ox-LDL, oxidized low density lipoprotein; RCT, reverse cholesterol transport; NLRP3, NOD-like receptor protein-3; ABCA1, ATP-binding cassette transporter A1; LXR, liver X receptor; HUVECs, human umbilical vein endothelial cells; MCP-1, monocyte chemoattractant protein-1; VCAM-1, vascular cell adhesion molecule-1; ICAM-1, intercellular adhesion molecule-1; LDH, lactate dehydrogenase; Bcl2, B-cell lymphoma-2; Bax, B-cell lymphoma 2 (BCL-2)-associated X protein; ICR, imprinting control region; STZ, streptozotocin; PGC-1α, proliferator-activated receptor-γ coactivator-1 alpha; PEPCK, phosphoenolpyruvate carboxykinase; G6Pase, glucose-6-phosphatase; ERS, endoplasmic reticulum stress; IRE1, inositol-requiring enzyme 1; PERK, protein kinase-like ER kinase; IRS-1, insulin receptor substrates -1; PI3K, phosphatidylinositol 3 kinase; BUN, blood urea nitrogen; Nox, NADPH oxidase; ASC, apoptosis-associated speck-like protein containing a CARD.

Similarly, Choi et al. showed the ameliorating effects of GBCK25 (fermented ginseng, rich in CK) on nonalcoholic steatohepatitis (NASH). They found that GBCK25 was capable of downregulating cytochrome P450 2E1 (CYP2E1) levels alongside reduced activation of cellular c-Jun N-terminal kinase (JNK) [55]. These findings indicate that CK can be used for liver disease prevention and/or treatment.

4.2. Anti-Inflammatory

From previous studies, the anti-inflammatory activity of CK was ascribed to decreased synthesis of pro-inflammatory cytokines ((interleukin (IL)-6, IL-1β, and tumor necrosis factor-alpha (TNF-α)), cyclooxygenase-2 (COX-2), and inducible nitric oxide synthase (iNOS) [11]. However, recent studies have strengthened our understanding of the mechanistic implications at molecular and cellular levels (Table 3). In one study, CK attenuated NF-κB by modulating the Akt1-mediated inflammatory gene expression in LPS-induced macrophages [2]. Compound K-rich fraction (BIOGF1K), consisted of 3.2 g of CK and 1.5 g of saponin F1, and was examined for its anti-inflammatory activity. Compound K-rich fraction has down-regulated LPS-stimulated nitric oxide (NO) production in RAW264.7 cells. Furthermore, expressions of iNOS and IFN-β were reduced by suppressing stimulation of NF-κB and interferon regulatory factor 3, respectively. The inhibitory mechanism of BIOGF1K was due to the blockage of an inhibitor of kB kinase (IKK) and TANK-binding kinase 1 (TBK1), leading to reduced production of NO and IFN-β [56]. Likewise, in another study BIOGF1K inhibited COX-2 and iNOS mRNA expressions in LPS-induced RAW264.7 cells. Mechanistically, BIOGF1 K blocked activation of activator protein-1 (AP-1) pathway by targeting mitogen-activated protein kinases (MAPKs) such as ERK (extracellular signal-regulated kinase) and p38, and MAPK kinases (MAPKKs) such as MAPK/ERK kinase 1/2 and MAPK kinase 3/6 [57]. Together, these findings indicate that BIOGF1 K plays a protective role in macrophage-mediated inflammatory responses. In addition, the use of CK as BSA-CK NPs [39] and CK-conjugated superparamagnetic iron oxide nanoparticles [58], has been shown to have anti-inflammatory activity against RAW 264.7 cells induced by LPS. In another study, CK-mediated modulation of sodium/glucose cotransporter one via the epidermal growth factor receptor (EGFR) pathway was found to reduce intestinal inflammation [59].

Inflammation commonly follows pain. In this line, the effect of CK on inflammation and pain was represented using *in vivo* models of xylene-induced ear swelling, and paw oedema stimulated with carrageen. The anti-inflammatory and pain-reducing effects of CK were due to the decreased production of prostaglandin E2 by downregulating COX-2 expression (Table 3) [60]. Referring to arthritis, the attenuating role of CK has been shown by inhibiting the production of inflammatory cytokines, suppressing T-cell activation, inhibiting the multiplication of B-cells, macrophages regulation, and reducing the level of autoantibodies [11]. Among T cells, the potential mechanism of CK treatment involves suppression of dendritic cells (DCs) priming of T-cell activation, suppression of chemokine CCL21 (with receptor CCR7) associated with DC movement and signaling between T cells and DCs in collagen-induced arthritis animal model. Notably, a positive correlation ($R^2 = 0.9830$, $p = 0.0009$) was found in percentages of activated T-cells and DCs, while a negative correlation ($R^2 = 0.8348$, $p = 0.03$) in percentages of naïve T cells and DCs [61]. In another study, CK suppressed humoral immune response of T helper type 1 (Th1) cells and significantly suppressed expressions of matrix metalloproteinases (MMP)-3 and-13 and receptor activator of NF-κB ligand (RANKL) [62]. Concerning effects on B cells, CK was described as reducing the percentage of memory B cells. Authors suggested that the reduction in memory B cells may be dependent upon T-cells [63]. Previously, CK displayed anti-arithic effects on multifunctional macrophages by reducing the development of pro-inflammatory cytokines. In a recent study, however, the function of CK was shown to inhibit β-arrestin2, thus hindering the transition of macrophages from type M1 to type M2 [64]. The protective role of CK was also reported against osteoarthritis using in vitro and silico studies. Compound K displayed high binding affinity to a cytokine-activated kinase (IKK) compared to other ginsenosides as revealed in the molecular docking analysis. Thus, the anti-osteoarthritic effect of CK was due to inhibition of IKK activity in vitro [65]. Interestingly, in a recent study, GNPs were made intracellularly using *Gluconacetobacter liquefaciens* kh-1 (a probiotic strain) and used for synthesizing peptide (CopA3) conjugated nanoparticle (GNP-CK-CopA3) hybrids. Compound K, as peptide-nanoparticle hybrids showed anti-inflammatory effects by inhibiting the activation of NF-kB and MAPK signaling pathways [66].

4.3. Anti-Atherosclerosis

Atherosclerosis is well known to be an inflammatory disease; the anti-inflammatory effects of CK are more or less directly linked to its anti-atherogenic effects. In terms of anti-atherosclerosis, an important feature of CK was found to be associated with liver X receptor alpha (LXRα) (Table 3). Targeting LXRα, a study showed that CK treatment resulted in a dose-dependent reduction of atherosclerotic plaques by activating the reverse cholesterol transport (RCT) pathway, reducing inflammatory cytokines, and inhibition of inflammasome activity with LXR activation in apoE-/- C57BL/6 mice. Compound K triggered the RCT pathway by upregulating ATP-binding cassette transporter (ABC) A1, ABCG1, LXRα, ABCG5, and ABCG8. In addition, CK supplementation increased the cholesterol efflux and reduced the inflammasome activity in peritoneal macrophages of mice [67]. Another research demonstrated the use of CK and its derivatives in the activation of LXRα. The study documented the synthesis of six CK derivatives by adding short-chain fatty acids into the carbohydrate chain of CK at different locations. Effects on the foam cell model were evaluated, and the biological activities of all derivatives were found to be at par or better than their parent CK. All derivatives were capable of activating LXRα. Compound K derivative 1 displayed the best potency amongst all [68].

Similarly, it was found that the CK prevents inflammation and apoptosis in human umbilical vein endothelial cells, induced through oxidized low-density lipoprotein (ox-LDL). In endothelial cells, lectin-like oxidized low-density lipoprotein receptor-1 (LOX-1) uptakes ox-LDL leading to pro-inflammatory effects. Compound K decreased LOX-1 expression and inhibited the nuclear translocation of NF-kB, and phosphorylation of JNK and p38 [69]. The results indicate that CK [67,69] and its derivatives [68] have the anti-atherosclerosis effect.

4.4. Anti-Diabetic

Ginsenosides play an important anti-diabetic role by modulating insulin resistance, regulating lipid and glucose metabolism, protecting from the inflammatory response, and oxidative stress. In this line, a study showed that CK administration suppressed liver gluconeogenesis by inhibiting glucose-6-phosphatase and phosphoenolpyruvate carboxykinase expressions in HFD-fed ICR mouse model and HepG2 cell line. Meanwhile, the expressions of hepatocyte nuclear factor 4 alpha, peroxisome proliferator-activated receptor 1-alpha, and forkhead transcription factor O1 were decreased while AMPK phosphorylation was increased significantly [70]. Furthermore, the management of insulin resistance is essential for controlling diabetes. In this line, CK was found to be able to inhibit inflammation and modulate insulin resistance in adipose tissue by repressing the activation of NOD-like receptor family, pyrin-containing protein 3 (NLRP3) associated with endoplasmic reticulum stress (ERS) (Table 3) [71]. In another study, beta-cyclodextrin-conjugated CK (β-CD) was used to modulate diabetes against an alloxan-induced zebrafish model. The recovery of affected pancreatic islets in CD-CK conjugate was significantly higher (EC_{50} = 2.16 µM) than in CK (EC_{50} = 7.22 µM) [72]. Furthermore, the protective effect of CK on diabetic nephropathy in HFD/ streptozotocin-induced mice has been demonstrated through significant reduction of oxidative stress and down-regulating expressions of NADPH oxidase (Nox)-1 and-4 proteins. Additionally, the reactive oxygen species (ROS)-mediated activation of the inflammasome assembly was reduced, and renal p38 MAPK phosphorylation was inhibited (Table 3) [73].

4.5. Anti-Cancer

The promising anti-cancer activity CK has been previously identified in various types of cell lines, including lung carcinoma, leukemia, breast cancer, colorectal cancer, prostate cancer, gastric carcinoma, nasopharyngeal carcinoma and pulmonary adenocarcinoma [11,74]. Among recent findings (Table 4), a study documented the suppressing effect of CK on COX-2 and Arg-1 genes linked to immunosuppression, apoptosis, and pro-inflammatory cytokines production by myeloid-derived suppressor cells (MDSCs) from the xenografted colorectal (CT26) cancer mice. Compound K could act as a promising therapeutic molecule by targeting MDSCs [75]. Another study elucidated the inhibitory action of CK on the development and metastasis of glioblastoma cell lines (U87MG and U373MG). The effects were due to cell cycle arrest, decreased cyclins (D1 and D3) levels, apoptosis through nuclear condensation, activation of apoptotic enzymes, increased production of ROS, and the depolarized potential of the mitochondrial membrane. The anti-proliferative effect was due to the blockage of the phosphatidylinositol three kinase (PI3K)/Akt signaling pathway in glioblastoma [76]. Likewise, CK was found to block glycogen synthase kinase 3β signaling [77] and the PI3K/Akt signaling pathway [78] in breast cancer cells (MCF-7). Additionally, the combined CK and cisplatin had better effects than either molecule alone [78]. A later study gave in vivo evidence of CK's protecting effects against hormone-independent breast cancer by degrading cyclin D1 protein [79] (Table 4). Recently, Li et al. synthesized ester derivatives (1c, 2c, 3c) of M1, and found that among all, compounds 2c, 3c had an effective growth inhibitory effect on MCF-7 cells [80]. Another study shed light on the biological mechanism of CK against breast cancer using SKBR3 cells. Compound K displayed anti-cancer effects in SKBR3 cells by enhancing apoptosis through downregulation of Akt-1. In addition, CK was found to reduce invasion and metastasis [81].

Compound K inhibited proliferation, augmented autophagy, and apoptosis of non-small cell lung cancer (NSCLC) (A549 and H1975) cells through the mammalian target of rapamycin (mTOR)/AMPK and JNK signaling pathways (Table 4) [82]. Furthermore, the suppression of the growth of NSCLC cells was studied by targeting the metabolism of glucose. Compound K suppressed the levels of hypoxia-inducible factor 1-alpha and its downstream glucose transporter1 gene [83]. Another study showed the anti-cancer effect of CK against HepG2 cells and xenografted (HepG2) BALB/c nude mice. Compound K resulted in cell cycle arrest, blocked cell cycle progression, and apoptosis induction by modulating B-cell lymphoma 2 (Bcl2) to Bcl2 associated X (an apoptosis regulator) ratio in HepG2 cells. Furthermore, a substantial reduction in tumor proliferation was observed in the CK-supplemented mice group [84]. Also, CK induced apoptosis and ERS in liver cancer cells and xenografted mice by modulating signal transducers and activators of transcription-3 (STAT3) activation [85]. Another study showed for the first time that CK targeted annexin A2, which leads to inhibition of NF-κB [86]. Compound K enhanced ERS and calcium release by ryanodine receptors leading to apoptosis in lung cancer cells of humans. In particular, the use of an ER stress inhibitor (4-phenylbutyrate) enhanced CK- mediated apoptosis [87]. Another research provided the first proof that the CK usage results in the TNF-related apoptosis-inducing ligand (TRAIL) sensitization in TRAIL-resistant HT-29 cells and potentiated TRAIL-stimulated apoptosis in HCT116 by autophagy-linked death receptor (DR) 5 stimulation. The upregulated expression of DR5 was dependent upon ROS mediated JNK-autophagy-activation and CCAAT/enhancer-binding protein (C/EBP) homologous protein/p53 pathway (autophagy-independent) [88]. In neuroblastoma cells, CK enhanced ROS-linked apoptosis and impaired the autophagic flux. In addition, CK with chloroquine (combination approach) stimulated apoptosis in cell line and mouse models and may, therefore, be a potential approach for treating neuroblastoma [16]. The protective role of CK was also investigated against glioma (inveterate brain tumor). Compound K was observed to inhibit the stromal cell-derived growth factor 1 migration of C6 glioma cells by controlling protein kinase C alpha, ERK1/2, and MMP signaling molecules (Table 4) [89]. Recent studies showed the bioactivity of CK against human osteosarcoma cell (MG63 and U2-OS) lines.

Table 4. Anti-cancer, neuroprotection, anti-aging/skin protection, and other activities of CK and its derivatives.

Material	ST	Model	Treatments	Major Findings	Ref.
Anti-cancer					
CK	In vivo	Balb/c mice with CT26 tumor cells		↓expression of Cox-2 and Arg-1; ↓ productions of IL-1β, IL-6, and IL-17; ↓ CT26 tumor growth	[75]
CK	In vitro	U87MG and U373MG cells	CK (50, 20, and 10 µM), 72 h	Significant growth reduction of target cells and inhibited cells mobility and invasion; G0/G1 phase arrest for U87MG (80.7%) and U373MG (77.3%); ↑ apoptosis; Negative regulation of PI3K/Akt/mTOR signaling pathway	[76]
CK	In vitro	MCF-7 cells	CK (70, 50, 30, and 10 µM), 24 h	Inhibited proliferation dose-and time-dependently; ↓ expressions of GSK3β, cyclin D1, and β-catenin	[77]
CK	In vitro	MCF-7 cells	CK (50 mmol/L) or cisplatin (10 mg/L), alone or in combination, 24–96 h	Anti-proliferation activity: CK (19.18 ± 2.25), cisplatin (21.34 ± 2.84), and both (43.37 ± 5.62); ↑ apoptosis in the combined treatment compared to individual treatments	[78]
CK	In vivo	Xenograft nude mice	CK (1 or 0.2 mg/kg), every other day, 3 weeks	Reduction in the tumor weight	[79]
CK	In vitro	MCF10DCIS.com and MCF10CA1a	CK (20, 10 µM), 24, 48, and 72 h	↓ viability in dose-and time-dependently; ↑ cell cycle blockage; ↓ cyclin D1 production and ↑ cyclin D1 degradation	
M1 and its derivatives	In vitro	MCF-7 and MDA–MB–231 cells	M1, 1c, 2c, and 3c (100, 50, 25, and 1 µM)	Derivatives 2c and 3c showed good inhibitory effects 80% inhibition for MCF-7 (lower con.); For MDA-MB-231, better effects on higher concentration; Derivatives 2c and 3c changed membrane permeability and promoted apoptosis of MCF-7	[80]
CK	In vitro	SKBR3 cells	CK (0–50 µM), 3–24 h	↑ anti-proliferative and apoptotic activities; ↑ levels of cleaved caspase-7, -8, and caspase-9; ↓ Bcl2 levels and AKT-1 levels, no effect on AKT-2 levels	[81]

Table 4. Cont.

Material	ST	Model	Treatments	Major Findings	Ref.
CK	In vitro	A549 and H1975	CK (20 μg/mL), 24 h	↑ anti-proliferative and apoptotic activities ↑ beclin-1 protein level ↓ p-JNK/JNK, p-c-Jun/c-Jun, LC3II/LC3I and p62 levels ↑ levels of caspase-3 and cleaved PARP in both cells AMPK/mTOR, JNK signaling pathways activated	[82]
CK	In vitro	NSCLC		Dose-dependent anti-proliferative effect Inhibited expression of PDK1, HK II, and LDHA Inhibited expressions of HIF-1α and GLUT1	[83]
CK	In vivo	Xenografted BALB/c mice	CK (10 mg/kg/day)	Reduced tumor volume and ↓ tumor weight (49.4%) ↓viabilities of HepG2 cells in dose-and time-dependently and ↑ apoptosis	[84]
CK	In vitro	HepG2 cells	CK (20, 10, 5, and 2.5 μmol/L), 48 h	↑ cell arrest at 5 μmol (68.61 ± 2.91%) and l0 μmol (78.29 ± 2.57%) ↓ expressions of cyclin D1 and CDK-4 ↑ expressions of cleaved-caspase-3, -9, Bax, p21^{Cip1} and p27^{Kip1} ↓ Bcl-2 and PARP (inactive)	
CK	In vivo	SMMC-7721 cells injected BALB/c nude mice	CK (20, 10, and 5 mg/kg/day), 15 days	Dose-dependent inhibition of tumor Significant ↓ in body weight of mice (20 mg/kg) ↓ p-STAT3 levels	[85]
CK	In vitro	HepG2 and SMMC-7721	CK (60, 40, and 20 μM) 48 h	↑apoptosis and ERS in cell lines ↓ DNA-binding ability of STAT3 ↓ p-STAT3 levels ↑ERS markers (CHOP and GRP78) expressions PERK and IRE1 signaling pathways activated	
CK	In vitro	HepG2 cells	CK (6 μM), 12 h	↓ interaction of and colocalization (nucleus) of p50 and annexin A2 NF- κB signaling pathways activation inhibited and ↓ downstream genes expressions	[86]
CK	In vitro	A549 and SK-MES-1	CK (15, 10, and 5 μM), 48 h and 15 μM, 6, 12, 24, 36, or 48 h	IC$_{50}$ for viabilities of A549 (17.78 μM) and SK-MES-1 (16.53 μM) ↑ caspase 12 dependent apoptosis Induced ERS by ↑ p-eIF2α expressions and protein levels of XBP-1S, GRP78(BiP), and IRE1α ↑ intracellular calcium levels and m-calpain activities	[87]

Table 4. Cont.

Material	ST	Model	Treatments	Major Findings	Ref.
CK	In vitro	HT-29 and HCT116 cells	CK (50 or 20 µM), 24 h	↓expressions of Mcl-1, survivin, Bcl-2, XIAP, and cFLIP ↑expressions of tBid, Bax, and cytochrome c, and DR5 ↑ in LC3-II and Atg7 levels and expressions of p53 and CHOP ↑ JNK phosphorylation	[88]
CK	In vivo	SK-N-BE(2) injected BALB/c nude mice	CK (30 mg/kg) and chloroquine (50 mg/kg), 3 times/week/60 days	↑TUNEL-positive cells and caspase-3 expression Compared to chloroquine, CK and CK+ chloroquine significantly reduced tumor size ↑ inhibition in the combination approach	[16]
CK	In vitro	SK-N-BE(2) and SH-SY5Y cells	CK (20, 15, 10, 5 and 2 µM), 24 h	↑ cell cycle arrest (at sub G1 phase), ROS production and P21 protein level a ↑ caspase-dependent apoptosis Induced early phase autophagy by ↑ BECN, Atg7, and LC3B expressions Inhibited late phase autophagy	
CK	In vitro	SDF-1 induced C6 glioma cells	CK (10, 3, 1, 0.3, 0.1, and 0.03 µM), 24 h	CK abridged scratch wound-healing and inhibited C6 cells migration ↓ phosphorylation of downstream targets PKCα (SDF-1 pathway) and ERK1/2 (CXCR4 pathway)	[89]
CK	In vitro	MG63 and U2-OS cells	CK (30, 25, 20, 15, 10, and 5 µM), 3 days	Anti-proliferative effect against osteosarcoma cells (IC$_{50}$ = 20 µM for 3 days) ↑apoptosis rate CK (20 µM): U2-OS (17.66 ± 1.37%), MG-63 (24.16 ± 2.25%) Suppressed invasion and migration Blocked PI3K/mTOR/p70S6K1 signaling pathway ↑PTEN levels in both cells ↓p-AKT and p-mTOR in both cells ↓expressions of p-mTOR, p-mTOR/mTOR ratio and p70S6K1 in U2-OS cells treated with RAD001 (mTOR inhibitor)	[90]
GCKT-liposomes	In vivo	Athymic nude mice	GCK (15 mg/kg), GCKT-liposomes (15 mg/kg)/ 5 times every 3 days	GCKT-liposomes group, ↓mean tumor size from 219.0 ± 17.0 mm^3 to 45.8 ± 3.2 mm^3 slow ↑ in body weight in the initial days later no change	[33]
	In vitro	A549	GCK + GCKT-liposomes different concentrations, 24 h	IC$_{50}$, GCKT-liposomes (16.3 ± 0.8 µg/ml) and CK (24.9 ± 1.0 µg/ml) No cytotoxicity to A549 with T-liposomes alone	

Table 4. Cont.

Material	ST	Model	Treatments	Major Findings	Ref.
CK-M (TPGS/PEG-PCL+CK)	In vivo	Male athymic nude mice	CK and CK-M (15 mg/kg) once every 3 days, 15 days	Tumor volume after treatment CK-M (2.67 ± 0.88), CK (4.27 ± 0.35) CK-M ↓ tumor growth (79.12 ± 0.60 to 52.04 ± 4.62%) Bodyweight: CK-M group (25.02 ± 2.42), control (22.83 ± 1.83) low toxicity of CK-M to the mouse model	[36]
	In vitro	A549 and PC-9 cells	CK or CK-M (100, 50, 25, 12.5, 6.25, and 3.125 µg/mL), 24 h	IC$_{50}$ for A549: CK (21.97 ± 1.50 µg/mL) CK-M (25.43 ± 2.18 µg/mL) IC$_{50}$ for PC-9: CK (14.46 ± 1.24 µg/mL) CK-M (18.35 ± 1.90µg/mL) ↑CK-M uptake by A549, PC-9 cells ↑ apoptosis ↓ inhibited tumor cell invasion and metastasis Regulated Bcl-2, Bax, MMP-2, and Caspase-3 levels	
CK-AP/TPGS	In vivo	Nude mice	CK-AP/TPGS (30 mg/kg) every 3 days until the 12th day	Maximum anti-tumor effect (66.24 ± 8.77%) by CK mixed micelles at 15th day low toxicity to kidney and liver ↑ apoptosis of tumor tissue ↑ Bax/Bcl-2 ratio (7.25-times) ↑ cellular uptake and tumor targeting	[37]
	In vitro	A549 cells	CK-AP/TPGS and CK (80, 40, 20, 10, and 5, µg/mL), 24 h	CK mixed micelles had a better effect on cell cycle arrest at G0/G1 phase than free CK IC$_{50}$ for A549: free CK (16.11 ± 1.23 µg/mL) and CK mixed micelles (10.29 ± 1.1 µg/mL) ↑ apoptosis, A549: CK mixed micelles (45 ± 5.25%) and CK (17.28 ± 2.25%)	
CK PC/DP micellar system	In vivo	Xenografted nude mice	CK or CK mixed micelles (30 mg/kg) every 3 days for 12 consecutive days	No damage to liver and kidney Significant apoptosis of tumor tissue ↑ Bax/Bcl-2 ratio ↑ expressions of caspase-3, -8, -9 and PARP	[38]
	In vitro	A549 cells	CK or CK mixed micelles (12.15 µg/mL), 24 h	IC$_{50}$ for A549: CK (18.31 µg/mL) and CK mixed micelles (12.15 µg/mL) Effective cell cycle arrest at G1 by CK PC/DP compared to CK Highest apoptosis rate in CK PC/DP compared to CK	

Table 4. Cont.

Material	ST	Model	Treatments	Major Findings	Ref.
BSA-CK NPs	In vitro	HaCaT, HepG2, A549, HT29 cancer cells. LPS- induced RAW264.7 cells	CK and BSA-CK (20, 15, 10, 5, and 1 µM), 24 h	Improved anti-cancer ability of BSA-CK NPs compared to CK Higher ↓ in NO production by BSA-CK NPs	[39]
DCY51T AuCKNps	In vitro	A549, HT29, AGS and RAW264.7 cells	DCY51T AuCKNps 0.1, 1, 5, 10, 15, and 20 µM Phototherapy- NPs+ AGS + 1 or 5 mg/mL, 24 h + laser at 800 nm, 10 min.	↑cytotoxicity for A549 and HT29 compared to CK ↑apoptosis after laser treatment in AGS	[40]
CK + chitosan NPs	In vitro	HepG2 cells	CK and CK-NPs (3.125, 6.25, 12.5, 25, and 30 µg/mL), 24 h	At 30 µg/mL, the apoptotic cell percentage, CK (39.02 ± 0.42%) and CK-NPs (47.57 ± 1.65%)	[41]
GK-OCMC NPs	In vitro	PC3 cells	CK and GK-OCMC NPs (30 µg/mL)	↑ apoptosis by GK-OCMC treatment ↑ levels of caspase-3 (29.93%) and caspase-9 (20.78%) compared to GK treatment.	[42]
APD-CK micelles	In vitro	HepG2 and Huh-7 cells	CK (30, 20, 10, 5, and 2.5 µg/mL), 24 h and 48 h	Time-dependent and dose-dependent cytotoxic effects of APD-CK ↑expressions of PARP, caspase-3, and -9 in HepG2 cells by APD-CK micelles	[43]
	In vivo	Nude mice	5 mg/kg, 24 h	Strong tumor inhibition with parthenolide/ CK tLyp-1 liposomes than combined	[91]
Parthenolide/ CK tLyp-1 liposomes	In vitro	A549	Parthenolide (1.5 µg/mL) + CK (30 µg/mL) in 5:1 ratio	↑ mitochondrial apoptosis: CK (8.2%), parthenolide (11.8%), CK+ parthenolide (34.7%), Parthenolide/ CK tLyp-1 liposomes (56.7%) ↑ROS levels: CK (3.7%), parthenolide (5.8%), CK+ parthenolide (24.6%), Parthenolide/ CK tLyp-1 liposomes (28.7 %) Marked structural changes in mitochondria and impaired mitochondrial membrane potential	
CKGal	In vitro	AGS, B16F10, HeLa, and U87MG	CKGal, CK, F12, and Rh2 each at (200, 100, 50, 25, 12.5, 6.25 µmol), 72 h	↓ cell viability: U87MG (13.7%), AGS (8.7%), B16F10 (2.6%), and HeLa (7.3%) IC$_{50}$ CKGal: HeLa (40.38 µmol), U87MG (40.38 µmol), B16F10 (22.4 µmol), and AGS (4.487 µmol) cells	[92]

Table 4. Cont.

Material	ST	Model	Treatments	Major Findings	Ref.
			Neuroprotection		
CK from RG	In vitro	Glutamate-induced HT22 (hippocampal) cells	CK (8, 4, 2, and 1 μM), 12 h	↓glutamate-induced cytotoxicity Induced Nrf2 growth in the nucleus ↑ expressions of HO-1, NQO1, and GR and ↓ Nrf2 and Keap1 expressions	[93]
	In vivo	Scopolamine-induced C57BL/6J mice	CK (10, 5, and 1 mg/kg) daily, 2 weeks	Restored memory and cognitive functions Modulated Nrf2-mediated cognitive functions	
CK	In vivo	Diabetic db/db mice	CK (10 mg/kg) per day, 12 weeks	Improved cognitive dysfunction, behavioral impairment, glucose tolerance and insulin sensitivity, and dyslipidemia ↓ fasting glucose levels and ↓ IL-1β, TNF-α, and IL-6 in the hippocampus ↓MDA levels ↑ SOD and GSH-Px activities ↓TXNIP, NLRP3 inflammasome, ASC, cleaved IL-1β, and cleaved caspase-1 ↓ CHOP, BiP p-PERK, p-IRE1α, and total ATF6 (Ameliorated ERS)	[94]
CK	In vivo	SD rats	Morphine (26 nmol/10 mL) per h, CK (10 mg/10 mL/h), 7 days + naloxone (10 mg/kg), 6 h	↓escape behavior and teeth chattering ↓p-ERK, p-NR1	[95]
		Cortical neurons from C57BL/6 mice	CK (5, 1, and 0.1 mM), 30 min + morphine (1 mM), 6 h	↓NR1, p-NR1 levels No significant effect on ERK	
CK	In vivo	SD rats	CK (120, 160, and 80 mg/kg), twice a day at 12 h interval, 5 days followed by lithium chloride-pilocarpine or PTZ	PTZ-induced behavioral seizures ↓reduced the seizure intensity and duration and prolonged latency (High dose) Lithium chloride-pilocarpine-induced behavioral seizures ↓reduced the seizure intensity and prolonged latency (High dose) ↑ GABA levels and GABAARα1 and KCC2 expressions ↓NKCC1 expressions	[96]
CK	In vivo	Kunming mice	CK (30, 10, and 3 mg/kg) since 8 to 14 day after partial hepatectomy	Improved MWM test scores of POCD mice ↓ TNF-α, IL-1β, and LDL-C serum levels ↑ HDL-C levels In Hippocampal tissues: ↓ IL-1β, TNF-α, and NF-κB P65 ↑ downstream targets of LXRα- ABCG1, ABCA1, and apoE	[97]

Table 4. Cont.

Material	ST	Model	Treatments	Major Findings	Ref.
CK	In vivo	Memory-impaired ICR mice induced with scopolamine hydrobromide	CK1 (CK 20 mg/kg + SCOP 2 mg/kg); CK2 (CK 40 mg/kg + SCOP 2 mg/kg), daily, 2 weeks	↑memory function ↓ neuronal apoptosis and its morphology restored Inhibited expression of Amyloid β ↑SOD and GPx levels and reduced ↓ MDA levels Activated Nrf2/Keap1 signaling pathway	[98]
CK	In vitro	Amyloid β peptide treated HT22 cells	CK (10, 5, and 2.5 μM), 24 h	↑ survival rate and restored growth and morphology of HT22 cells ↓apoptosis and expression of amyloid β peptide ↑ expressions of GLUT3, GLUT1, IRS2, and IDE ↓ expressions of CDK5, GSK3β, and tau	[99]
CK	In vivo	SD rats	CK (200,100, and 50 mg/kg), 8 weeks	↓ cognitive discrepancies in vascular dementia rats at 200 mg/kg Ameliorated neuronal damage Significant ↓ of amyloid β1-42 ↑Akt or protein kinase B activity, involved in the PI3K/Akt pathway leading to ↑GSK3β and IDE levels	[100]
CK	In vivo	Wistar rats	CK (60 and 30 mg/kg/day), 15 days	Significant ↓ in neurobehavioral scores ↓water content in brain tissue at 60 mg/kg/day ↓ brain infarct volume ratio ↑SOD and GSH-Px activities and ↓MDA levels ↓expressions of inflammatory molecules	[101]
CK	In vivo	Kunming mice SD rats	CK (30, 10, and 3 mg/kg), daily once, 4 weeks CK (30, 10, and 3 mg/kg), daily once, 2 weeks	Improved depressive-like activities in mice In rats, ↑sucrose preference and body weight Improved food consumption and crossings in CUMS rats ↑dopamine and 5-HT (serotonin) levels and no effect on norepinephrine ↓ expression of neurotransmitter degrading enzymes ↑BDNF, NGF levels and SOD, GPx, and GSH activities	[102]
CK	In vivo	Kunming mice	CK (30, 10 and 3 mg/kg), 4 weeks	Prevented depressive-and anxiety-like behaviors ↓ MDA level and ↑ SOD expression ↓ IL-1β and IL-18 Inhibited expressions of NLRP3 and cleaved caspase-1	[103]

Table 4. Cont.

Material	ST	Model	Treatments	Major Findings	Ref.
CK	In vitro	Thrombin-induced EnNSCs	CK (10 µM)	Improved sphere-forming ability ↓apoptosis of EnNSCs ↑proliferation of Ki67-positive EnNSCs cells ↑neurogenesis of Doublecortin-positive EnNSCs cells Activated LXRα signaling by ↑expressions of HMGB3 and RBBP7	[104]
CK	In vivo	Thrombin-induced C57BLC/6	CK (10 mg/kg)	Improved the neurobehavioral function ↑neurogenesis in cerebral subventricular zone	
CK	In vivo	C57BL/6 mice 2 months and 24 months old treated	CK (15, 10, and 5 mg/kg), 3 days. Last CK dose, EdU treatment for 24 h for cell proliferation. Neuronal survival: Last CK dose, followed by EdU for 3 days sacrificed after 4 weeks	↑EdU-incorporated cells in 2 months' dose (dose-dependent) and 24 months at 15 mg/Kg ↑number of cells: PCNA labeled/EdU+PCNA labelled and Ki-67/EdU+Ki-67 positive cells ↑new cells survival and their differentiation into neurons (observed in cells labeled with EdU+ NeuN) ↑BDNF and NT3 levels Induced phosphorylation of Akt and ERK1/2 at 10 mg/Kg (2 months) and 15 mg/Kg (24 months)	[105]
Anti-aging/skin protection					
CK	In vitro	HaCaT	CK (0.01–1 µM), 3 h	↑hyaluronic acid production ↑phosphorylation of ERK and Akt	[106]
CK	In vitro	Pretreated NIH3T3 cells HaCaT cells B16F10 cells	CK (0–10 µM) +UV (30 mJ/cm²) irradiation followed by CK, 24 h	↓MMP1 and COX-2 levels Restored collagen (I) level ↑TGM, FLG, and HAS-1 and -2 (slight) levels ↑melanin content but no effect on melanin secretion and tyrosinase activity Modulated phosphorylation of IκBα MAPKs, JNK, and ERK	[107]
BIOGF1K	In vitro	UVB-treated (30 mJ/cm2) NIH3T3 cells	BIOGF1K 30, or 15 mg/mL, 24 h	No cytotoxicity, Inhibited apoptosis Repressed morphological changes ↓melanin secretion and restored sirtuin 1 and type I procollagen levels ↓levels of MMP-1, MMP-2, COX-2 and ↓activity of AP-1 and MAPK	[108]

Table 4. Cont.

Material	ST	Model	Treatments	Major Findings	Ref.
CK	In vitro	HaCaT cells	CK (5 μM), maclurin (15 μM), and maclurin/CK, 24 h	No cytotoxicity to HaCaT cells ↓MMP-1 level in combination than in individual treatments	[109]
CK	In vivo	UV-treated (100 mJ/cm^2) SKH-1 (hairless) mice DNCB-induced atopic dermatitis	CK (0.3%), daily two times, 2 weeks CK (0.3%), daily two times, 2 weeks	TEWL value: in UVB treated group (85 g/m^2/h) and CK + UVB group (57 g/m^2/h) and in DNCB-treated group (65 g/m2/h) decreased to (42 g/m2/h) in CK + DNCB group Improved skin hydration: 37% from 31% (UV-treated) and 28% from 20% (DNCB-treated) CK improved epidermal hyperkeratosis Suppressed skin thickness to 73.5% in the UV model and 50.5% in the DNCB model ↑ SPINK5 levels and ↓ KLK-5 and PAR2 in both models	[110]
CK	In vitro	HaCaT cells UV-treated (15 mJ/cm^2)	CK (30, 10, 3, and 1 μM), 24 h	↓ SPINK expression by decreasing KLK-7, -5 and PAR2	
CK	In vivo	Imiquimod (IMQ)-induced psoriasis-like dermatitis C57BL/6 female mice	CK (0.1% and 1%), next three days	CK (1%) suppressed imiquimod-induced keratinocyte proliferation ↓ epidermal thicknesses ↓ RegIIIγ expression in IMQ-treated mouse keratinocytes	[111]
CK	In vitro	HaCaT cells	CK (2, 1.6, 1.2, 0.8, and 0.4 μg/mL) + IL-36γ (μg/mL)	Dose-dependent inhibition of proliferation No effect on apoptosis CK (0.4 μg/ml) inhibited REG3A expression induced by IL-36γ	

Others

Material	ST	Model	Treatments	Major Findings	Ref.
CK	In vivo	UUO C57BL/6 mice after) UUO induction I/R injury with unilateral NX model	CK (30 mg/kg body wt.) therapeutic group (1 day before), preventive group (3 days) + one day after ligation of renal vessels	UUO model, ↓NLRP3 inflammasome activation in kidney↑ribosome-governed activation Prevented renal tubulointerstitial lesions in the kidney ↓TNF-α, IL-6, IL-1β, and MCP-1 in urine Inhibited activation of T-cells and NF-κB Improvement kidney pathology and kidney function in NX + I/R model (Therapeutic effects)	[112]

Table 4. *Cont.*

Material	ST	Model	Treatments	Major Findings	Ref.
CK (M1)	In vitro	M-1 under MICP J774A.1 macrophages	CK (10 μM), 30 min CK (0–10 μM), 30 min + LPS, 5.5 h	↓ caspase-1, IL-1β NF-κB p65, and NLRP3 in M-1 cells Suppressed NLRP3 expression by ↓NF-κB activation in macrophages ↓ phosphorylation and activity of STAT3 in activated macrophages	[113]
	In vivo	LPS-induced NZB/WF1 mice	M1 (50 mg/kg)	↓levels of BUN, Cr, albuminuria, and anti-dsDNA autoantibodies ↓glomerulonephritis activity scores ↓IL-1β, TNF-α, IFN-γ, IL-6, MCP-1, and IL-12p70 ↓T-cell proliferation, number of Th cells (expressed IL-4 or IFN-γ), CD3$^+$CD69$^+$ cells, and CD4$^+$CD69$^+$ cells	
	In vitro	LPS-treated BMDCs, podocytes	M1 (10 μM), 30 min + with or without LPS (100 ng/mL), 6 h	↓ ROS production and inhibited activation of NLRP3 inflammasome	
CK analogues	In vivo	OVA-sensitized asthmatic mouse	CK and its analogues (20 mg/kg) for 7 days	Comparable anti-asthmatic effects of CK analogues T1, T2, T3, T8 and T12 IgE (ng/mL) value = CK (1501.85 ± 184.66), T1 (1237.11 ± 106.28), T2 (975.82 ± 160.32), T3 (1136.96 ± 121.85), T8 (1191.08 ± 107.59) and T12 (1258.27 ± 148.70)	[114]

Table 4. Cont.

Material	ST	Model	Treatments	Major Findings	Ref.
CK	In vitro	H9c2 cells	CK (2, 4, and 8 µM), 48 h	↑cell survival and ↓cell damage ↓ROS production and mitochondrial damage ↓ production of phagocytic precursors ↓ Bax/Bcl-2 ratio, cleaved caspase-3 and PARP ↓ p-Beclin-1/beclin-1ratio, Atg5, Atg7, LC3II/I ↑ P62 expression	[115]

CK, compound K; ST, study type; COX-2, cyclooxygenase-2; IL, interleukin; PI3K, phosphatidylinositol 3 kinase; Akt, protein kinase B; mTOR, mammalian target of rapamycin; GSK3β, glycogen synthase kinase 3β; Bcl2, B-cell lymphoma-2; JNK, c-Jun N-terminal kinase; AP-1 (also known as c-jun); LC3, microtubule-associated protein 1A/1B-light chain 3; PARP, poly (ADP-ribose) polymerase; AMPK, 5′ AMP-activated protein kinase; NSCLC, non-small cell lung cancer; PDK1, 3-Phosphoinositide-dependent protein kinase 1; HKII, mitochondrial hexokinase II; LDHA, lactate dehydrogenase A; HIF-1α, hypoxia-inducible factor 1; GLUT, glucose transporter; CDK-4, cyclin-dependent kinase-4; Bax, B-cell lymphoma 2 (BCL-2)-associated X protein; ERS, endoplasmic reticulum stress; STAT3, signal transducer and activator of transcription 3; p-STAT3, phosphorylated-STAT3; CHOP, C/EBP homologous protein; GRP78, glucose-regulated protein-78; PERK, protein kinase-like endoplasmic reticulum kinase; IRE1, inositol-requiring enzyme 1; NF-kB, nuclear factor-kB; p-eIF2α, phospho-eukaryotic translation initiation factor 2 subunit α; XBP-1S, X-box binding protein-1S; Bip, binding immunoglobulin protein; Mcl-1, myeloid cell leukemia 1; XIAP, X-linked inhibitor of apoptosis protein; cFLIP, fas-associated death domain-like IL-1-converting enzyme-inhibitory protein; tBid, truncated BID; DR5, death receptor 5; Atg7, autophagy-related 7; TUNEL, TdT-mediated dUTP nick end labelling; ROS, reactive oxygen species; BECN, Beclin-1; SDF-1, stromal cell-derived growth factor 1; PKCα, protein kinase Cα; ERK, extracellular signal-regulated kinase; CXCR-4, C-X-C chemokine receptor type 4; IC$_{50}$, half maximal inhibitory concentration; p70S6K1, ribosomal protein S6 kinase β 1; PTEN, phosphatase and tensin homolog; GCK, ginsenoside CK; GCKT, GCK with TPGS; TPGS, D-α-tocopheryl polyethylene glycol 1000 succinate; PEG, polyethylene glycol; PCL, polycaprolactone; MMP, matrix metalloproteinase; AP, ascorbyl palmitate; PC, phosphatidylcholine; DP 1,2-distearoyl-sn-glycero-3-phosphoethanolamine polyethylene glycol 2000; BSA, bovine serum albumin; NP, nanoparticles; NO, nitric oxide; OCMC, O-carboxymethyl chitosan; APD-CK, A54-PEG-DA–OCMC polymer CK-loaded micelle; ROS, reactive oxygen species; tLyP-1, truncated form of the cyclic tumor-homing peptide LyP-1; RG, red ginseng; Nrf2, nuclear factor (erythroid-derived 2)-like 2; HO-1, heme oxygenase-1; NQO1, NAD(P)H dehydrogenase [quinone] 1; GR, glutathione reductase; Keap1, Kelch-like ECH associated protein 1; TNF-α, tumor necrosis factor alpha; MDA, malondialdehyde; iNOS, inducible nitric oxide synthase; MAPKs, mitogen-activated protein kinases; SOD, superoxide dismutase; GSH, glutathione; TXNIP, thioredoxin-interacting protein; NLRP3, NOD-like receptor protein-3; ASC, apoptosis-associated speck-like protein containing a CARD; p-IRE1α, phospho-IRE1 alpha; ATF6, activating transcription factor 6; SD, Sprague-Dawley; p-PERK, phospho-PERK; p-NR1, phospho-N-methyl-D-aspartate acid receptor subunit 1; p-ERK, phospho-ERK; PTZ, pentylenetetrazole; GABA, gamma amino-butyric acid; GABA$_A$Rα1, GABA type A receptor subunit alpha1; KCC2, K-Cl cotransporter isoform 2; NKCC1, Na-K-2Cl cotransporter isoform 1; MWM, Morris water-maze; POCD, post-operative cognitive dysfunction; LDL-C, low density lipoprotein-cholesterol; HDL-C, high density lipoprotein-cholesterol; LXRα, liver X receptor alpha; ABCG1/A1, ATP-binding cassette transporter G1/A1; apoE, apolipoprotein E; ICR, imprinting control region; GPx, glutathione peroxidase; IRS2, insulin receptor substrates 2; IDE, insulin-degrading enzyme; CDK, cyclin-dependent kinase; CUMS, chronic unpredictable mild stress; BDNF, brain derived neurotrophic factor; NGF, nerve growth factor; EnNSCs, endogenous neural stem cells; HMGB3, High mobility group protein B3; RBBP7, RB binding protein 7; EdU, 5-ethynyl-2′-deoxyuridine; PCNA, proliferating cell nuclear antigen; NT3, neurotrophin-3; NeuN, neuronal nuclear protein; TGM, transglutaminase; FLG, filaggrin; HAS, hyaluronic acid synthases; IκBα, inhibitor of NF-κB; DNCB, 1-chloro-2,4-dinitrobenzene; TEWL, transepidermal water loss; SPINK5, serine protease inhibitor Kazal type-5; KLK, kallikrein; PAR2, protease activated receptor 2; REG3A, regenerating islet-derived protein 3-alpha; UUO, unilateral ureteral obstruction; MCP-1, monocyte chemoattractant protein-1; NX, nephrectomy; I/R, ischaemia reperfusion; MICP, mechanically induced constant pressure; LPS, lipopolysaccharide; BMDCs, bone marrow-derived dendritic cells; OVA, ovalbumin.

The bioactivity of CK has been described by inhibiting viability and proliferation, inducing apoptosis, by blocking the PI3K/mTOR/p70S6K1 signaling pathway (Table 4) [90]. Recently, many studies have been published comparing the health-promoting activities of CK and its derivatives (Table 4). Yang et al. identified the liposomal mediated improved anti-cancer activity of CK. They found that using GCKT-liposomes, the cellular uptake of GCK by lung adenocarcinoma (A549) cell line increased by enhancing time treatments (1, 2, and 4 h). The anti-tumor efficacy of GCKT-liposomes was observed to be more compared to CK. The use of GCKT-liposomes was advocated to overcome problems such as insufficient drug packaging, instable nature, rapid drug discharge, and poor blood circulation of conventional liposomes [33].

Similarly, CK-M described earlier in this review, were used for in vitro (A549 and PC-9) and in vivo models. The apoptosis percentage of CK-M was higher than free CK. Meanwhile, CK-M also displayed an improved tumor inhibitory effect in vivo [36]. The anti-lung cancer effects (in vitro and in vivo) of CK AP/TPGS mixed micelles [37] and CK PC/DP micellar system [38] have also been documented. Moreover, using in vitro models, BSA-CK NPs showed more significant cytotoxic effects in the liver carcinoma (HepG2), skin cell line (HaCaT), A549 cells, and colon cancer cell line (HT29) compared to monomer CK. However, for in vivo application, authors advocated the use of human serum albumin as an alternative to BSA to evade plausible immunologic concerns in humans [39]. In addition, CK-loaded GNPs have been identified as effectual photothermal and chemotherapeutic agents [40]. On a similar line, a higher dose-dependent inhibitory effect of chitosan nanoparticles loaded with CK (CK-NPs) was observed compared to CK. Authors described a lower (IC_{50} = 16.58 μg/mL) value for CK-NPs compared to CK (IC_{50} = 23.33 μg/mL) in HepG2 cells [41]. Likewise, CK loaded O-OCMC nanoparticles showed inhibitory effects against prostate cancer (PC3) cells through enhanced cytotoxicity and uptake of CK [42]. Chitosan polymer micelles decorated using A54 peptide, known as APD-CK, were utilized against Huh-7 and HepG2 cells. APD-CK showed higher cytotoxicity compared to CK and promoted apoptosis of HepG2 cells (Table 4) [43]. In another study, tLyp-1 (tumor-homing peptide) decorated liposomes loaded with parthenolide (active anti-tumor agent isolated from *Tanacetum parthenium*) and CK have been evaluated as lung cancer-targeting system. Enhanced anti-tumor activity was observed against both the cell line and animal model with limited adverse effects. In A549 cells, CK/parthenolide tLyp-1 liposomes decreased mitochondrial membrane potential and allowed greater Ca^{2+} efflux as well as significant inhibition of cell migration. From in vivo study, it was found that the complex has greater anti-tumor activity than the combination of these substances [91].

In another study, a derivative of CK, known as CKGal (20-O-β-D-lactopyranosyl-20(S)-protopanaxadiol) have been produced using β-1,4-galactosyltransferase, a regiospecific enzyme. The anti-proliferative action of CKGal was evaluated on skin melanoma (B16F10), brain carcinoma (U87MG), gastric cancer cell lines (AGS), and cervical carcinoma (HeLa). The CKGal displayed the best cytotoxicity against skin melanoma and cervical carcinoma compared to CK, Rh2, and F12 [92].

4.6. Neuroprotection

Several studies have documented the therapeutic effects of ginseng and ginsenosides in many central nervous system (CNS) ailments, for instance, Alzheimer's disease, Parkinson's disease, depression, and other ailments [6]. The protection could be ascribed to reducing neuroinflammation, neuroprotection, and regulating neurotransmitter release. In previous articles, the cognitive and neuroprotective role of CK has been described [3,11]. The current review summarizes the recent progress in neuroprotection effects of CK (Table 4).

In a study, CK (derived from red ginseng) was able to exert neuroprotective effects in memory-impaired mouse (scopolamine-induced) model by inducing nuclear factor (erythroid-derived 2)-like 2 (Nrf2)-facilitated antioxidants. No effect was observed on the acetylcholine esterase (AChE) activity. In addition to that, CK defense against glutamate-induced cytotoxicity was also observed in HT-22 cells [93]. Recently, CK was found to be protective against memory and cognitive impairment in db/db mice by suppressing inflammation and oxidative stress, ameliorating dyslipidemia, insulin sensitivity, glucose tolerance as well as modulating ER stress and NLRP3 inflammasome pathway (Table 4) [94]. Moreover, in another study, CK minimized the morphine dependency by decreasing N-methyl-D-aspartate acid receptor subunit 1 activation in cultured cortical neurons from mice and frontal cortex of rat brains [95]. Another recent research documented the protective effects of CK against epilepsy in status epilepticus (SE) rat model. Compound K stimulated the release of gamma amino-butyric acid (GABA) and enhanced the GABA type A receptor subunit alpha1-facilitated inhibitory synaptic transmission [96]. In addition to the anti-atherosclerosis effects of CK and its derivatives as described above [68], the role of LXRα in immunomodulation has also been described in continuous research. Researchers demonstrated that CK was able to mitigate post-operative cognitive dysfunction (POCD). They found that CK inhibited hippocampal inflammation by activating LXRα. CK attenuated memory dysfunction by modulating Morris water-maze (MWM) test scores in an aged mouse model (Table 4) [97].

Regulation of aggregated amyloid-β (Aβ) is an important part of Alzheimer's disease (AD) treatment. Concerning this, CK was found to enhance memory function, reduce Aβ expression and aggregation, and neuronal apoptosis by activating the Nrf2/Kelch-like ECH-associated protein-1 signaling pathway in ICR mice with diminished memory. Furthermore, the defensive effects were also due to the activation of the antioxidant system [98]. Likewise, the influence of the CK was elucidated using Aβ peptide-induced HT22 cells by improving viability, growth, and apoptosis of HT22 cells, as well as localization and expression of Aβ peptide in cells. Besides, ATP levels of cells were enhanced by increasing the activity of glucose transporters. Compound K restored abnormal energy metabolism (Aβ induced) by modulating the expressions of several enzymes (Table 4) [99]. Zong et al. first found that the CK mitigates cerebral discrepancies and $Aβ_{1-42}$ accumulation in the hippocampus of chronic cerebral hypoperfusion-induced vascular dementia SD rats by enhancing the pSer9Glycogen synthase kinase-3b expression. To add further, CK upregulated PI3K/Akt pathway, resulting in increased insulin-degrading enzyme activity, a central enzyme accountable for degrading $Aβ_{1-42}$ in the brain (Table 4) [100].

In an in vivo research, CK pretreatment resulted in the reduction of neurobehavioral score, water in brain tissue, and the cerebral infarct volume ratio against cerebral ischemia/reperfusion (I/R) injury in Wistar rats. Compound K enhanced activities of antioxidant enzymes, decreased levels of IL-1β, TNF-α, and declined level of high mobility group box 1 protein. Generally, the protective effects of CK against cerebral I/R damage may be due to anti-inflammatory and antioxidant bioactivities [101]. The earlier reviews have described the neuroprotective role of CK [3]. However, its antidepressant effect has been described recently. Depression is a global societal health concern. Concerning the effect of CK on depression, a study used two models: behavioral despair model (mice) and the chronic unpredictable mild stress (CUMS, rats) model. The antidepressant role may be due to regulation of the concentration of monoamine neurotransmitters, enhanced antioxidant capacity, and increased expressions of neuronal growth factor and brain-derived neurotrophic factor in the CNS [102]. In a follow-up study, the defensive effect of CK on CUMS depression was evaluated by inhibiting oxidative stress, inflammatory cytokines and NLRP3 expression using a mouse model [103].

Amongst others, recent work on explaining the beneficial effects of CK on hippocampal neurogenesis has been published. In one study, CK was found to induce neurogenesis and decrease apoptosis in thrombin-induced endogenous neural stem cells (EnNSCs) and improve animal prognosis by stimulating LXRα activation [104]. In another study, CK treatment triggered the proliferation of fresh cells and substantially increased their differentiation in the hippocampus (dentate gyrus) by activating brain derived neurotrophic factor (BDNF) signaling. The higher dose of CK was found to be more effective in aged mice compared to young ones (Table 4) [105].

4.7. Anti-Aging/Skin Protection

It is well-known that the production and synthesis of hyaluronic acid (HA) decreases with age. A study by Lim et al. identified that CK led to increased production of HA by activating Src (tyrosine kinase)-dependent Akt and ERK [106]. Ultraviolet type B (UVB) radiation induces photo- aging due to collagen degradation (type I and III) and increased production of iNOS, COX-2, and MMPs. Compound K supplementation diminished production of COX-2 and MMP-1 in NIH3T3 cells treated with UVB, and expression of type I collagen was modulated. Compound K also displayed the ability to improve the skin's moisture level. The study also found skin hydration effects of CK in HaCaT cells (Table 4) [107]. Compound K-rich fraction applied to UVB-treated cells was equally successful in the prevention of UVB-mediated aging [108]. Interestingly, the effectiveness against reducing mRNA expression of MMP-1 was more in a synergistic approach by CK and maclurin (a natural compound) compared to individual compounds [109]. Another study assessed the role of CK in improving skin barrier function by upregulating the expression of serine protease inhibitor Kazal type-5 in atopic dermatitis-like mice and UVB-irradiated mouse model [110]. In recent research, CK improved imiquimod-induced psoriasis by inhibiting regenerating islet-derived protein 3 (RegIII) gamma expression in the mouse model and IL-36γ-induced Reg3A expression in human keratinocytes (Table 4) [111]. These findings advocate that CK plays a key role in the defense and anti-aging effects.

4.8. Others

Recently, a patented study investigating the beneficial effects of CK on renal tubulointerstitial lesions in C57BL/6 mice with unilateral ureteral obstruction identified the kidney-protective effects of CK. The results showed reduced production of pro-inflammatory cytokines and the prevention of leukocytes infiltration and fibrosis in the kidney. The positive outcomes were showcased by inhibiting NF-κB-associated priming, and by modulating STAT3 signaling and NLRP3 inflammasome activation (Table 4) [112]. Likewise, another study showed the protecting effects of CK on accelerated and severe lupus nephritis by hindering activation of NLRP3 inflammasome [113]. Ren and coworkers evaluated the protecting effects of CK and its analogues against asthma. Compound K and its analogues displayed a significant impact by reducing IgE and airway resistance [114]. Compound K pretreatment was reported to protect against cardiac I/R by activating the PI3K-Akt signaling pathway, which is crucial for autophagy-triggered apoptosis (Table 4) [115].

4.9. Clinical Studies

4.9.1. Anti-Diabetic

Clinical studies evaluated the bioactivities of hydrolyzed ginseng extract. Recently, a double-blind, randomized controlled trial assessed the anti-glycaemic effects of hydrolyzed ginseng extract (GINST15, rich in CK) on prediabetic participants for 12 months. GINST15 resulted in improved fasting and 1-hour postprandial glucose levels. No effect was observed on 2-hour postprandial glucose levels [116]. An earlier clinical study also confirmed these results in which fermented red ginseng extract supplementation decreased fasting glucose, postprandial glucose levels and improved insulin levels in type 2 diabetic subjects compared to placebo [117].

4.9.2. Neuroprotection

Flanagan et al. have documented the effects of GINST15 on hypo-pituitary-adrenal (HPA) and antioxidant activity clinically. In this double-blind, placebo-controlled, counterbalanced within-group study design different doses (high dose-960 mg and low dose-160 mg) of CK were given for 2 weeks. They found that, in response to severe exercise, CK supplementation resulted in dose-dependent declines in circulating cortisol and augmented antioxidant activity. This study first provided insights into the impact of ginseng treatment on the reactions to the stress associated with work [118]. A recent continued study by the same research group demonstrated direct evidence on task-related brain activity by evaluating CK's treatment on behavioral performance and electroencephalography measures of cortical activity. After exercise, the upper and lower body response times were improved. Compound K augmented activity in cortical regions accountable for sustained attention, whereas exercise-triggered increases in arousal were diminished. In short, CK has been found to have inducible effects on the activity of the brain [119].

4.9.3. Liver Protection

As mentioned above, in an in vivo study, GBCK25 has been found to have defensive effects against NASH [55]. On a similar line, recent research evaluated the protective effects of GBCK25 on liver function in a 12-week, randomized, double-blind clinical trial. The supplementation includes GBCK25 tablets (high (500) and low (125) mg/day) and placebo. Treatment at a low dose significantly reduced gamma-glutamyl transferase and high-sensitivity C-reactive protein levels in male participants, while high dose abridged fatigue score significantly. No side effects were observed for the supplementation. The study indicated that GBCK25 is safe and can improve liver function [120].

5. Concluding Remarks

The review aimed at providing current information concerning the pharmacokinetics, safety, and health-promoting activities of CK and its derivatives for preventing and managing diseases. It is well known that the CK is more bioavailable than its parent saponins and has several health benefits. Although more bioavailable than major ginsenosides, CK has certain drawbacks that restrict its clinical use. The use of CK derivatives as nanocarriers were shown to have better permeability, solubility, and efflux, including enhanced health-promoting activities. The review provides new insight into CK derivatives to increase the metabolic proficiency of CK. Most health-promoting activities were in vitro and in vivo, including hepatoprotective, anti-inflammatory, anti-atherosclerosis, anti-cancer, neuroprotection, skin protection, and anti-aging. Besides, the limited number of clinical studies have also been documented. The diverse bioactivities of CK were based on modulating complicated signaling pathways and targeting various molecules. Compound K has been found to attenuate the activities of AMPK, MAPK, NF-kB, PI3K/Akt, mTOR/AMPK, JNK PI3K/mTOR/p70S6K1 signaling pathways. Overall, pharmacokinetic studies on monomer CK and its preclinical and clinical safety information data are limited. Further investigations are warranted to appraise the efficacy and safety of CK and its derivatives, especially in clinical studies.

Author Contributions: H.-J.L. was responsible for the conceptualization, writing, editing, supervision, project management, and funding; H.-J.L. and A.S. designed the study. A.S. wrote the manuscript; H.-J.L. reviewed the manuscript intensively; H.-J.L. and A.S. edited the manuscript. Both authors have read and agreed to the published version of the manuscript.

Funding: This study was supported by a grant "Cooperative Research Program of Center for Companion Animal Research (Project No. PJ01398402)" Rural Development Administration and partly supported by Korea Food Research Institute (E0164500-05), Republic of Korea.

Conflicts of Interest: The authors declare no conflict of interest.

References

1. Yun, T.-K. Panax ginseng—A non-organ-specific cancer preventive? *Lancet Oncol.* **2001**, *2*, 49–55. [CrossRef]
2. Lee, J.-O.; Choi, E.; Shin, K.K.; Hong, Y.H.; Kim, H.G.; Jeong, D.; Hossain, M.A.; Kim, H.S.; Yi, Y.-S.; Kim, D.; et al. Compound K, a ginsenoside metabolite, plays an antiinflammatory role in macrophages by targeting the AKT1-mediated signaling pathway. *J. Ginseng Res.* **2018**, *43*, 154–160. [CrossRef] [PubMed]
3. Oh, J.; Kim, J.-S. Compound K derived from ginseng: Neuroprotection and cognitive improvement. *Food Funct.* **2016**, *7*, 4506–4515. [CrossRef] [PubMed]
4. Yang, L.; Zou, H.; Gao, Y.; Luo, J.; Xie, X.; Meng, W.; Zhou, H.; Tan, Z. Insights into gastrointestinal microbiota-generated ginsenoside metabolites and their bioactivities. *Drug Metab. Rev.* **2020**, *52*, 125–138. [CrossRef]
5. Lee, I.-S.; Kang, K.; Kim, S.-Y. Panax ginseng Pharmacopuncture: Current Status of the Research and Future Challenges. *Biomolecules* **2019**, *10*, 33. [CrossRef]

6. Kim, K.H.; Lee, D.; Lee, H.L.; Kim, C.-E.; Jung, K.; Kang, K. Beneficial effects of Panax ginseng for the treatment and prevention of neurodegenerative diseases: Past findings and future directions. *J. Ginseng Res.* **2018**, *42*, 239–247. [CrossRef]
7. Noh, K.-H.; Oh, D.-K. Production of the Rare Ginsenosides Compound K, Compound Y, and Compound Mc by a Thermostable β-Glycosidase from Sulfolobus acidocaldarius. *Biol. Pharm. Bull.* **2009**, *32*, 1830–1835. [CrossRef]
8. Akao, T.; Kida, H.; Kanaoka, M.; Hattori, M.; Kobashi, K. Drug Metabolism: Intestinal Bacterial Hydrolysis is Required for the Appearance of Compound K in Rat Plasma after Oral Administration of Ginsenoside Rb1 from Panax ginseng. *J. Pharm. Pharmacol.* **1998**, *50*, 1155–1160. [CrossRef]
9. Zhou, L.; Chen, L.; Zeng, X.; Liao, J.; Ou-Yang, D.-S. Ginsenoside compound K alleviates sodium valproate-induced hepatotoxicity in rats via antioxidant effect, regulation of peroxisome pathway and iron homeostasis. *Toxicol. Appl. Pharmacol.* **2020**, *386*, 114829. [CrossRef]
10. Christensen, L.P. Ginsenosides: Chemistry, biosynthesis, analysis, and potential health effects. *Adv. Food Nutr. Res.* **2008**, *55*, 1–99.
11. Yang, X.-D.; Yang, Y.-Y.; Ou-Yang, D.-S.; Yang, G.-P. A review of biotransformation and pharmacology of ginsenoside compound K. *Fitoterapia* **2015**, *100*, 208–220. [CrossRef] [PubMed]
12. Hasegawa, H.; Sung, J.-H.; Matsumiya, S.; Uchiyama, M. Main Ginseng Saponin Metabolites Formed by Intestinal Bacteria. *Planta Medica* **1996**, *62*, 453–457. [CrossRef] [PubMed]
13. Kim, D.-H. Chemical Diversity of Panax ginseng, Panax quinquifolium, and Panax notoginseng. *J. Ginseng Res.* **2012**, *36*, 1–15. [CrossRef] [PubMed]
14. Upadhyaya, J.; Kim, M.-J.; Kim, Y.-H.; Ko, S.-R.; Park, H.-W.; Kim, M.-K. Enzymatic formation of compound-K from ginsenoside Rb1 by enzyme preparation from cultured mycelia of Armillaria mellea. *J. Ginseng Res.* **2015**, *40*, 105–112. [CrossRef]
15. Li, D.; Wu, Y.; Zhang, C.; Sun, J.; Zhou, Z.; Lu, W. Production of Triterpene Ginsenoside Compound K in the Non-conventional Yeast Yarrowia lipolytica. *J. Agric. Food Chem.* **2019**, *67*, 2581–2588. [CrossRef]
16. Oh, J.-M.; Kim, E.; Chun, S. Ginsenoside Compound K Induces Ros-Mediated Apoptosis and Autophagic Inhibition in Human Neuroblastoma Cells In Vitro and In Vivo. *Int. J. Mol. Sci.* **2019**, *20*, 4279. [CrossRef]
17. Kim, K.-A.; Yoo, H.H.; Gu, W.; Yu, D.-H.; Jin, M.J.; Choi, H.-L.; Yuan, K.; Guérin-Deremaux, L.; Kim, D.-H. A prebiotic fiber increases the formation and subsequent absorption of compound K following oral administration of ginseng in rats. *J. Ginseng Res.* **2014**, *39*, 183–187. [CrossRef]
18. Lee, J.; Lee, E.; Kim, N.; Lee, J.; Yoo, J.; Koh, B. Studies on absorption, distribution and metabolism of ginseng in humans after oral administration. *J. Ethnopharmacol.* **2009**, *122*, 143–148. [CrossRef]
19. Choi, I.-D.; Ryu, J.-H.; Lee, N.-E.; Lee, M.-H.; Shim, J.-J.; Ahn, Y.-T.; Sim, J.-H.; Huh, C.-S.; Shim, W.-S.; Yim, S.-V.; et al. Enhanced Absorption Study of Ginsenoside Compound K (20-O-β-(D-Glucopyranosyl)-20(S)-protopanaxadiol) after Oral Administration of Fermented Red Ginseng Extract (HYFRG™) in Healthy Korean Volunteers and Rats. *Evidence-Based Complement. Altern. Med.* **2016**, *2016*, 3908142. [CrossRef]
20. Dong, W.-W.; Han, X.-Z.; Zhao, J.; Zhong, F.-L.; Ma, R.; Wu, S.; Li, D.; Quan, L.-H.; Jiang, J. Metabolite profiling of ginsenosides in rat plasma, urine and feces by LC-MS/MS and its application to a pharmacokinetic study after oral administration of Panax ginseng extract. *Biomed. Chromatogr.* **2017**, *32*, e4105. [CrossRef]
21. Igami, K.; Ozawa, M.; Inoue, S.; Iohara, D.; Miyazaki, T.; Shinoda, M.; Anraku, M.; Hirayama, F.; Uekama, K. The formation of an inclusion complex between a metabolite of ginsenoside, compound K and ?-cyclodextrin and its dissolution characteristics. *J. Pharm. Pharmacol.* **2015**, *68*, 646–654. [CrossRef]
22. Kim, J.S.; Kim, Y.; Han, S.-H.; Jeon, J.-Y.; Hwang, M.; Im, Y.-J.; Lee, S.Y.; Chae, S.-W.; Kim, M.-G.; Kim, J.H. Development and validation of an LC-MS/MS method for determination of compound K in human plasma and clinical application. *J. Ginseng Res.* **2013**, *37*, 135–141. [CrossRef] [PubMed]
23. Jin, H.; Seo, J.-H.; Uhm, Y.-K.; Jung, C.-Y.; Lee, S.-K.; Yim, S.-V. Pharmacokinetic comparison of ginsenoside metabolite IH-901 from fermented and non-fermented ginseng in healthy Korean volunteers. *J. Ethnopharmacol.* **2012**, *139*, 664–667. [CrossRef] [PubMed]
24. Fukami, H.; Ueda, T.; Matsuoka, N. Pharmacokinetic Study of Compound K in Japanese Subjects After Ingestion of Panax ginseng Fermented by Lactobacillus paracasei A221 Reveals Significant Increase of Absorption into Blood. *J. Med. Food* **2019**, *22*, 257–263. [CrossRef] [PubMed]

25. Shimojo, Y.; Ozawa, Y.; Toda, T.; Igami, K.; Shimizu, T. Probiotic Lactobacillus paracasei A221 improves the functionality and bioavailability of kaempferol-glucoside in kale by its glucosidase activity. *Sci. Rep.* **2018**, *8*, 9239. [CrossRef]
26. Jin, S.; Jeon, J.-H.; Lee, S.; Kang, W.Y.; Seong, S.J.; Yoon, Y.-R.; Choi, M.-K.; Song, I.-S. Detection of 13 Ginsenosides (Rb1, Rb2, Rc, Rd, Re, Rf, Rg1, Rg3, Rh2, F1, Compound K, 20(S)-Protopanaxadiol, and 20(S)-Protopanaxatriol) in Human Plasma and Application of the Analytical Method to Human Pharmacokinetic Studies Following Two Week-Repeated Administration of Red Ginseng Extract. *Molecules* **2019**, *24*, 2618. [CrossRef]
27. Choi, M.-K.; Jin, S.; Jeon, J.-H.; Kang, W.Y.; Seong, S.J.; Yoon, Y.-R.; Han, Y.-H.; Song, I.-S. Tolerability and pharmacokinetics of ginsenosides Rb1, Rb2, Rc, Rd, and compound K after single or multiple administration of red ginseng extract in human beings. *J. Ginseng Res.* **2018**, *44*, 229–237. [CrossRef]
28. Chen, L.; Zhou, L.; Wang, Y.; Yang, G.; Huang, J.; Tan, Z.; Wang, Y.; Zhou, G.; Liao, J.; Ou-Yang, D.-S. Food and Sex-Related Impacts on the Pharmacokinetics of a Single-Dose of Ginsenoside Compound K in Healthy Subjects. *Front. Pharmacol.* **2017**, *8*, 636. [CrossRef]
29. Chen, Y.; Lu, Y.; Yang, Y.; Chen, X.; Zhu, L.; Zhong, D. Determination of ginsenoside compound K in human plasma by liquid chromatography-tandem mass spectrometry of lithium adducts. *Acta Pharm. Sin. B* **2015**, *5*, 461–466. [CrossRef]
30. Yang, L.; Wang, C.-Y.; Xie, X.-N.; Wang, Y.-C.; Peng, J.-B.; Huang, W.-H.; Chen, Y.; Ouyang, D.-S.; Tan, Z.-R. LC-MS/MS determination of ginsenoside compound K and its metabolite 20 (S)-protopanaxadiol in human plasma and urine: Applications in a clinical study. *Bioanalysis* **2019**, *11*, 365–380. [CrossRef]
31. Zhou, L.; Chen, L.; Wang, Y.; Huang, J.; Yang, G.; Tan, Z.; Wang, Y.; Liao, J.; Zhou, G.; Hu, K.; et al. Impact of NR1I2, adenosine triphosphate-binding cassette transporters genetic polymorphisms on the pharmacokinetics of ginsenoside compound K in healthy Chinese volunteers. *J. Ginseng Res.* **2018**, *43*, 460–474. [CrossRef] [PubMed]
32. Lee, P.S.; Han, J.-Y.; Song, T.W.; Sung, J.H.; Kwon, O.-S.; Song, S.; Chung, Y. Physicochemical characteristics and bioavailability of a novel intestinal metabolite of ginseng saponin (IH901) complexed with β-cyclodextrin. *Int. J. Pharm.* **2006**, *316*, 29–36. [CrossRef] [PubMed]
33. Yang, L.; Xin, J.; Zhang, Z.; Yan, H.; Wang, J.; Sun, E.; Hou, J.; Jia, X.; Lv, H. TPGS-modified liposomes for the delivery of ginsenoside compound K against non-small cell lung cancer: Formulation design and its evaluationin vitroandin vivo. *J. Pharm. Pharmacol.* **2016**, *68*, 1109–1118. [CrossRef] [PubMed]
34. Sawant, R.R.; Torchilin, V.P. Challenges in Development of Targeted Liposomal Therapeutics. *AAPS J.* **2012**, *14*, 303–315. [CrossRef]
35. Song, I.S.; Cha, J.-S.; Choi, M.-K. Characterization, in Vivo and in Vitro Evaluation of Solid Dispersion of Curcumin Containing d-α-Tocopheryl Polyethylene Glycol 1000 Succinate and Mannitol. *Molecules* **2016**, *21*, 1386. [CrossRef] [PubMed]
36. Yang, L.; Zhang, Z.; Hou, J.; Jin, X.; Ke, Z.; Liu, D.; Du, M.; Jia, X.; Lv, H. Targeted delivery of ginsenoside compound K using TPGS/PEG-PCL mixed micelles for effective treatment of lung cancer. *Int. J. Nanomed.* **2017**, *12*, 7653–7667. [CrossRef] [PubMed]
37. Zhang, Y.; Tong, D.; Che, D.; Pei, B.; Xia, X.; Yuan, G.; Jin, X. Ascorbyl palmitate/d-α-tocopheryl polyethylene glycol 1000 succinate monoester mixed micelles for prolonged circulation and targeted delivery of compound K for antilung cancer therapy in vitro and in vivo. *Int. J. Nanomed.* **2017**, *12*, 605–614. [CrossRef]
38. Jin, X.; Yang, Q.; Cai, N. Preparation of ginsenoside compound-K mixed micelles with improved retention and antitumor efficacy. *Int. J. Nanomed.* **2018**, *13*, 3827–3838. [CrossRef]
39. Singh, P.; Singh, H.; Castro-Aceituno, V.; Ahn, S.; Kim, Y.-J.; Yang, D.-C. Bovine serum albumin as a nanocarrier for the efficient delivery of ginsenoside compound K: Preparation, physicochemical characterizations and in vitro biological studies. *RSC Adv.* **2017**, *7*, 15397–15407. [CrossRef]
40. Kim, Y.-J.; Perumalsamy, H.; Markus, J.; Balusamy, S.R.; Wang, C.; Kang, S.H.; Lee, S.; Park, S.Y.; Kim, S.; Castro-Aceituno, V.; et al. Development of Lactobacillus kimchicus DCY51T-mediated gold nanoparticles for delivery of ginsenoside compound K: In vitro photothermal effects and apoptosis detection in cancer cells. *Artif. Cells Nanomed. Biotechnol.* **2019**, *47*, 30–44. [CrossRef]
41. Zhang, J.; Wang, Y.; Jiang, Y.; Liu, T.; Luo, Y.; Diao, E.; Cao, Y.; Chen, L.; Zhang, L.; Gu, Q.; et al. Enhanced cytotoxic and apoptotic potential in hepatic carcinoma cells of chitosan nanoparticles loaded with ginsenoside compound K. *Carbohydr. Polym.* **2018**, *198*, 537–545. [CrossRef] [PubMed]

42. Zhang, J.; Zhou, J.; Yuan, Q.; Zhan, C.; Shang, Z.; Gu, Q.; Zhang, J.; Fu, G.; Hu, W. Characterization of ginsenoside compound K loaded ionically cross-linked carboxymethyl chitosan–calcium nanoparticles and its cytotoxic potential against prostate cancer cells. *J. Ginseng Res.* **2020**. [CrossRef]
43. Zhang, J.; Jiang, Y.; Li, Y.; Li, W.; Zhou, J.; Chen, J.; Shang, Z.; Gu, Q.; Wang, W.; Shen, T.; et al. Micelles modified with a chitosan-derived homing peptide for targeted intracellular delivery of ginsenoside compound K to liver cancer cells. *Carbohydr. Polym.* **2019**, *230*, 115576. [CrossRef] [PubMed]
44. Li, G.; Yang, M.; Hao, X.; Li, C.; Gao, Y.; Tao, J. Acute toxicity of sodium formononetin-3′-sulphonate (Sul-F) in Sprague-Dawley rats and Beagle dogs. *Regul. Toxicol. Pharm.* **2015**, *73*, 629–633. [CrossRef] [PubMed]
45. Gao, Y.; Wang, T.; Wang, G.; Li, G.; Sun, C.; Jiang, Z.; Yang, J.; Li, Y.; You, Y.; Wu, X.; et al. Preclinical safety of ginsenoside compound K: Acute, and 26-week oral toxicity studies in mice and rats. *Food Chem. Toxicol.* **2019**, *131*, 110578. [CrossRef]
46. Li, C.; Wang, Z.; Wang, T.; Wang, G.; Li, G.; Sun, C.; Lin, J.; Sun, L.; Sun, X.; Cho, S.; et al. Repeated-dose 26-week oral toxicity study of ginsenoside compound K in Beagle dogs. *J. Ethnopharmacol.* **2019**, *248*, 112323. [CrossRef]
47. Chen, L.; Zhou, L.; Huang, J.; Wang, Y.; Yang, G.; Tan, Z.; Wang, Y.; Zhou, G.; Liao, J.; Ou-Yang, D.-S. Single- and Multiple-Dose Trials to Determine the Pharmacokinetics, Safety, Tolerability, and Sex Effect of Oral Ginsenoside Compound K in Healthy Chinese Volunteers. *Front. Pharmacol.* **2018**, *8*, 965. [CrossRef]
48. Lee, I.K.; Kang, K.A.; Lim, C.M.; Kim, K.C.; Kim, H.S.; Kim, D.-H.; Kim, B.J.; Chang, W.Y.; Hyun, J.-W.; Hyun, J.W. Compound K, a Metabolite of Ginseng Saponin, Induces Mitochondria-Dependent and Caspase-Dependent Apoptosis via the Generation of Reactive Oxygen Species in Human Colon Cancer Cells. *Int. J. Mol. Sci.* **2010**, *11*, 4916–4931. [CrossRef]
49. Xie, T.; Li, Z.; Li, B.; Sun, R.; Zhang, P.; Lv, J. Characterization of ginsenoside compound K metabolites in rat urine and feces by ultra-performance liquid chromatography with electrospray ionization quadrupole time-of-flight tandem mass spectrometry. *Biomed. Chromatogr.* **2019**, *33*, e4643. [CrossRef]
50. Li, W.; Zhang, M.; Zheng, Y.-N.; Li, J.; Wang, Y.-P.; Wang, Y.-J.; Gu, J.; Jin, Y.; Wang, H.; Chen, L. Snailase Preparation of Ginsenoside M1 from Protopanaxadiol-Type Ginsenoside and Their Protective Effects Against CCl4-Induced Chronic Hepatotoxicity in Mice. *Molecules* **2011**, *16*, 10093–10103. [CrossRef]
51. Lee, H.-U.; Bae, E.-A.; Han, M.J.; Kim, N.-J.; Kim, D.-H. Hepatoprotective effect of ginsenoside Rb1 and compound K on tert-butyl hydroperoxide-induced liver injury. *Liver Int.* **2005**, *25*, 1069–1073. [CrossRef] [PubMed]
52. Igami, K.; Shimojo, Y.; Ito, H.; Miyazaki, T.; Kashiwada, Y. Hepatoprotective effect of fermented ginseng and its major constituent compound K in a rat model of paracetamol (acetaminophen)-induced liver injury. *J. Pharm. Pharmacol.* **2014**, *67*, 565–572. [CrossRef] [PubMed]
53. Chen, X.-J.; Liu, W.-J.; Wen, M.-L.; Liang, H.; Wu, S.-M.; Zhu, Y.-Z.; Zhao, J.-Y.; Dong, X.-Q.; Li, M.-G.; Bian, L.; et al. Ameliorative effects of Compound K and ginsenoside Rh1 on non-alcoholic fatty liver disease in rats. *Sci. Rep.* **2017**, *7*, 41144. [CrossRef] [PubMed]
54. Hwang, Y.-C.; Oh, D.-H.; Choi, M.C.; Lee, S.Y.; Ahn, K.-J.; Chung, H.-Y.; Lim, S.-J.; Chung, S.H.; Jeong, I.-K. Compound K attenuates glucose intolerance and hepatic steatosis through AMPK-dependent pathways in type 2 diabetic OLETF rats. *Korean J. Intern. Med.* **2018**, *33*, 347–355. [CrossRef] [PubMed]
55. Choi, N.; Kim, J.W.; Jeong, H.; Shin, D.G.; Seo, J.H.; Kim, J.H.; Lim, C.W.; Han, K.M.; Kim, B. Fermented ginseng, GBCK25, ameliorates steatosis and inflammation in nonalcoholic steatohepatitis model. *J. Ginseng Res.* **2019**, *43*, 196–208. [CrossRef] [PubMed]
56. Hossen, M.J.; Hong, Y.D.; Baek, K.-S.; Yoo, S.; Hong, Y.H.; Kim, J.H.; Lee, J.-O.; Kim, D.; Park, J.; Cho, J.Y. In vitro antioxidative and anti-inflammatory effects of the compound K-rich fraction BIOGF1K, prepared from Panax ginseng. *J. Ginseng Res.* **2017**, *41*, 43–51. [CrossRef]
57. Kim, E.; Yi, Y.-S.; Son, Y.-J.; Han, S.Y.; Kim, N.H.; Nam, G.; Hossain, M.A.; Kim, J.-H.; Park, J.; Cho, J. BIOGF1K, a compound K-rich fraction of ginseng, plays an antiinflammatory role by targeting an activator protein-1 signaling pathway in RAW264.7 macrophage-like cells. *J. Ginseng Res.* **2018**, *42*, 233–237. [CrossRef]
58. Singh, H.; Du, J.; Singh, P.; Mavlonov, G.T.; Yi, T.-H. Development of superparamagnetic iron oxide nanoparticles via direct conjugation with ginsenosides and its in-vitro study. *J. Photochem. Photobiol. B Biol.* **2018**, *185*, 100–110. [CrossRef]

59. Wang, C.W.; Huang, Y.C.; Chan, F.N.; Su, S.C.; Kuo, Y.H.; Huang, S.F.; Hung, M.W.; Lin, H.C.; Chang, W.L.; Chang, T.C. A gut microbial metabolite of ginsenosides, compound K, induces intestinal glucose absorption and Na+/glucose cotransporter 1 gene expression through activation of cAMP response element binding protein. *Mol. Nutr. Food Res.* **2015**, *59*, 670–684. [CrossRef]
60. Chen, J.; Si, M.; Wang, Y.; Liu, L.; Zhang, Y.; Zhou, A.; Wei, W. Ginsenoside metabolite compound K exerts anti-inflammatory and analgesic effects via downregulating COX2. *Inflammopharmacology* **2018**, *27*, 157–166. [CrossRef]
61. Chen, J.; Wu, H.; Wang, Q.; Chang, Y.; Liu, K.; Wei, W. Ginsenoside Metabolite Compound K Suppresses T-Cell Priming via Modulation of Dendritic Cell Trafficking and Costimulatory Signals, Resulting in Alleviation of Collagen-Induced Arthritis. *J. Pharmacol. Exp. Ther.* **2015**, *353*, 71–79. [CrossRef] [PubMed]
62. Lee, Y.J.; Song, K.Y.; Lee, E.Y.; Kang, H.S.; Song, Y. Compound K, a Metabolite of Ginsenosides, Attenuates Collagen-induced Arthritis in Mice. *J. Rheum. Dis.* **2015**, *22*, 154–166. [CrossRef]
63. Chen, J.; Wang, Q.; Wu, H.; Liu, K.; Wu, Y.; Chang, Y.; Wei, W. The ginsenoside metabolite compound K exerts its anti-inflammatory activity by downregulating memory B cell in adjuvant-induced arthritis. *Pharm. Biol.* **2016**, *54*, 1–9. [CrossRef] [PubMed]
64. Wang, R.; Zhang, M.; Hu, S.; Liu, K.; Tai, Y.; Tao, J.; Zhou, W.; Zhao, Z.; Wang, Q.; Wei, W. Ginsenoside metabolite compound-K regulates macrophage function through inhibition of β-arrestin2. *Biomed. Pharmacother.* **2019**, *115*, 108909. [CrossRef]
65. Kang, S.; Siddiqi, M.H.; Yoon, S.J.; Ahn, S.; Noh, H.-Y.; Kumar, N.S.; Kim, Y.-J.; Yang, D.-C. Therapeutic potential of compound K as an IKK inhibitor with implications for osteoarthritis prevention: An in silico and in vitro study. *Vitr. Cell. Dev. Biol. Anim.* **2016**, *52*, 895–905. [CrossRef] [PubMed]
66. Liu, Y.; Perumalsamy, H.; Kang, C.H.; Kim, S.H.; Hwang, J.-S.; Koh, S.-C.; Yi, T.-H.; Kim, Y.-J. Intracellular synthesis of gold nanoparticles by Gluconacetobacter liquefaciens for delivery of peptide CopA3 and ginsenoside and anti-inflammatory effect on lipopolysaccharide-activated macrophages. *Artif. Cell. Nanomed. B* **2020**, *48*, 777–788. [CrossRef] [PubMed]
67. Zhou, L.; Zheng, Y.; Li, Z.; Bao, L.; Dou, Y.; Tang, Y.; Zhang, J.; Zhou, J.; Liu, Y.; Jia, Y.; et al. Compound K Attenuates the Development of Atherosclerosis in ApoE−/− Mice via LXRα Activation. *Int. J. Mol. Sci.* **2016**, *17*, 1054. [CrossRef]
68. Huang, Y.; Liu, H.; Zhang, Y.; Li, J.; Wang, C.; Zhou, L.; Jia, Y.; Li, X. Synthesis and Biological Evaluation of Ginsenoside Compound K Derivatives as a Novel Class of LXRα Activator. *Molecules* **2017**, *22*, 1232. [CrossRef]
69. Lu, S.; Luo, Y.; Zhou, P.; Yang, K.; Sun, G.; Sun, X. Ginsenoside compound K protects human umbilical vein endothelial cells against oxidized low-density lipoprotein-induced injury via inhibition of nuclear factor-κB, p38, and JNK MAPK pathways. *J. Ginseng Res.* **2017**, *43*, 95–104. [CrossRef]
70. Wei, S.; Li, W.; Yu, Y.; Yao, F.; Lixiang, A.; Lan, X.; Guan, F.; Zhang, M.; Chen, L. Ginsenoside Compound K suppresses the hepatic gluconeogenesis via activating adenosine-5' monophosphate kinase: A study in vitro and in vivo. *Life Sci.* **2015**, *139*, 8–15. [CrossRef]
71. Chen, W.; Wang, J.; Luo, Y.; Wang, T.; Li, X.; Li, A.; Li, J.; Liu, K.; Liu, B. Ginsenoside Rb1 and compound K improve insulin signaling and inhibit ER stress-associated NLRP3 inflammasome activation in adipose tissue. *J. Ginseng Res.* **2015**, *40*, 351–358. [CrossRef] [PubMed]
72. Nam, Y.H.; Le, H.T.; Rodriguez, I.; Kim, E.Y.; Kim, K.; Jeong, S.Y.; Woo, S.H.; Lee, Y.R.; Castañeda, R.; Hong, J.; et al. Enhanced antidiabetic efficacy and safety of compound K/β-cyclodextrin inclusion complex in zebrafish. *J. Ginseng Res.* **2016**, *41*, 103–112. [CrossRef] [PubMed]
73. Song, W.; Wei, L.; Du, Y.; Wang, Y.; Jiang, S. Protective effect of ginsenoside metabolite compound K against diabetic nephropathy by inhibiting NLRP3 inflammasome activation and NF-κB/p38 signaling pathway in high-fat diet/streptozotocin-induced diabetic mice. *Int. Immunopharmacol.* **2018**, *63*, 227–238. [CrossRef] [PubMed]
74. Metwaly, A.M.; Lianlian, Z.; Huang, L.-Q.; Dou, D. Black Ginseng and Its Saponins: Preparation, Phytochemistry and Pharmacological Effects. *Molecules* **2019**, *24*, 1856. [CrossRef]
75. Wang, R.; Li, Y.; Wang, W.; Zhou, M.; Cao, Z. [Compound K suppresses myeloid-derived suppressor cells in a mouse model bearing CT26 colorectal cancer xenograft]. *Nan fang yi ke da xue xue bao = J. South. Med. Univ.* **2015**, *35*, 748–752.

76. Lee, S.; Kwon, M.C.; Jang, J.-P.; Sohng, J.K.; Jung, H.J. The ginsenoside metabolite compound K inhibits growth, migration and stemness of glioblastoma cells. *Int. J. Oncol.* **2017**, *51*, 414–424. [CrossRef]
77. Kwak, C.W.; Son, Y.M.; Gu, M.J.; Kim, G.; Lee, I.K.; Kye, Y.C.; Kim, H.W.; Song, K.D.; Chu, H.; Park, B.-C.; et al. A Bacterial Metabolite, Compound K, Induces Programmed Necrosis in MCF-7 Cells via GSK3β. *J. Microbiol. Biotechnol.* **2015**, *25*, 1170–1176. [CrossRef]
78. Zhang, K.; Li, Y. Effects of ginsenoside compound K combined with cisplatin on the proliferation, apoptosis and epithelial mesenchymal transition in MCF-7 cells of human breast cancer. *Pharm. Biol.* **2015**, *54*, 561–568. [CrossRef]
79. Lee, S.J.; Lee, J.S.; Lee, E.; Lim, T.-G.; Byun, S. The ginsenoside metabolite compound K inhibits hormone-independent breast cancer through downregulation of cyclin D1. *J. Funct. Foods* **2018**, *46*, 159–166. [CrossRef]
80. Li, K.-K.; Yan, X.-M.; Li, Z.-N.; Yan, Q.; Gong, X.-J. Synthesis and antitumor activity of three novel ginsenoside M1 derivatives with 3′-ester modifications. *Bioorg. Chem.* **2019**, *90*, 103061. [CrossRef]
81. Choi, E.; Kim, E.; Kim, J.H.; Yoon, K.; Kim, S.; Lee, J.; Cho, J. AKT1-targeted proapoptotic activity of compound K in human breast cancer cells. *J. Ginseng Res.* **2019**, *43*, 692–698. [CrossRef] [PubMed]
82. Li, C.; Dong, Y.; Wang, L.; Xu, G.; Yang, Q.; Tang, X.; Qiao, Y.; Cong, Z. Ginsenoside metabolite compound K induces apoptosis and autophagy in non-small cell lung cancer cells via AMPK–mTOR and JNK pathways. *Biochem. Cell Biol.* **2019**, *97*, 406–414. [CrossRef] [PubMed]
83. Chen, H.-F.; Wu, L.-X.; Li, X.-F.; Zhu, Y.-C.; Wang, W.-X.; Xu, C.-W.; Huang, Z.-Z.; Du, K.-Q. Ginsenoside compound K inhibits growth of lung cancer cells via HIF-1α-mediated glucose metabolism. *Cell. Mol. Biol.* **2019**, *65*, 48–52. [CrossRef]
84. Dong, X.; Han, H.; Shi, H.; Wang, T.; Wang, B.; Zhao, J. Compound K, a metabolite of ginseng saponin, induces apoptosis of hepatocellular carcinoma cells through the mitochondria-mediated caspase-dependent pathway. *Int. J. Clin. Exp. Med.* **2017**, *10*, 11146–11156.
85. Zhang, X.; Zhang, S.; Sun, Q.; Jiao, W.; Yan, Y.; Zhang, X. Compound K Induces Endoplasmic Reticulum Stress and Apoptosis in Human Liver Cancer Cells by Regulating STAT3. *Molecules* **2018**, *23*, 1482. [CrossRef]
86. Wang, Y.-S.; Zhu, H.; Li, H.; Li, Y.; Zhao, B.; Jin, Y.-H. Ginsenoside compound K inhibits nuclear factor-kappa B by targeting Annexin A2. *J. Ginseng Res.* **2018**, *43*, 452–459. [CrossRef]
87. Shin, D.-H.; Leem, D.-G.; Shin, J.-S.; Kim, J.-I.; Kim, K.-T.; Choi, S.Y.; Lee, M.-H.; Choi, J.-H.; Lee, K.-T. Compound K induced apoptosis via endoplasmic reticulum Ca2+ release through ryanodine receptor in human lung cancer cells. *J. Ginseng Res.* **2017**, *42*, 165–174. [CrossRef]
88. Chen, L.; Meng, Y.; Sun, Q.; Zhang, Z.; Guo, X.; Sheng, X.; Tai, G.; Cheng, H.; Zhou, Y. Ginsenoside compound K sensitizes human colon cancer cells to TRAIL-induced apoptosis via autophagy-dependent and -independent DR5 upregulation. *Cell Death Dis.* **2016**, *7*, e2334. [CrossRef]
89. Kim, H.; Roh, H.S.; Kim, J.E.; Park, S.D.; Park, W.H.; Moon, J.-Y. Compound K attenuates stromal cell-derived growth factor 1 (SDF-1)-induced migration of C6 glioma cells. *Nutr. Res. Pr.* **2016**, *10*, 259–264. [CrossRef]
90. Chen, K.; Jiao, J.; Xue, J.; Chen, T.; Hou, Y.; Jiang, Y.; Qian, L.; Wang, Y.; Ma, Z.; Liang, Z.; et al. Ginsenoside CK induces apoptosis and suppresses proliferation and invasion of human osteosarcoma cells through the PI3K/mTOR/p70S6K1 pathway. *Oncol. Rep.* **2020**, *43*, 886–896. [CrossRef]
91. Jin, X.; Zhou, J.; Zhang, Z.; Lv, H. The combined administration of parthenolide and ginsenoside CK in long circulation liposomes with targeted tLyp-1 ligand induce mitochondria-mediated lung cancer apoptosis. *Artif. Cells Nanomed. Biotechnol.* **2018**, *46*, S931–S942. [CrossRef] [PubMed]
92. Darsandhari, S.; Shrestha, B.; Pandey, R.P.; Lee, S.; Jung, H.J.; Kim, Y.-J.; Sohng, J.K. Enzymatically Synthesized Ginsenoside Exhibits Antiproliferative Activity in Various Cancer Cell Lines. *Appl. Sci.* **2019**, *9*, 893. [CrossRef]
93. Seo, J.Y.; Ju, S.H.; Oh, J.; Lee, S.K.; Kim, J.-S. Neuroprotective and Cognition-Enhancing Effects of Compound K Isolated from Red Ginseng. *J. Agric. Food Chem.* **2016**, *64*, 2855–2864. [CrossRef] [PubMed]
94. Li, C.-W.; Deng, M.-Z.; Gao, Z.-J.; Dang, Y.-Y.; Zheng, G.-D.; Yang, X.-J.; Chao, Y.-X.; Cai, Y.-F.; Wu, X.-L. Effects of compound K, a metabolite of ginsenosides, on memory and cognitive dysfunction in db/db mice involve the inhibition of ER stress and the NLRP3 inflammasome pathway. *Food Funct.* **2020**, *11*, 4416–4427. [CrossRef] [PubMed]
95. Yayeh, T.; Yun, K.; Jang, S.; Oh, S. Morphine dependence is attenuated by red ginseng extract and ginsenosides Rh2, Rg3, and compound K. *J. Ginseng Res.* **2016**, *40*, 445–452. [CrossRef]

96. Zeng, X.; Hu, K.; Chen, L.; Zhou, L.; Luo, W.; Li, C.; Zong, W.; Chen, S.; Gao, Q.; Zeng, G.; et al. The Effects of Ginsenoside Compound K Against Epilepsy by Enhancing the γ-Aminobutyric Acid Signaling Pathway. *Front. Pharmacol.* **2018**, *9*, 9. [CrossRef]
97. Liu, Q.; Liu, L.; Liu, H.; Jiang, J.; Guo, S.; Wang, C.; Jia, Y.; Tian, Y. Compound K attenuated hepatectomy-induced post-operative cognitive dysfunction in aged mice via LXRα activation. *Biomed. Pharmacother.* **2019**, *119*, 109400. [CrossRef]
98. Yang, Q.; Lin, J.; Zhang, H.; Liu, Y.; Kan, M.; Xiu, Z.; Chen, X.; Lan, X.; Li, X.; Shi, X.; et al. Ginsenoside compound K regulates amyloid β via the Nrf2/Keap1 signaling pathway in mice with scopolamine hydrobromide-induced memory impairments. *J. Mol. Neurosci.* **2019**, *67*, 62–71. [CrossRef]
99. Chen, X.; Li, H.; Yang, Q.; Lan, X.; Wang, J.; Cao, Z.; Shi, X.; Li, J.; Kan, M.; Qu, X.; et al. Ginsenoside compound K ameliorates Alzheimer's disease in HT22 cells by adjusting energy metabolism. *Mol. Biol. Rep.* **2019**, *46*, 5323–5332. [CrossRef]
100. Zong, W.; Zeng, X.; Chen, S.; Chen, L.; Zhou, L.; Wang, X.; Gao, Q.; Zeng, G.; Hu, K.; Ou-Yang, D.-S. Ginsenoside compound K attenuates cognitive deficits in vascular dementia rats by reducing the Aβ deposition. *J. Pharmacol. Sci.* **2019**, *139*, 223–230. [CrossRef]
101. Jiang, S.; Zhang, H.; Qian, M.; Su, X.; Sun, X.; Wu, T.; Song, W. Effects of ginsenoside CK pretreatment on oxidative stress and inflammation in rats with cerebral ischemia/reperfusion injury. *Biotechnol. Biotechnol. Equip.* **2018**, *32*, 1606–1612. [CrossRef]
102. Song, W.; Guo, Y.; Jiang, S.; Wei, L.; Liu, Z.; Wang, X.; Su, Y. Antidepressant Effects of the Ginsenoside Metabolite Compound K, Assessed by Behavioral Despair Test and Chronic Unpredictable Mild Stress Model. *Neurochem. Res.* **2018**, *43*, 1371–1382. [CrossRef] [PubMed]
103. Song, W.; Li, G.; Tang, Y.; Wei, L.; Song, D.; Wang, X.; Zhang, C.; Jin, X.; Jiang, S. Ginsenoside compound K inhibits oxidative stress and NLRP3 inflammasome activity in mice exposed to chronic unpredictable mild stress. *Biotechnol. Biotechnol. Equip.* **2019**, *33*, 1372–1379. [CrossRef]
104. Zhou, L.; Yang, F.; Yin, J.-W.; Gu, X.; Xu, Y.; Liang, Y.-Q. Compound K induces neurogenesis of neural stem cells in thrombin induced nerve injury through LXRα signaling in mice. *Neurosci. Lett.* **2020**, *729*, 135007. [CrossRef]
105. Oh, J.-M.; Jeong, J.H.; Park, S.Y.; Chun, S. Ginsenoside Compound K Induces Adult Hippocampal Proliferation and Survival of Newly Generated Cells in Young and Elderly Mice. *Biomolecules* **2020**, *10*, 484. [CrossRef]
106. Lim, T.-G.; Jeon, A.J.; Yoon, J.H.; Song, D.; Kim, J.-E.; Kwon, J.Y.; Kim, J.R.; Kang, N.J.; Park, J.-S.; Yeom, M.H.; et al. 20-O-β-D-glucopyranosyl-20(S)-protopanaxadiol, a metabolite of ginsenoside Rb1, enhances the production of hyaluronic acid through the activation of ERK and Akt mediated by Src tyrosin kinase in human keratinocytes. *Int. J. Mol. Med.* **2015**, *35*, 1388–1394. [CrossRef]
107. Kim, E.; Kim, N.; Yoo, S.; Hong, Y.H.; Han, S.Y.; Jeong, S.; Jeong, D.; Kim, J.-H.; Cho, J.; Park, J. The skin protective effects of compound K, a metabolite of ginsenoside Rb1 from Panax ginseng. *J. Ginseng Res.* **2017**, *42*, 218–224. [CrossRef]
108. Hong, Y.H.; Kim, N.; Nam, G.; Yoo, S.; Han, S.Y.; Jeong, S.-G.; Kim, E.; Jeong, D.; Yoon, K.; Kim, S.; et al. Photoaging protective effects of BIOGF1K, a compound-K-rich fraction prepared from Panax ginseng. *J. Ginseng Res.* **2017**, *42*, 81–89. [CrossRef]
109. Lee, S.Y. Synergistic effect of maclurin on ginsenoside compound K induced inhibition of the transcriptional expression of matrix metalloproteinase-1 in HaCaT human keratinocyte cells. *J. Ginseng Res.* **2017**, *42*, 229–232. [CrossRef]
110. Park, N.-J.; Bong, S.-K.; Lee, S.; Jung, Y.; Jegal, H.; Kim, J.; Kim, S.-K.; Kim, Y.K.; Kim, S.-N. Compound K improves skin barrier function by increasing SPINK5 expression. *J. Ginseng Res.* **2019**. [CrossRef]
111. Fan, H.; Wang, Y.; Zhang, X.; Chen, J.; Zhou, Q.; Yu, Z.; Chen, Y.; Chen, Z.; Gu, J.; Shi, Y. Ginsenoside compound K ameliorates imiquimod-induced psoriasis-like dermatitis through inhibiting REG3A/RegIIIγ expression in keratinocytes. *Biochem. Biophys. Res. Commun.* **2019**, *515*, 665–671. [CrossRef] [PubMed]
112. Hsu, W.-H.; Hua, K.-F.; Tuan, L.-H.; Tsai, Y.-L.; Chu, L.J.; Lee, Y.-C.; Wong, W.-T.; Lee, S.-L.; Lai, J.-H.; Chu, C.-L.; et al. Compound K inhibits priming and mitochondria-associated activating signals of NLRP3 inflammasome in renal tubulointerstitial lesions. *Nephrol. Dial. Transplant.* **2019**, *35*, 74–85. [CrossRef]
113. Lin, T.-J.; Wu, C.-Y.; Tsai, P.-Y.; Hsu, W.-H.; Hua, K.-F.; Chu, C.-L.; Lee, Y.-C.; Chen, A.; Lee, S.-L.; Lin, Y.-J.; et al. Accelerated and Severe Lupus Nephritis Benefits From M1, an Active Metabolite of Ginsenoside, by Regulating NLRP3 Inflammasome and T Cell Functions in Mice. *Front. Immunol.* **2019**, *10*, 1951. [CrossRef]

114. Ren, S.; Liu, R.; Wang, Y.; Ding, N.; Li, Y. Synthesis and biological evaluation of Ginsenoside Compound K analogues as a novel class of anti-asthmatic agents. *Bioorg. Med. Chem. Lett.* **2019**, *29*, 51–55. [CrossRef]
115. Li, X.; Huang, Q.; Wang, M.; Yan, X.; Song, X.; Ma, R.; Jiang, R.; Zhao, D.; Sun, L. Compound K Inhibits Autophagy-Mediated Apoptosis Through Activation of the PI3K-Akt Signaling Pathway Thus Protecting Against Ischemia/Reperfusion Injury. *Cell. Physiol. Biochem.* **2018**, *47*, 2589–2601. [CrossRef]
116. Bessell, E.; Fuller, N.R.; Markovic, T.P.; Burk, J.; Picone, T.; Hendy, C.; Tan, M.M.C.; Caterson, I.D. Effects of alpha-cyclodextrin on cholesterol control and Compound K on glycaemic control in people with pre-diabetes: Protocol for a Phase III randomized controlled trial. *Clin. Obes.* **2019**, *9*, e12324. [CrossRef] [PubMed]
117. Oh, M.-R.; Park, S.-H.; Kim, S.-Y.; Baek, H.-I.; Kim, M.-G.; Jeon, J.-Y.; Ha, K.-C.; Na, W.-T.; Cha, Y.-S.; Park, B.-H.; et al. Postprandial glucose-lowering effects of fermented red ginseng in subjects with impaired fasting glucose or type 2 diabetes: A randomized, double-blind, placebo-controlled clinical trial. *BMC Complement. Altern. Med.* **2014**, *14*, 237. [CrossRef] [PubMed]
118. Flanagan, S.D.; Dupont, W.H.; Caldwell, L.K.; Hardesty, V.H.; Barnhart, E.C.; Beeler, M.K.; Post, E.M.; Volek, J.S.; Kraemer, W.J. The Effects of a Korean Ginseng, GINST15, on Hypo-Pituitary-Adrenal and Oxidative Activity Induced by Intense Work Stress. *J. Med. Food* **2018**, *21*, 104–112. [CrossRef] [PubMed]
119. Flanagan, S.D.; Proessl, F.; Dunn-Lewis, C.; Canino, M.C.; Sterczala, A.J.; Connaboy, C.; Dupont, W.H.; Caldwell, L.K.; Kraemer, W.J. Constitutive and Stress-Induced Psychomotor Cortical Responses to Compound K Supplementation. *Front. Neurosci.* **2020**, *14*, 315. [CrossRef] [PubMed]
120. Jung, S.-J.; Hwang, J.-H.; Park, S.-H.; Choi, E.-K.; Ha, K.-C.; Baek, H.-I.; Shin, D.-G.; Seo, J.-H.; Chae, S.-W. A 12-week, randomized, double-blind study to evaluate the efficacy and safety of liver function after using fermented ginseng powder (GBCK25). *Food Nutr. Res.* **2020**, *64*, 3517. [CrossRef]

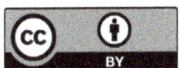

© 2020 by the authors. Licensee MDPI, Basel, Switzerland. This article is an open access article distributed under the terms and conditions of the Creative Commons Attribution (CC BY) license (http://creativecommons.org/licenses/by/4.0/).

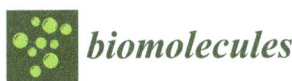

Review

Effects of Red and Fermented Ginseng and Ginsenosides on Allergic Disorders

Myung Joo Han [1] and Dong-Hyun Kim [2],*

[1] Department of Food and Nutrition, Kyung Hee University, Seoul 02447, Korea; mjhan@khu.ac.kr
[2] Neurobiota Research Center, Department of Pharmacy, Kyung Hee University, Seoul 02447, Korea
* Correspondence: dhkim@khu.ac.kr; Tel.: +82-2-961-0374

Received: 21 February 2020; Accepted: 15 April 2020; Published: 20 April 2020

Abstract: Both white ginseng (WG, dried root of *Panax* sp.) and red ginseng (RG, steamed and dried root of *Panax* sp.) are reported to exhibit a variety of pharmacological effects such as anticancer, antidiabetic, and neuroprotective activities. These ginsengs contain hydrophilic sugar-conjugated ginsenosides and polysaccharides as the bioactive constituents. When taken orally, their hydrophilic constituents are metabolized into hydrophobic ginsenosides compound K, Rh1, and Rh2 that are absorbable into the blood. These metabolites exhibit the pharmacological effects more strongly than hydrophilic parental constituents. To enforce these metabolites, fermented WG and RG are developed. Moreover, natural products including ginseng are frequently used for the treatment of allergic disorders. Therefore, this review introduces the current knowledge related to the effectiveness of ginseng on allergic disorders including asthma, allergic rhinitis, atopic dermatitis, and pruritus. We discuss how ginseng, its constituents, and its metabolites regulate allergy-related immune responses. We also describe how ginseng controls allergic disorders.

Keywords: *Panax* sp.; ginsenosides; polysaccharides; allergy; immune system

1. Introduction

Allergies including asthma, allergic rhinitis, atopic dermatitis (AD), atopic conjunctivitis, and anaphylaxis are common, persistent, and incorrigible disorders [1,2]. The prevalence of allergies ranges from 10% to 40% of the population worldwide [2]. A variety of drugs, including immune modulators and biological agents, have been developed for the treatment of allergies [3,4]. However, they have certain limitations due to their side effects: glucocorticoids often induce the adrenal insufficiency and cause infections and skin atrophy; calcineurin inhibitors cause neurotoxicity, nephrotoxicity, infections, and skin cancers; and biological agents such as omalizumab increase infections and tumor development [5,6]. Therefore, natural products with fewer adverse effects such as red ginseng and radix glycyrrhizae have been frequently used as the functional foods and traditional Chinese medicines [7,8]. Many studies have been conducted on their anti-allergic effects. Of these, we focused on the anti-allergic effects of ginseng and the constituent ginsenosides and polysaccharides in the present review.

2. Chemistry of Ginseng

The term ginseng is used to represent the dried root of the *Panax* spp. (family Araliaceae), including *Panax ginseng* Meyer (Korean ginseng), *Panax quiquifolium* L. (American Ginseng), and *Panax notoginseng* (Burk.) FHChen (notoginseng) [9,10]. When the fresh roots of these *Panax* spp., particularly Korean ginseng, are dried or steamed/dried, they are named white ginseng (WG) or red ginseng (RG), respectively. Ginseng has been used world-wide as herbal medicine or functional food for promoting vitality, increasing the resistance to stress, and modulating immune responses [11,12]. The bioactive constituents are considered to be ginsenosides, such as protopanxadiol-type, protopanaxatriol-type, and oleanane-type ginsenosides, and polysaccharides such as ginsan [13] (Figure 1). Of protopanaxadiol-type ginsenosides, ginsenosides Rb1, Rb2, Rc, Rd, and Rg3 and quinquenosides I and II are highly isolated from ginseng [14,15]. Of protopanaxatriol-type ginsenosides, ginsenosides Rg1 and Re are frequently isolated [16,17]. Of oleanane-type ginsenosides, ginsenoside Ro and chikusetsusaponin are isolated [10,18,19].

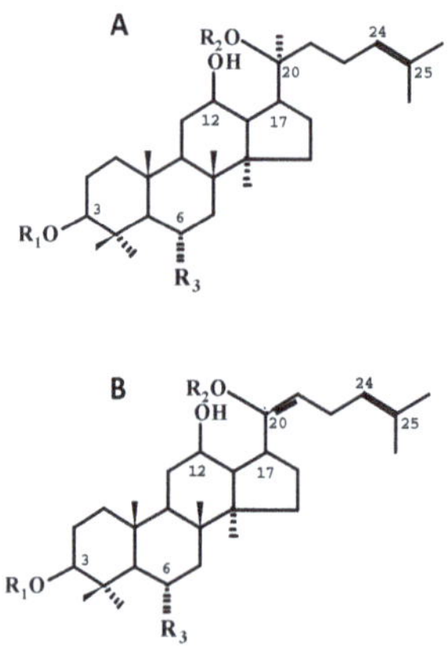

Ginsenoside	M	R1	R2	R3
Ginsenoside Rb1	A	Glc-Glc-	Glc-Glc-	H
Ginsenoside Rb2	A	Glc-Glc-	Ara(p)-Glc-	H
Ginsenoside Rc	A	Glc-Glc-	Ara(f)-Glc-	H
Ginsenoside Rd	A	Glc-Glc-	Glc-	H
Ginsenoside Rg3	A	Glc-Glc-	H	H
Ginsenoside Rg5	B	Glc-Glc-	H	H
Ginsenoside F2	A	Glc-	Glc-	H
Ginsenoside Rh2	A	Glc-	H	H
Compound K	A	H	Glc-	H
Protopanaxdiol	A	H	H	H
Ginsenoside Re	A	H	Glc-	Rha- Glc-O-
Ginsenoside Rf	A	H	H	Glc-Glc-O-
Ginsenoside Rg1	A	H	Glc-	Glc-O-
Ginsenoside Rg2	A	H	H	Rha- Glc-O-
Ginsenoside Rh1	A	H	H	Glc-O-
Ginsenoside F1	A	H	Glc-	OH
protopanaxatriol	A	H	H	OH

Figure 1. The Representative Ginsenosides Contained in WG and RG.

3. The Role of Gut-Microbiota-Mediated Metabolism in the Mediation of Biological Effects of Ginseng

Korean ginseng, American ginseng, and notoginseng all contain hydrophilic sugar-conjugated ginsenosides and polysaccharides as the bioactive components [13]. Of ginsenosides, hydrophilic ginsenosides Rb1, Rb2, Rc, and Re have a variety of pharmacological activities such as anti-inflammatory, antidiabetic, hepatoprotective, and anticancer activities in the in vivo studies [13,20]. However, when these ginsenosides or ginseng extracts are orally gavaged, these ginsenosides such as Rb1 and Re are not easily absorbed into the blood [21,22] (Figure 2). Therefore, these contact with gut microbiota, which transform hydrophobic metabolites such as compound K (CK) and ginsenoside Rh1. These metabolites such as CK are detected in the blood rather than parental constituents [21,22]. In addition, when ginsenoside Rb1 was orally administered in germ-free rats, Rb1 and CK both were not detected in the blood [23]. To understand the reason for this, when ginsenosides were incubated with fecal bacteria, they were strongly and quickly transformed into CK [24]. Orally administered ginsenoside Rb1, a main constituent of *Panax ginseng*, is transformed to CK through ginsenosides Rd and F2 in humans and animals by gut bacteria, such as *Bifidobacterium* sp. and *Bacteroides* sp., and thereafter these metabolites are detected in the blood and urine [25–27]. The absorption of gut-microbiota-mediated metabolites from ginseng constituent ginsenosides are significantly affected by intestinal environmental factors such as diets and antibiotics [28–31]. The biological activities of ginsenosides Rb1 and Re, such as anti-inflammatory and anti-allergic activities, are attenuated in mice by oral gavage of antibiotics [30,31]. When RG extract is orally administered in humans and mice, ginsenoside Rd is the most highly detected, followed by ginsenoside Rg3, ginsenoside

Rg1, and protopanaxatriol [32,33]. However, when bifidobacteria-fermented red ginseng (fRG) is orally administered, ginsenoside Rd is the most highly detected, followed by ginsenoside Rg1, CK, ginsenoside Rg3, and protopanaxtriol [32,33]. The contents of these ginsenosides except ginsenoside Rg3 absorbed into the blood are significantly higher in the fRG-treated volunteers and mice than in the RG-treated volunteers and mice. However, when notoginseng extract, whose which main constituents are ginsenosides Ra3, Rb1, Rd, Re, and Rg1 and notoginsenoside R1, is orally administered to rats, the compounds mainly absorbed to the blood are ginsenosides Ra2, Rb1, and Rd, including CK [34]. This is controversial. Nevertheless, of parental ginsenosides and their metabolites, CK, ginsenosides Rh1, Rh2 and protopanaxtriol, which are hydrophobic metabolites of ginsenosides by gut microbiota, exhibit the most potent biological effects compared to those of parental compounds [31–33,35–40]. These results suggest that when ginseng extracts are orally administered, their hydrophilic constituents are metabolized by gut microbiota and their metabolites absorbable into the blood can express pharmacological effects: the pharmacological activities of ginseng extracts may be dependent on the absorbable metabolites produced by gut microbiota.

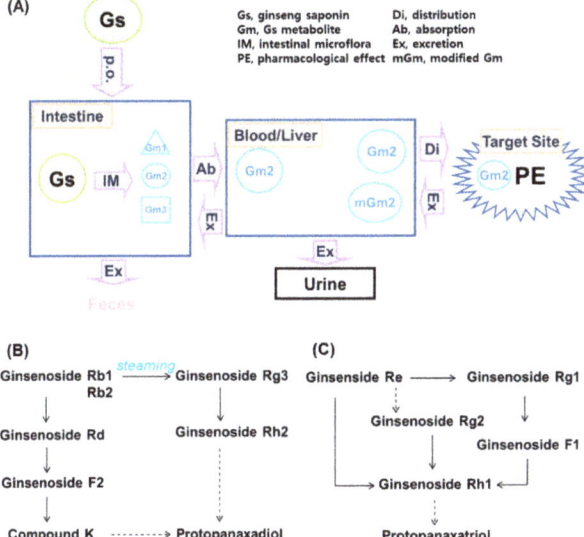

Figure 2. The proposed metabolic pathway of ginseng and its constituent ginsenosides by gut microbiota. (**A**) The fate of orally administered ginseng saponins in vivo. (**B**) The metabolic pathway of protopanaxadiol-type ginsenosides. (**C**) The metabolic pathway of protopanaxatriol-type ginsenosides. Solid arrows, potently proceeded; dashed arrows, weakly proceeded.

4. Anti-Allergic Effects of Ginseng

Ginseng extracts including RG extracts have been used in the traditional Chinese medicine for the treatment of allergic diseases including asthma, rhinitis, and AD [7,8,41]. Actually, many studies have been performed to support their anti-allergic effects in vitro, in animals, and in patients with allergic disorders.

4.1. The In Vitro and In Vivo Anti-Allergic Effects of Ginseng

The anti-allergic effects of ginseng have been mainly studied in vitro, in animals, and in patients with allergic disorders (Table 1). First, Kim and Yang evaluated the effects of WG on ovalbumin-induced asthma in mice [42]. They found that intraperitoneally injected RG restored the ovalbumin-induced expression of eosinophil major basic protein (EMBP), interleukin (IL)-1β, IL-4, IL-5, and tumor necrosis factor (TNF)-α expression in lung tissues. RG inhibited the ovalbumin-induced numbers of goblet cells and mitogen-activated protein kinases (MAPKs) in the bronchoalveolar lavage fluid of mice. Babayigit et al. reported that orally administered RG extract suppressed the chronic airway inflammation and mast cell populations in ovalbumin-sensitized mice [43]. Oral administration of WG or RG alleviated IL-4, IL-5, and IL-13 expression and immune cell infiltration in the bronchoalveolar regions of mice with ovalbumin-induced asthma [44]. They also suppressed IgE levels. Of these, RG more strongly lowered IgE level. Lee et al. reported that RG and fRG reduced serum IgE and ovalbumin-specific IgE levels and intestinal mucosal mast cell protease (MMCP)-1, IL-4, TNF-α, cyclooxygenase (COX)-2, and inducible NO synthase (iNOS) expression in ovalbumin-sensitized mice [45]. Furthermore, RG and fRG inhibited IL-4 expression in phorbol 12-myristate-13-acetate/A23187-stimulated RBL-2H3 cells and alleviated ovalbumin-induced allergic rhinitis in mice [46]. In particular, fRG potently reduced nasal allergy symptoms; IgE level in the blood; IL-4 and IL-5 levels in nasal mucosa; and mast cell, eosinophil, and Th2 cell populations in bronchoalveolar lavage fluid and restored ovalbumin-induced gut dysbiosis. The inhibitory effects of fRG in the treatment of allergic rhinitis were better than those of RG. Jung et al. reported that RG suppressed IL-4 and IL-5 levels and eosinophil populations in the nasal lavage fluid of ovalbumin-sensitized mice [47]. RG increased ovalbumin-suppressed splenic IL-12 expression; IFN-γ-to-IL-4 ratio; and small intestinal CD8-, IFNγ-, and IgA-positive cell populations in ovalbumin-sensitized mice [48]. Furthermore, fRG treatment improved the activities and emotions of quality of life. These results suggest that RG and fRG can alleviate allergic rhinitis in mice by suppressing IgE, IL-4, IL-5, and IL-13 expression and restoring altered gut microbiota and that fRG may display anti-allergic rhinitis activity more strongly than RG did due to the richness of absorbable ginsenosides.

Table 1. Summary of ginseng extract effects on allergic disorders.

Ginseng	Effect	Dosage/Ad. Route	Ref
RG	*in mice with OVA-sensitized asthma/rhinitis* • Suppressed IgE, MMCP-1, IL-1β, IL-4, IL-5, IL-13, TNF-α, COX-2, and iNOS expression; MMPK and NF-κB activation; and mast cell, eosinophil, and Th2 cell populations • Increased ovalbumin-suppressed splenic IL-12 expression; IFN-γ-to-IL-4 ratio; and small intestinal CD8-, IFNγ-, and IgA-positive cell populations • Alleviated chronic airway inflammation, nasal allergy symptoms, and gut microbiota dysbiosis	B, 2 g/kg, *p.o.* 7 d B, 30 m/kg, *p.o.* 7 d B, 0.2%, in diet 8 w B, 50 mg/kg, *p.o.* 6 d B, 2 g/kg, *p.o.* 14 d B, 60 mg/kg, *p.o.* 37 d	[43] [44] [45] [46] [47] [48]
	in NC/Nga mice with TNCB-induced AD • Suppressed IgE, IL-4, IL-10, IL-31, TNF-α, and TSLP expression; MAPKs activity; and NF-κB-independent Ikaros activation. • Suppressed mast cell, Treg cell, and Langerhans cell populations. • Suppressed ear thickness, clinical skin severity, and pruritic sensation	200 mg/kg, *p.o.* 10 d 200 mg/kg, *p.o.* 3 w 200 mg/kg, *p.o.* 5 d 0.1%, s.a. 21 d	[49] [50] [51] [52]
	in mice with DNCB/DNFB-induced AD • Decreased IgE, IL-4, IL-6, IL-10, TSLP, TNF-α, nerve growth factor, and TARC expression and MAPK and p70S6K signaling Decreased ear swelling and dermatitis score	B, 0.1%, s.a. 2 w B, 400 mg/kg, *p.o.* 6 w B, 1%, s.a. 8 d B, 1%, s.a. 8 d	[53] [54] [55] [56]
	in mice with oxazolone-induced AD • Inhibited IL-1β, TNF-α, and COX-2 expression Suppressed ear skin edema	I, 0.1%, s.a. 7 d	[57]

Table 1. Cont.

Ginseng	Effect	Dosage/Ad. Route	Ref
	in mice with pruritus • Inhibited chloroquine-induced scratching, histamine-induced scratching, and compound 48/80-induced scratching behaviors Inhibited histamine receptor type 1/TRPV1 pathway and Ca^{2+} influx	I, 100 mg/m, *p.o.* I, 50 mg/m, *p.o.* I, 200 mg/kg, *p.o.* B, 200 mg/kg, *p.o.*	[58] [59] [60] [61]
	in mice with PCA reaction • Inhibited IgE/antigen-induced PCA reaction • Inhibited the IgE/antigen-stimulated degranulation, IL-4 expression, NF-κB activation in basophils	B, 200 mg/kg, *p.o.* I, 50 mg/kg, *p.o.*	[61] [62]
WG	*in mice with OVA-sensitized asthma/rhinitis* • Suppressed EMBP, IL-1β, IL-4, and IL-5 expression and MMPK activity • Suppressed IL-4, IL-5, and IL-13 expression and immune cell infiltration	B, 20 mg/kg, *i.p.* 3 d B, 30 m/kg, *p.o.* 7 d	[42] [44]
fRG	*in mice with OVA-sensitized asthma/rhinitis* • Inhibited nasal allergy symptoms and gut dysbiosis • Suppressed IgE, IL-4, and IL-5 expression and mast cell, eosinophil, Th2 cell, Th2/Th1 populations	B, 0.2%, in diet, 8 w B, 50 mg/kg, *p.o.* 6 d B, 60 mg/kg, *p.o.* 37 d	[45] [46] [48]
	in mice with PCA reaction • Inhibited IgE-DNP-stimulated passive cutaneous anaphylaxis in mice • Inhibited IgE-DNP-stimulated IL-4 expression in RBH-2H3 mast cells	B, 50 mg/kg, *p.o.*	[63]
CG	*in NC/Nga mice with DNCB-induced AD* • Inhibited IgE; TNF-α/IFN-γ-induced TARC, TNF-α, IFN-γ, IL-4, IL-5; and IL-13 expression • Ameliorated dermatitis severity	20 mg/kg, *s.a.* 4 w	[64]
BG	*in mice with DNCB-induced AD* • Reduced IgE and IL-4 expression and leukocyte populations • Alleviated the AD-like skin symptoms	B, 100 mg/kg, *s.a.* 4 w	[65]

AD, atopic dermatitis; Ad, administered; B, Balb/c; BG, γ-irradiated black ginseng; CG, cultivated ginseng; COX, cyclooxygenase; d, day; DNCB, 1-chloro-2,4-dinitrobenzene; DNFB, 2,4-dinitrofluorobenzene; EMBP, eosinophil major basic protein; fRG, fermented red ginseng; I, ICR; IFN, interferon; iNOS, inducible NO synthase; m, mouse; MAPK, mitogen-activated protein kinase; MMCP, mucosal mast cell protease; OVA, ovalbumin; PCA, passive cutaneous anaphylaxis; p.o., per oral; s.a., skin application; TARC, thymus and activation-regulated chemokine; TNCB, 2,4,6-trinitro-1-chrolobenzene; TNF, tumor necrosis factor; Treg, regulatory T; TSLP, thymic stromal lymphopoietin; w, week; WG, white ginseng.

In addition, Lee and Cho reported that RG suppressed mast cell populations, pruritic sensation, and IL-31 expression in NC/Nga mice with 2, 4, 6-trinitro-1-chrolobenzene (TNCB)-induced AD [49]. They also found that RG extract suppressed the ear thickness, IgE levels in the blood, and regulatory (FOXP3+) T cell and Langerhans cell (CD1a+) populations in the lesions of TNCB-sensitized NC/Ng mice [50]. Treatment with RG inhibited thymic stromal lymphopoietin (TSLP) and TNF-α expression and Langerhans cell populations in NC/Nga mice with TNCB-induced AD [51]. Kim et al. reported that topical application of RG significantly suppressed the clinical skin severity score in NC/Nga mice with TNCB-induced AD [52]. Furthermore, RG treatment decreased the mast cell infiltration and TNF-α and IL-4 expression in the TNCB-exposed lesions but did not affect IgE levels in the blood. Sohn et al. reported that RG decreased IgE levels in the blood and IL-4 and IL-10 expression, MAPKs activity, and NF-κB-independent Ikaros activation in the dorsal surface of mice with 1-chloro-2, 4-dinitrobenzene

(DNCB)-induced AD [53]. RG decreased the IL-6, thymic stromal lymphopoietin (TSLP), and TNF-α, and thymus and activation-regulated chemokine (TARC) expression; MAPKs activation; and dermatitis score in DNCB sensitized mice [54]. The topical pretreatment with RG prevented the induction of ear swelling, nerve growth factor expression, and nerve fiber extension in mice by exposure to 2, 4-dinitrofluorobenzene (DNFB) [55]. RG treatment suppressed mammalian target of rapamycin (mTOR)/p70 ribosomal protein S6 kinase (p70S6K) signaling in anti-FcεRIa antibody-stimulated human basophil KH812 cells and DNFB-sensitized mice [56]. Choi et al. reported that cultivated Korean ginseng (CG) inhibited TNF-α/IFN-γ-induced thymus and activation-regulated chemokine (TARC) expression through NF-κB-dependent signaling in HaCaT cells [64]. Furthermore, CG ameliorated DNCB-induced atopic dermatitis severity; IgE and TARC expression in the blood; and TARC, TNF-α, IFN-γ, IL-4, IL-5, and IL-13 expression in the skin lesions of mice. Bae et al. reported that RG suppressed oxazolone-induced ear skin edema, IL-1β, TNF-α, and COX-2 expression in mice and inhibited iNOS and COX-2 expression in lipopolysaccharide-induced RAW264.7 cells [57]. Kang et al. reported that γ-irradiated black ginseng extract reduced the IgE/antigen-complex-induced degranulation in RBL-2H3 mast cells and alleviated the AD-like skin symptoms, IgE and IL-4 expression, and leukocyte populations in the blood [65]. These findings suggest that ginseng including RG and CG can suppress allergen-induced IgE level, TNF-α, TSLP, IL-4, and IL-6 expression, resulting in the attenuation of AD.

Lee et al. reported that RG strongly inhibited chloroquine-induced scratching in mice [58]. Furthermore, RG inhibited chloroquine-induced Ca^{2+} influx in the primary culture of mouse dorsal root ganglia. RG also showed an anti-pruritic effect in mice with histamine-induced scratching by blocking the histamine-induced histamine receptor type 1/TRPV1 pathway in sensory neurons [59]. Trinh et al. reported that RG extract inhibited IgE/antigen-induced passive cutaneous anaphylaxis reaction in mice and inhibited the IgE/antigen-stimulated degranulation and IL-4 expression in basophils [60]. They also found that ginseng and RG extracts inhibited compound 48/80-induced scratching behaviors, IL-4 expression, and NF-κB activation in mice [61]. Hwang et al. reported that the fermentation of ginseng with *Lactobacillus plantarum* inhibited the IgE-DNP-stimulated IL-4 expression in RBH-2H3 mast cells and passive cutaneous anaphylaxis in mice [63]. Park and Park evaluated the effects of RG on the regeneration of the full-thickness skin wounds in rat [66]. They also found that oral or topical treatments with RG significantly suppressed the wound size and accelerated tissue regeneration rate. RG significantly increased the gene expression levels of transforming growth factor-β1 and vascular endothelial growth factor during the early stages of wound healing. RG treatment increased matrix metalloproteinase (MMP)-1 and MMP-9 expression. Kim et al. reported that RG alleviated epidermal growth factor (EGF)-induced damage by blocking NF-κB and ERK in NCI-H292 cells and EGF-stimulated human airway epithelial cells [67]. These results suggest that RG and fRG can alleviate anaphylaxis and pruritus by suppressing IgE level, IL-4 and IL-5 expression, and NF-κB activation.

Based on these findings, ginseng including RG and fRG alleviates the acute and chronic phases of allergic diseases by modulating the innate and adaptive immune cells. Thus, ginseng can suppress IgE, IL-4, and IL-5 expression and Th2-to-Th1 cell ratio through the modulation of mast cell, basophil, and eosinophil activation, resulting in the attenuation of AD, allergic rhinitis, asthma, and pruritus. The anti-allergic effects of WG and RG were enforced by the fermentation. Their constituents may affect several pathways involved in allergic diseases by specific and nonspecific action mechanisms. However, their anti-allergic effects can be influenced by the quality and quantity of anti-allergic constituents found in the ginseng and the administered route. Therefore, the preparation of ginseng products must be standardized and well-characterized.

4.2. Efficacy of Ginseng in Patients with Allergic Disorders

A few reports are available on the clinical effectiveness of ginsengs against allergic disorders (Table 2). Kim et al. reported that in an 8-week, open, noncomparative clinical study of patients with AD, RG decreased eczema area and severity index score, transepidermal water loss, visual analogue scale, and sleep disturbance [68]. Jung et al. reported that in an open, noncomparative clinical study of patients with allergic rhinitis, RG alleviated rhinorrhea, nasal itching, and eye itching and suppressed IgE, IL-4 levels and eosinophil counts [69]. Park et al. reported that in a randomized, double-blind, placebo-controlled trial of patients with cold hypersensitivity in the hands and feet (CHHF), RG increased skin temperature of the hands and feet and decreased visual analog scale score of CHHF severity [70]. Jung et al. reported that in a 4-week, double-blind, placebo-controlled study of patients with persistent perennial allergic rhinitis, there was no significant difference in the total nasal symptom score between the fRG-treated and placebo groups in the experimental period, while the fRG-treated group, but not placebo group, showed the alleviation of nasal congestion [71]. These results suggest that RG and fRG may alleviate AD, allergic rhinitis, and cold hypersensitivity. Although several clinical trials have demonstrated effects of ginsengs in patients with allergic disorders, further controlled studies are required to clearly elucidate these effects.

Table 2. Summary of ginseng extract effects on allergic disorders.

Ginseng	Effect	Ref
RG	*in an 8-week, open, noncomparative clinical study of patients with AD (1–2 g/day)* • decreased eczema area and severity index score, transepidermal water loss, visual analogue scale • decreased sleep disturbance	[68]
	in an open, noncomparative clinical study of patients with allergic rhinitis (3 mg/kg/day, 4 weeks) • alleviated rhinorrhea, nasal itching, and eye itching • suppressed IgE, IL-4 levels and eosinophil counts	[69]
	in a randomized, double-blind, placebo-controlled trial of patients with cold hypersensitivity in the hands and feet (CHHF) (1 g/day, 8 weeks) • increased skin temperature of the hands and feet • decreased visual analog scale score of CHHF severity	[70]
fRG	*in double-blind, placebo-controlled study of patients with persistent perennial allergic rhinitis (750 mg/day, 4 weeks)* • Alleviated nasal congestion and the activities and emotions of quality of life.	[71]

AD, atopic dermatitis; fRG, fermented red ginseng; RG, red giseng.

5. Anti-Allergic Effects of Ginseng Constituents

In order to search for bioactive constituents of ginseng to treat allergic disorders, many researchers have examined the anti-allergic effectiveness of their constituent ginsenosides and polysaccharides in in vitro and in vivo studies [7,72,73] (Table 3). Of the ginsenosides, Rb1 inhibited IL-4 and GATA3 expression, airway resistance, and eosinophil population in the bronchoalveolar lavage fluid of ovalbumin-sensitized mice, while interferon-γ (IFNγ) and T-bet expression were increased [74]. Rb1 also inhibited compound 48/80-induced scratching behaviors in mice, while the IgE/complex-induced degranulation and IL-4 expression were not affected in RBL-2H3 cells [60,61]. Ginsenoside Rd suppressed ovalbumin-induced expression of IgE, IL-4, IL-5, and IL-13 in nasal mucosa and bronchoalveolar lavage fluid and alleviated gut dysbiosis in mice, resulting in the attenuation of allergic rhinitis [46]. Ginsenoside Rd enhanced Th1-response to *Candida albicans* surface mannan extract in mice [75]. Wang et al. reported that, of tested ginsenosides Rb1, Rd, F2, CK, and 20(S)-protopanaxadiol, ginsenoside F2 most potently inhibited the compound 48/80-stimulated degranulation of mast cells and RBL-2H3 cells [76]. Oh et al. found that ginsenoside Rg1 significantly reduced ovalbumin-induced increases in TSLP, IL-1β, and IL-4 expression; histamine and IgE levels; and eosinophil and mast cell populations in mice, while interferon-γ expression was enhanced [77]. Ginsenoside Rg1 inhibited NF-κB signaling pathways in cultured mast cells in vitro [77]. The combination of ginsenoside Rg1 with aluminum hydroxide strongly induced immune responses to ovalbumin in mice [78]. Lee et al. reported that ginsenoside Rg3 inhibited chloroquine-induced Ca^{2+} influx in primary culture of mouse dorsal root ganglia [58]. Furthermore, ginsenoside Rg3 significantly reduced chloroquine-induced scratching in mice. Lee et al. reported that ginsenoside Rg3 inhibited NF-κB activation and COX-2 expression in IL-1β-stimulated human asthmatic airway epithelial tissues [79]. Ginsenoside Rh2 attenuates allergic airway inflammation in ovalbumin-sensitized mice by regulating NF-κB activation and p38 MAPK phosphorylation [80]. RG saponin fraction and ginsenosides Rg3 and Rh2 inhibited compound 48/80- or histamine-induced scratching behavior and vascular permeability [61]. Ginsenosides Rg3 and Rh2 inhibited IL-4 and TNF-α expression in IgE/antigen-complex-stimulated RBL-2H3 cells [61,81].

Bae et al. examined the inhibitory effects of ginsenosides Rg3, Rf, and Rh2 on IgE/antigen-complex-induced passive cutaneous anaphylaxis in mice [82]. Of these, ginsenoside Rh2 most potently inhibited the IgE/antigen-complex-induced passive cutaneous anaphylaxis reaction. Ginsenoside Rh2 strongly inhibited the IgE/antigen-complex-induced RBL-2H3 cell degranulation [82]. Ginsenoside Rh2 also inhibited oxazolone-induced expression of COX-2, IL-1β, and TNF-α in the ears of mice, while the IL-4 expression was not affected [83]. Kim et al. reported that topical application of ginsenosides Rh2 or Rh2 plus Rg3 significantly reduced the clinical skin severity scores, ear thickness, mast cell populations, and TNF-α and IL-4 expression in the skin lesions of mice with TNCB-sensitized AD [52], while IFNγ expression and IgE levels were not affected.

Oral administration of ginsenoside Rh1 reduced AD-like clinical symptoms, ear swelling, IL-4, and IgE levels in the skin lesions of hairless mice with oxazolone-induced AD, while IFNγ and Foxp3 expression were increased [38]. Ginsenoside Rh1 also inhibited the release of histamine from rat peritoneal mast cells and the IgE/antigen-complex-induced passive cutaneous anaphylaxis reaction in mice. Ginsenoside Rh1 increased the membrane-stabilizing action in mast cells and inhibited COX-2 expression and NF-κB activation in RAW 264.7 cells. Park et al. reported that CK, a metabolite of ginsenoside Rb1, inhibited NO and prostaglandin E2 production in lipopolysaccharide-induced RAW 264.7 cells more strongly than the parental ginsenoside Rb1 [84]. CK also reduced the COX-2 expression and NF-κB activation. CK inhibited the IgE/antigen-complex-induced cell degranulation in RBL-2H3 cells and oxazolone-induced chronic dermatitis in mice [36]. Lin et al. reported that CK improved the accelerated and severe lupus nephritis in mice by blunting NLRP3 inflammasome activation and regulating T cell functions [85]. CK and its derivatives inhibited IgE production in mice with ovalbumin-sensitized asthma [86]. Shin et al. examined the anti-pruritic and vascular-permeability-inhibitory effects of ginsenoside Rb1 and its metabolite CK in mice with compound 48/80-, substance P-, or histamine-induced scratching behaviors [87]. When orally administered, ginsenoside Rb1 and CK both suppressed pruritic behaviors and skin vascular permeability. However, the intraperitoneal injection of ginsenoside Rb1 did not inhibit compound 48/80-induced scratching behaviors, while CK potently inhibited scratching behavior. Moreover, CK-fortified ginseng extract alleviated *Dermatophagoides farinae* body extract induced dermatitis score, ear thickness, scratching time, severity of skin lesions, and eosinophil and mast cell populations in NC/Nga mice [88]. These results suggest that ginsenosides and their metabolites can alleviate asthma, allergic rhinitis, AD, and scratching behavior by inhibiting IgE and IL-4 expression, NF-κB activation, and Ca^{2+} influx; increasing IFNγ expression; and stabilizing the degranulation of mast cells and basophils. Of ginsenosides and their metabolites, the most absorbable ginsenosides Rh1 and CK the most potently can alleviate AD, allergic rhinitis, pruritus, and anaphylaxis in vivo and in vitro, followed by Rd.

Ginseng polysaccharides isolated from *Panax japonicus* or *Panax ginseng*, the immunity-potentiating anti-cancer agents, stimulated immune response; thus, they activate phagocytosis, natural killer cell activity, and cytotoxic T cell activity [89]. Furthermore, they activate the phagocytosis of neutrophils and macrophages [90]. Ginsan isolated from *Panax ginseng* reduced ovalbumin-sensitized IL-5 expression and airway hyperresponsiveness, remodeling, and eosinophilia in mice, resulting in the attenuation of asthma [91]. RG-II isolated from *Panax ginseng* induced the Th1/Th2 immune response and IFNγ expression in mice with ovalbumin-induced asthma, while IL-4 and GATA3 expression and eosinophil populations were decreased in the bronchoalveolar lavage fluid [92]. CVT-E002 derived from North American Ginseng also activated Th1 responses and increased IL-10 expression, resulting in the attenuation of allergic airway inflammation and airway hyperresponsiveness [93]. These suggest that ginseng polysaccharides can stimulate the Th1 cell immune responses, resulting in the attenuation of asthma with the suppression of Th2 cell activation.

In addition, Lee et al. reported that oral intake of Korean ginseng could induce anaphylaxis in occupational settings by non-IgE-dependently activating basophil/mast cells [94]. Hon and Leung et al. reported that urticarial could occur in a feeding neonate, whose mother took American ginseng [95]. Erdle et al. reported that a child experienced anaphylaxis after inhaling powered American ginseng [96]. These results suggest that ginseng must be carefully used in clinic, because it can cause side effects due to its allergic reactions.

Table 3. Summary of ginseng constituent effects on allergic disorders.

Constituent	Effect	Ref
Ginsenoside Rb1	• Suppressed IL-4 and GATA3 expression, airway resistance, and eosinophil cell population and increased IFNγ and T-bet expression in ovalbumin-sensitized mice • Inhibited compound 48/80-induced scratching behaviors in mice • Inhibited NO and prostaglandin E2 production in LPS-induced RAW 264.7 cells • Inhibited IgE/antigen-induced degranulation of RBL-2H3 cells and PCA reaction in mice • Inhibited compound 48/80-stimulated degranulation of mast cells and RBL-2H3 cells.	[36,60,62,74,84]
Ginsenoside Re	• Suppressed histamine-induced IL-4 and TNF-α expression, NF-κB and c-jun activation, and scratching behaviors in mice	[38,97]
Ginsenoside Rd	• Suppressed IgE, IL-4, IL-5, and IL-13 expression and allergic rhinitis and gut dysbiosis in ovalbumin-sensitized mice • Enhanced Th1-response to *Candida albicans* surface mannan extract in mice • Inhibited compound 48/80-stimulated degranulation of mast cells and RBL-2H3 cells	[46,75]
Ginsenoside Rg1	• Reduced TSLP, IL-1β, and IL-4 expression; histamine and IgE secretion; and eosinophil and mast cell populations and increased IFNγ expression in ovalbumin-induced mice • Inhibited NF-κB signaling pathways in cultured mast cells • Induced immune responses to OVA in mice by the combination with aluminum hydroxide	[77,78]

Table 3. Cont.

Constituent	Effect	Ref
Ginsenoside Rg3	• Inhibited chloroquine-induced Ca^{2+} influx in primary culture of mouse dorsal root ganglia • Reduced chloroquine-induced scratching in mice • Inhibited NF-κB activation and COX-2 expression in IL-1β-induced human asthmatic airway epithelial tissues • Alleviated allergic airway inflammation and suppressed NF-κB activation and p38 MAPK phosphorylation in OVA-sensitized mice • Inhibited compound 48/80- or histamine-induced scratching behavior and vascular permeability • Inhibited IL-4 and TNF-α expression in IgE/antigen-complex-stimulated RBL-2H3 cell • Inhibited the IgE/antigen-complex-induced PCA reaction in mice • Inhibited the IgE/antigen-complex-induced RBL-2H3 cell degranulation • Reduced the clinical skin severity scores, ear thickness, mast cell populations, and TNF-α and IL-4 expression in the skin lesions of mice with TNCB-sensitized AD by the combination with Rh2	[52,58,79,82]
Ginsenoside Rh2	• Suppressed allergic airway inflammation and suppressed NF-κB activation and p38 MAPK phosphorylation in OVA-sensitized mice • Inhibited compound 48/80- or histamine-induced scratching behavior and vascular permeability • Inhibited IL-4 and TNF-α expression in IgE/antigen-complex-stimulated RBL-2H3 cell • Inhibited the IgE/antigen-complex-induced PCA reaction in mice • Inhibited the IgE/antigen-complex-induced RBL-2H3 cell degranulation • Inhibited oxazolone-induced expression of COX-2, IL-1β, and TNF-γ in the ears of mice • Reduced the clinical skin severity scores, ear thickness, mast cell populations, and TNF-α and IL-4 expression in the skin lesions of mice with TNCB-sensitized AD	[52,61,80–83]
Ginsenoside Rh1	• Reduced AD-like clinical symptoms, ear swellings, IL-4, and IgE expression and increased IFNγ and Foxp3 in mice with oxazolone-induced AD • Inhibited the release of histamine from rat peritoneal mast cells and the IgE/antigen-complex-induced PCA reaction in mice • Increased the membrane-stabilizing action in mast cells • Inhibited COX-2 expression and NF-κB activation in RAW 264.7 cells • Inhibited histamine-induced IL-4 and TNF-α expression, NF-κB and c-jun activation, and scratching behaviors in mice	[38,97]

Table 3. *Cont.*

Constituent	Effect	Ref
Compound K (CK)	• Inhibited NO and prostaglandin E2 production, COX-2 expression, and NF-κB activation in LPS-induced RAW 264.7 cells • Inhibited IgE/antigen-complex-induced cell degranulation in RBL-2H3 cells and oxazolone-induced chronic dermatitis in mice • Improved the accelerated and severe lupus nephritis in mice • Inhibited IgE production in mice with ovalbumin-sensitized asthma • Inhibited compound 48/80-, substance P-, or histamine-induced scratching behaviors and vascular permeability in mice • Inhibited IgE/antigen-induced degranulation of RBL-2H3 cells and PCA reaction in mice • Inhibited compound 48/80-stimulated degranulation of mast cells and RBL-2H3 cells • (CK-fortified ginseng extract) Alleviated *Dermatophagoides farinae* body extract induced dermatitis score, ear thickness, scratching time, severity of skin lesions, and eosinophil and mast cell populations in NC/Nga mice	[36,62,84–88]
Polysaccharide	*Ginsan* • Reduced ovalbumin-sensitized IL-5 expression and airway hyperresponsiveness, remodeling, and eosinophilia (asthma) in mice *RG-II* • Induced the Th1/Th2 immune response and IFNγ expression and suppressed IL-4 and GATA3 expression and eosinophil populations in mice with ovalbumin-induced asthma *CVT-E002* • Activated Th1 responses, increased IL-10 expression, suppressed allergic airway inflammation and airway hyperresponsiveness	[91–93]

AD, atopic dermatitis; CK, compound K; COX, cyclooxygenase; IFN, interferon; LPS, lipopolysaccharide; MAPK, mitogen-activated protein kinase; OVA, ovalbumin; PCA, passive cutaneous anaphylaxis; TNCB, 2, 4, 6-trinitro-1-chrolobenzene; Th, helper T cell.

6. Gut Microbiota Enforce Anti-Allergic Activities of Ginseng Constituents

Ginseng extracts and their constituents, particularly ginsenosides, showed anti-allergic effects in the in vivo studies. However, the absorption of these ginsenosides into the blood is not easy due to their hydrophilicity. Therefore, they are metabolized by gut microbiota in the intestine, which transform hydrophilic ginsenosides such as ginsenosides Rb1, Rb2, and Re into hydrophobic ginsenosides such as CK and Rh1 [13,20,97,98]. Comparing the anti-allergic activities of naïve ginsenosides Rb1, Rg3, and Re to those of their metabolite ginsenosides CK, Rh2, and Rh1, metabolites (ginsenosides CK, Rh2, and Rh1) suppress allergic reactions such as passive cutaneous anaphylaxis, scratching, and asthma more potently than parental ginsenosides Rb1, Rg3, and Re, respectively [38,62,81,82,93]. However, oral gavage of antibacterials suppresses their biotransformations and attenuates anti-allergic activities in mice. For example, when antibiotics (cefadroxil, oxytetracycline, and erythromycin mixture; COE), are orally gavaged, the fecal ginsenoside Re-metabolizing β-glucosidase and α-rhamnosidase activities and production of the metabolite ginsenoside Rh1 production are significantly suppressed [98]. The metabolism of ginsenoside Rb1 by gut microbiota is also inhibited by antibiotic treatment [31,97,98]. Furthermore, the anti-allergic activity of orally gavaged ginsenoside Re is significantly attenuated in mice treated with COE, but that of orally gavaged ginsenoside Rh1 are not affected. Oral gavage of ginsenoside Rh1 inhibits IL-4 and TNF-α expression and NF-κB and c-jun activation in mice with histamine-stimulated scratching more potently than parental ginsenoside Re. These results suggest that orally administered ginseng extracts and their hydrophilic ginsenosides should be metabolized to hydrophobic ginsenosides by gut microbiota, which enhances their anti-allergic activity, and, when simultaneously treated with antibacterials, their anti-allergic activities are attenuated. In addition, ginseng extract has been reported to rarely activate allergic responses rather than attenuate allergic disorders [95–97]. However, the mechanism should be clarified to safely use ginseng for the treatment of allergic disorders in clinics.

7. Conclusions

Herein, we discussed the current knowledge related to the effectiveness of ginseng on allergic disorders including asthma, allergic rhinitis, AD, and pruritus. Many studies are limited in examining the effectiveness of ginseng, including red ginseng and fRG and their constituent ginsenosides Rb1, Rd, and Rg3, against allergic disorders. Nevertheless, ginseng extracts alleviate allergic disorders such as asthma, allergic rhinitis, AD, and pruritus by inhibiting IgE, IL-4, and IL-5 expression through the modulation of mast cells, eosinophils, and Th1-to-Th2 ratio (Figure 3). Of ginseng extracts, fRG most potently alleviates allergic disorders, followed by RG and WG. Of their ginsenosides, CK, Rh1, and Rh2, which are the metabolites from hydrophilic parental ginsenosides by gut microbiota, strongly alleviated allergic disorders. To enforce these metabolites, fRG was developed. These ginseng constituents, absorbable into the blood, should express pharmacological effects, and the pharmacological activities of ginseng extracts may be dependent on the absorbable metabolites produced by gut microbiota. Ginseng itself can be allergen. Moreover, the great part of these results are inconclusive in the quality and quantity of anti-allergic constituents found in the ginseng and the administered route. Therefore, the anti-allergic effects of ginseng must be supported by further clinical and in-depth in vitro and in vivo studies.

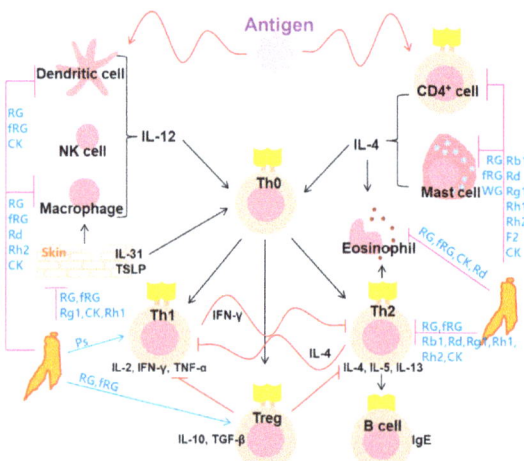

Figure 3. The hypothetical antiallergic action mechanisms of ginseng and ginsenosides. CK, compound K; fRG, fermented red ginseng; RG, red ginseng; WG, white ginseng.

Author Contributions: M.J.H. and D.-H.K. conceived the idea for this study. M.J.H. and D.-H.K. designed the study. M.J.H. and D.-H.K. analyzed the data. M.J.H. and D.-H.K. wrote the main manuscript text. All authors reviewed and approved the contents of the manuscript.

Conflicts of Interest: The authors declare no conflict of interest. The funders had no role in the design of the study, in the collection, analyses, or interpretation of data, in the writing of the manuscript, or in the decision to publish the results.

References

1. Stephani, J.; Radulović, K.; Niess, J.H. Gut Microbiota, Probiotics and Inflammatory Bowel Disease. *Arch. Immunol. Ther. Exp.* **2011**, *59*, 161–177. [CrossRef]
2. Skoner, D.P. Allergic rhinitis: Definition, epidemiology, pathophysiology, detection, and diagnosis. *J. Allergy Clin. Immunol.* **2001**, *108*, S2–S8. [CrossRef] [PubMed]
3. Braido, F.; Sclifò, F.; Ferrando, M.; Canonica, G.W. New Therapies for Allergic Rhinitis. *Curr. Allergy Asthma Rep.* **2014**, *14*, 422. [CrossRef]
4. Ricketti, P.A.; Alandijani, S.; Lin, C.H.; Casale, T. Investigational new drugs for allergic rhinitis. *Expert Opin. Investig. Drugs* **2017**, *26*, 279–292. [CrossRef] [PubMed]
5. Aaronson, D.W. Side effects of rhinitis medications. *J. Allergy Clin. Immunol.* **1998**, *101*, S379–S382. [CrossRef]
6. Cox, L.S. How safe are the biologicals in treating asthma and rhinitis? *Allergy Asthma Clin. Immunol.* **2009**, *5*, 4. [CrossRef]
7. Bielory, L. Complementary and alternative interventions in asthma, allergy, and immunology. *Ann. Allergy Asthma Immunol.* **2004**, *93*, S45–S54. [CrossRef]
8. Kulka, M. The potential of natural products as effective treatments for allergic inflammation: Implications for allergic rhinitis. *Curr. Top. Med. Chem.* **2009**, *9*, 1611–1624. [CrossRef]
9. Attele, A.S.; Wu, J.A.; Yuan, C.-S. Ginseng pharmacology: Multiple constituents and multiple actions. *Biochem. Pharmacol.* **1999**, *58*, 1685–1693. [CrossRef]
10. Kim, D.-H. Chemical Diversity of Panax ginseng, Panax quinquifolium, and Panax notoginseng. *J. Ginseng Res.* **2012**, *36*, 1–15. [CrossRef]
11. Mancuso, C.; Santangelo, R. Panax ginseng and Panax quinquefolius: From pharmacology to toxicology. *Food Chem. Toxicol.* **2017**, *107*, 362–372. [CrossRef] [PubMed]
12. Nocerino, E.; Amato, M.; Izzo, A.A. The aphrodisiac and adaptogenic properties of ginseng. *Fitoterapia* **2000**, *71*, S1–S5. [CrossRef]
13. Zhao, B.; Lv, C.; Lu, J. Natural occurring polysaccharides from Panax ginseng C. A. Meyer: A review of isolation, structures, and bioactivities. *Int. J. Boil. Macromol.* **2019**, *133*, 324–336. [CrossRef] [PubMed]
14. Shibata, S. Chemistry and cancer preventing activities of ginseng saponins and some related triterpenoid compounds. *J. Korean Med Sci.* **2001**, *16*, S28–S37. [CrossRef] [PubMed]
15. Yoshikawa, M.; Murakami, T.; Yashiro, K.; Yamahara, J.; Matsuda, H.; Saijoh, R.; Tanaka, O. Bioactive saponins and glycosides. XI. Structures of new dammarane-type triterpene oligoglycosides, quinquenosides I, II, III, IV, and V, from American ginseng, the roots of Panax quinquefolium L. *Chem. Pharm. Bull.* **1998**, *46*, 647–654. [CrossRef]
16. Zhu, G.-Y.; Li, Y.-W.; Hau, D.K.-P.; Jiang, Z.-H.; Yu, Z.-L.; Fong, W.-F. Protopanaxatriol-Type Ginsenosides from the Root of Panax ginseng. *J. Agric. Food Chem.* **2011**, *59*, 200–205. [CrossRef]
17. Zhang, S.; Chen, C.; Lu, W.; Wei, L. Phytochemistry, pharmacology, and clinical use of Panax notoginseng flowers buds. *Phytother. Res.* **2018**, *32*, 2155–2163. [CrossRef]
18. Yang, W.; Hu, Y.; Wu, W.-Y.; Ye, M.; Guo, D.-A. Saponins in the genus *Panax*, L. (*Araliaceae*): A systematic review of their chemical diversity. *Phytochemistry* **2014**, *106*, 7–24. [CrossRef]
19. Liu, Y.; Zhao, J.; Chen, Y.; Li, W.; Li, B.; Jian, Y.; Sabir, G.; Cheng, S.; Tuo, Q.; Khan, I.; et al. Polyacetylenic Oleanane-Type Triterpene Saponins from the Roots of Panax japonicus. *J. Nat. Prod.* **2016**, *79*, 3079–3085. [CrossRef]
20. Choi, K.-T. Botanical characteristics, pharmacological effects and medicinal components of KoreanPanax ginsengC A Meyer. *Acta Pharmacol. Sin.* **2008**, *29*, 1109–1118. [CrossRef]
21. Akao, T.; Kanaoka, M.; Kobashi, K. Appearance of compound K, a major metabolite of ginsenoside Rb1 by intestinal bacteria, in rat plasma after oral administration–measurement of compound K by enzyme immunoassay. *Boil. Pharm. Bull.* **1998**, *21*, 245–249. [CrossRef] [PubMed]

22. Abdel-Tawab, M.; Bahr, U.; Karas, M.; Wurglics, M.; Schubert-Zsilavecz, M. DEGRADATION OF GINSENOSIDES IN HUMANS AFTER ORAL ADMINISTRATION. *Drug Metab. Dispos.* **2003**, *31*, 1065–1071. [CrossRef] [PubMed]
23. Akao, T.; Kida, H.; Kanaoka, M.; Hattori, M.; Kobashi, K. Drug Metabolism: Intestinal Bacterial Hydrolysis is Required for the Appearance of Compound K in Rat Plasma after Oral Administration of Ginsenoside Rb1 from Panax ginseng. *J. Pharm. Pharmacol.* **1998**, *50*, 1155–1160. [CrossRef]
24. Kobashi, K.; Akao, T. Relation of Intestinal Bacteria to Pharmacological Effects of Glycosides. *Biosci. Microflora* **1997**, *16*, 1–7. [CrossRef]
25. Kim, D.H. Herbal medicines are activated by intestinal microflora. *Nat. Prod. Sci.* **2002**, *8*, 35–43.
26. Bae, E.-A.; Park, S.-Y.; Kim, D.-H. Constitutive beta-glucosidases hydrolyzing ginsenoside Rb1 and Rb2 from human intestinal bacteria. *Boil. Pharm. Bull.* **2000**, *23*, 1481–1485. [CrossRef]
27. Bae, E.-A.; Han, M.J.; Kim, E.-J.; Kim, D.-H. Transformation of ginseng saponins to ginsenoside Rh2 by acids and human intestinal bacteria and biological activities of their transformants. *Arch. Pharmacal Res.* **2004**, *27*, 61–67. [CrossRef]
28. Kim, D.-H. Gut microbiota-mediated pharmacokinetics of ginseng saponins. *J. Ginseng Res.* **2018**, *42*, 255–263. [CrossRef]
29. Kim, K.-A.; Yoo, H.H.; Gu, W.; Yu, D.-H.; Jin, M.J.; Choi, H.-L.; Yuan, K.; Guérin-Deremaux, L.; Kim, D.-H. A prebiotic fiber increases the formation and subsequent absorption of compound K following oral administration of ginseng in rats. *J. Ginseng Res.* **2014**, *39*, 183–187. [CrossRef]
30. Kim, D.-H. Gut Microbiota-Mediated Drug-Antibiotic Interactions. *Drug Metab. Dispos.* **2015**, *43*, 1581–1589. [CrossRef]
31. Xu, R.; Peng, Y.; Wang, M.; Fan, L.; Li, X. Effects of broad-spectrum antibiotics on the metabolism and pharmacokinetics of ginsenoside Rb1: A study on rats' gut microflora influenced by lincomycin. *J. Ethnopharmacol.* **2014**, *158*, 338–344. [CrossRef] [PubMed]
32. Kim, J.-K.; Kim, J.-Y.; Jang, S.-E.; Choi, M.-S.; Jang, H.-M.; Yoo, H.-H.; Kim, N.-H. Fermented Red Ginseng Alleviates Cyclophosphamide-Induced Immunosuppression and 2,4,6-Trinitrobenzenesulfonic Acid-Induced Colitis in Mice by Regulating Macrophage Activation and T Cell Differentiation. *Am. J. Chin. Med.* **2018**, *46*, 1879–1897. [CrossRef] [PubMed]
33. Kim, J.-K.; Choi, M.S.; Jeung, W.; Ra, J.; Yoo, H.H.; Kim, D.-H. Effects of gut microbiota on the pharmacokinetics of protopanaxadiol ginsenosides Rd, Rg3, F2, and compound K in healthy volunteers treated orally with red ginseng. *J. Ginseng Res.* **2019**. [CrossRef]
34. Liu, H.; Yang, J.; Du, F.; Gao, X.; Ma, X.; Huang, Y.; Xu, F.; Niu, W.; Wang, F.; Mao, Y.; et al. Absorption and Disposition of Ginsenosides after Oral Administration of Panax notoginseng Extract to Rats. *Drug Metab. Dispos.* **2009**, *37*, 2290–2298. [CrossRef] [PubMed]
35. Lee, H.-U.; Bae, E.-A.; Han, M.J.; Kim, N.-J.; Kim, D.-H. Hepatoprotective effect of ginsenoside Rb1 and compound K on tert-butyl hydroperoxide-induced liver injury. *Liver Int.* **2005**, *25*, 1069–1073. [CrossRef] [PubMed]
36. Shin, Y.-W.; Bae, E.-A.; Kim, S.-S.; Lee, Y.-C.; Kim, N.-H. Effect of ginsenoside Rb1 and compound K in chronic oxazolone-induced mouse dermatitis. *Int. Immunopharmacol.* **2005**, *5*, 1183–1191. [CrossRef]
37. Kim, T.W.; Choi, H.-J.; Kim, N.-J.; Kim, N.-H. Anxiolytic-like Effects of Ginsenosides Rg3 and Rh2 from Red Ginseng in the Elevated Plus-Maze Model. *Planta Med.* **2009**, *75*, 836–839. [CrossRef]
38. Park, E.-K.; Choo, M.-K.; Han, M.J.; Kim, D.-H. Ginsenoside Rh1 Possesses Antiallergic and Anti-Inflammatory Activities. *Int. Arch. Allergy Immunol.* **2004**, *133*, 113–120. [CrossRef]
39. Gu, W.; Kim, K.-A.; Kim, D.-H. Ginsenoside Rh1 ameliorates high fat diet-induced obesity in mice by inhibiting adipocyte differentiation. *Boil. Pharm. Bull.* **2013**, *36*, 102–107. [CrossRef]
40. Lee, S.-Y.; Jeong, J.-J.; Eun, S.-H.; Kim, D.-H. Anti-inflammatory effects of ginsenoside Rg1 and its metabolites ginsenoside Rh1 and 20(S)-protopanaxatriol in mice with TNBS-induced colitis. *Eur. J. Pharmacol.* **2015**, *762*, 333–343. [CrossRef]
41. Inoue, K.-I. Korean red ginseng for allergic rhinitis. *Immunopharmacol. Immunotoxicol.* **2013**, *35*, 693. [CrossRef] [PubMed]
42. Kim, D.Y.; Yang, W.M. Panax ginseng ameliorates airway inflammation in an ovalbumin-sensitized mouse allergic asthma model. *J. Ethnopharmacol.* **2011**, *136*, 230–235. [CrossRef] [PubMed]

43. Babayigit, A.; Olmez, D.; Karaman, O.; Bagriyanik, H.A.; Yilmaz, O.; Kivcak, B.; Erbil, G.; Uzuner, N. Ginseng ameliorates chronic histopathologic changes in a murine model of asthma. *Allergy Asthma Proc.* **2008**, *29*, 493–498. [CrossRef] [PubMed]
44. Lim, C.-Y.; Moon, J.-M.; Kim, B.-Y.; Lim, S.-H.; Lee, G.-S.; Yu, H.-S.; Cho, S. Comparative study of Korean White Ginseng and Korean Red Ginseng on efficacies of OVA-induced asthma model in mice. *J. Ginseng Res.* **2014**, *39*, 38–45. [CrossRef] [PubMed]
45. Lee, E.-J.; Song, M.-J.; Kwon, H.-S.; Ji, G.E.; Sung, M.-K. Oral administration of fermented red ginseng suppressed ovalbumin-induced allergic responses in female BALB/c mice. *Phytomedicine* **2012**, *19*, 896–903. [CrossRef]
46. Kim, H.I.; Kim, J.-K.; Kim, J.-Y.; Han, M.J.; Kim, D.-H. Fermented red ginseng and ginsenoside Rd alleviate ovalbumin-induced allergic rhinitis in mice by suppressing IgE, interleukin-4, and interleukin-5 expression. *J. Ginseng Res.* **2019**, *43*, 635–644. [CrossRef]
47. Jung, J.H.; Kang, I.G.; Kim, D.; Hwang, Y.J.; Kim, S.T. The effect of Korean red ginseng on allergic inflammation in a murine model of allergic rhinitis. *J. Ginseng Res.* **2013**, *37*, 167–175. [CrossRef]
48. Sumiyoshi, M.; Sakanaka, M.; Kimura, Y. Effects of Red Ginseng extract on allergic reactions to food in Balb/c mice. *J. Ethnopharmacol.* **2010**, *132*, 206–212. [CrossRef]
49. Lee, H.J.; Cho, S.H. Therapeutic Effects of Korean Red Ginseng Extract in a Murine Model of Atopic Dermatitis: Anti-pruritic and Anti-inflammatory Mechanism. *J. Korean Med Sci.* **2017**, *32*, 679–687. [CrossRef]
50. Lee, J.H.; Cho, S.H. Korean red ginseng extract ameliorates skin lesions in NC/Nga mice: An atopic dermatitis model. *J. Ethnopharmacol.* **2011**, *133*, 810–817. [CrossRef]
51. Cho, E.; Cho, S.H. Effects of Korean red ginseng extract on the prevention of atopic dermatitis and its mechanism on early lesions in a murine model. *J. Ethnopharmacol.* **2013**, *145*, 294–302. [CrossRef] [PubMed]
52. Kim, H.S.; Kim, N.H.; Kim, B.K.; Yoon, S.K.; Kim, M.H.; Lee, J.Y.; Kim, H.O.; Park, Y.M. Effects of topically applied Korean red ginseng and its genuine constituents on atopic dermatitis-like skin lesions in NC/Nga mice. *Int. Immunopharmacol.* **2011**, *11*, 280–285. [CrossRef] [PubMed]
53. Sohn, E.-H.; Jang, S.-A.; Lee, C.-H.; Jang, K.-H.; Kang, S.-C.; Park, H.-J.; Pyo, S. Effects of Korean Red Ginseng Extract for the Treatment of Atopic Dermatitis-Like Skin Lesions in Mice. *J. Ginseng Res.* **2011**, *35*, 479–486. [CrossRef] [PubMed]
54. Park, J.-H.; Ahn, E.-K.; Ko, H.-J.; Lee, J.Y.; Hwang, S.-M.; Ko, S.; Oh, J.S. Korean red ginseng water extract alleviates atopic dermatitis-like inflammatory responses by negative regulation of mitogen-activated protein kinase signaling pathway in vivo. *Biomed. Pharmacother.* **2019**, *117*, 109066. [CrossRef] [PubMed]
55. Samukawa, K.; Izumi, Y.; Shiota, M.; Nakao, T.; Osada-Oka, M.; Miura, K.; Iwao, H. Red ginseng inhibits scratching behavior associated with atopic dermatitis in experimental animal models. *J. Pharmacol. Sci.* **2012**, *118*, 391–400. [CrossRef]
56. Osada-Oka, M.; Hirai, S.; Izumi, Y.; Misumi, K.; Samukawa, K.; Tomita, S.; Miura, K.; Minamiyama, Y.; Iwao, H. Red ginseng extracts attenuate skin inflammation in atopic dermatitis through p70 ribosomal protein S6 kinase activation. *J. Pharmacol. Sci.* **2018**, *136*, 9–15. [CrossRef] [PubMed]
57. Bae, E.A.; Han, M.J.; Shin, Y.W.; Kim, D.H. Antiallergic and antipsoriatic effects of Korean red ginseng. *J. Ginseng Res.* **2005**, *29*, 80–85.
58. Lee, W.J.; Kim, Y.S.; Shim, W.S. Korean Red Ginseng extract and ginsenoside Rg3 have anti-pruritic effects on chloroquine-induced itch by inhibition of MrgprA3/TRPA1-mediated pathway. *J. Ginseng Res.* **2018**, *42*, 470–475. [CrossRef]
59. Jang, Y.; Lee, W.-J.; Hong, G.-S.; Shim, W.-S. Red ginseng extract blocks histamine-dependent itch by inhibition of H1R/TRPV1 pathway in sensory neurons. *J. Ginseng Res.* **2015**, *39*, 257–264. [CrossRef] [PubMed]
60. Trinh, H.T.; Bae, E.A.; Han, M.J.; Shin, Y.W.; Kim, D.H. Inhibitory effects of red ginseng on passive cutaneous anaphylaxis and scratching behavior reactions in mice. *J. Ginseng Res.* **2007**, *31*, 137–141.
61. Trinh, H.-T.; Han, M.; Shin, Y.-W.; Han, S.-J.; Kim, N.-H. Evaluation of Antipruritic Effects of Red Ginseng and Its Ingredients in Mice. *Planta Med.* **2008**, *74*, 210–214. [CrossRef] [PubMed]
62. Choo, M.-K.; Park, E.-K.; Han, M.J.; Kim, N.-H. Antiallergic Activity of Ginseng and its Ginsenosides. *Planta Med.* **2003**, *69*, 518–522. [CrossRef] [PubMed]

63. Hwang, S.-W.; Sun, X.; Han, J.-H.; Kim, T.-Y.; Koppula, S.; Kang, T.-B.; Hwang, J.-K.; Lee, K.H. Fermentation-Mediated Enhancement of Ginseng's Anti-Allergic Activity against IgE-Mediated Passive Cutaneous Anaphylaxis In Vivo and In Vitro. *J. Microbiol. Biotechnol.* **2018**, *28*, 1626–1634. [CrossRef] [PubMed]

64. Choi, J.H.; Jin, S.W.; Park, B.H.; Kim, H.G.; Khanal, T.; Han, H.J.; Hwang, Y.P.; Choi, J.M.; Chung, Y.C.; Hwang, S.K.; et al. Cultivated ginseng inhibits 2,4-dinitrochlorobenzene-induced atopic dermatitis-like skin lesions in NC/Nga mice and TNF-α/IFN-γ-induced TARC activation in HaCaT cells. *Food Chem. Toxicol.* **2013**, *56*, 195–203. [CrossRef]

65. Kang, J.A.; Song, H.-Y.; Byun, E.-H.; Ahn, N.-G.; Kim, H.-M.; Nam, Y.R.; Lee, G.H.; Jang, B.-S.; Choi, D.S.; Lee, D.-E.; et al. Gamma-irradiated black ginseng extract inhibits mast cell degranulation and suppresses atopic dermatitis-like skin lesions in mice. *Food Chem. Toxicol.* **2018**, *111*, 133–143. [CrossRef]

66. Park, K.-S.; Park, D.H. The effect of Korean Red Ginseng on full-thickness skin wound healing in rats. *J. Ginseng Res.* **2018**, *43*, 226–235. [CrossRef]

67. Kim, J.-H.; Kang, J.W.; Kim, M.; Lee, D.-H.; Kim, H.; Choi, H.-S.; Kim, E.J.; Chung, I.-M.; Chung, I.-Y.; Yoon, D. The Liquid Panax ginseng Inhibits Epidermal Growth factor–induced metalloproteinase 9 and cyclooxygenase 2 expressions via inhibition of inhibitor factor kappa-B-alpha and extracellular signal-regulated kinase in NCI-H292 human airway epithelial cells. *Am. J. Rhinol. Allergy* **2011**, *25*, e55–e59. [CrossRef]

68. Kim, H.; Park, C.W.; Cho, S.H. The Beneficial Effect of Korean Red Ginseng Extract on Atopic Dermatitis Patients: An 8 Weeks Open, Noncomparative Clinical Study. *Ann. Dermatol.* **2018**, *30*, 304–308. [CrossRef]

69. Jung, J.H.; Kang, T.K.; Oh, J.H.; Jeong, J.U.; Ko, K.P.; Kim, S.T. The Effect of Korean Red Ginseng on Symptoms and Inflammation in Patients With Allergic Rhinitis. *Ear Nose Throat J.* **2020**, 145561320907172. [CrossRef]

70. Park, K.-S.; Park, K.-I.; Kim, J.-W.; Yun, Y.-J.; Kim, S.-H.; Lee, C.-H.; Park, J.-W.; Lee, J.-M. Efficacy and safety of Korean red ginseng for cold hypersensitivity in the hands and feet: A randomized, double-blind, placebo-controlled trial. *J. Ethnopharmacol.* **2014**, *158*, 25–32. [CrossRef]

71. Jung, J.-W.; Kang, H.-R.; Ji, G.-E.; Park, M.-S.; Song, W.-J.; Kim, M.-H.; Kwon, J.-W.; Kim, T.-W.; Park, H.-W.; Cho, S.-H.; et al. Therapeutic Effects of Fermented Red Ginseng in Allergic Rhinitis: A Randomized, Double-Blind, Placebo-Controlled Study. *Allergy, Asthma Immunol. Res.* **2011**, *3*, 103–110. [CrossRef] [PubMed]

72. Koda, A.; Nishiyori, T.; Nagai, H.; Matsuura, N.; Tsuchiya, H. Anti-allergic actions of traditional oriental medicine–actions against types I and IV hypersensitivity reactions. *Folia Pharmacol. Jpn.* **1982**, *80*, 31–41. [CrossRef]

73. Kobayashi, H.; Mizuno, N.; Teramae, H.; Kutsuna, H.; Ueoku, S.; Onoyama, J.; Yamanaka, K.; Fujita, N.; Ishii, M. Diet and Japanese herbal medicine for recalcitrant atopic dermatitis: Efficacy and safety. *Drugs Exp. Clin. Res.* **2004**, *30*, 197–202.

74. Chen, T.; Xiao, L.; Zhu, L.; Ma, S.; Yan, T.; Ji, H. Anti-Asthmatic Effects of Ginsenoside Rb1 in a Mouse Model of Allergic Asthma Through Relegating Th1/Th2. *Inflammation* **2015**, *38*, 1814–1822. [CrossRef]

75. Han, Y.; Rhew, K.Y. Ginsenoside Rd induces protective anti-Candida albicans antibody through immunological adjuvant activity. *Int. Immunopharmacol.* **2013**, *17*, 651–657. [CrossRef]

76. Wang, L.; Zhang, F.; Cao, Z.-Y.; Xiao, Y.; Li, S.; Yu, B.; Qi, J. Ginsenoside F2 induces the release of mediators associated with Anaphylactoid reactions. *Fitoterapia* **2017**, *121*, 223–228. [CrossRef]

77. Oh, H.-A.; Seo, J.-Y.; Jeong, H.-J.; Kim, H.-M. Ginsenoside Rg1 inhibits the TSLP production in allergic rhinitis mice. *Immunopharmacol. Immunotoxicol.* **2013**, *35*, 678–686. [CrossRef]

78. Sun, J.; Song, X.; Hu, S. Ginsenoside Rg1 and Aluminum Hydroxide Synergistically Promote Immune Responses to Ovalbumin in BALB/c Mice. *Clin. Vaccine Immunol.* **2007**, *15*, 303–307. [CrossRef]

79. Lee, I.-S.; Uh, I.; Kim, K.-S.; Kim, K.-H.; Park, J.; Kim, Y.; Jung, J.-H.; Jung, H.-J.; Jang, H.-J. Anti-Inflammatory Effects of Ginsenoside Rg3 via NF-κB Pathway in A549 Cells and Human Asthmatic Lung Tissue. *J. Immunol. Res.* **2016**, *2016*, 1–11. [CrossRef]

80. Li, L.C.; Piao, H.M.; Zheng, M.Y.; Lin, Z.H.; Choi, Y.H.; Yan, G.H. Ginsenoside Rh2 attenuates allergic airway inflammation by modulating nuclear factor-?B activation in a murine model of asthma. *Mol. Med. Rep.* **2015**, *12*, 6946–6954. [CrossRef]

81. Park, E.-K.; Choo, M.-K.; Kim, E.-J.; Han, M.J.; Kim, D.-H. Antiallergic activity of ginsenoside Rh2. *Boil. Pharm. Bull.* **2003**, *26*, 1581–1584. [CrossRef] [PubMed]

82. Bae, E.-A.; Han, M.J.; Shin, Y.-W.; Kim, N.-H. Inhibitory effects of Korean red ginseng and its genuine constituents ginsenosides Rg3, Rf, and Rh2 in mouse passive cutaneous anaphylaxis reaction and contact dermatitis models. *Boil. Pharm. Bull.* **2006**, *29*, 1862–1867. [CrossRef] [PubMed]
83. Zheng, H.; Jeong, Y.; Song, J.; Ji, G.E. Oral administration of ginsenoside Rh1 inhibits the development of atopic dermatitis-like skin lesions induced by oxazolone in hairless mice. *Int. Immunopharmacol.* **2011**, *11*, 511–518. [CrossRef] [PubMed]
84. Park, E.-K.; Shin, Y.-W.; Lee, H.-U.; Kim, S.-S.; Lee, Y.-C.; Lee, B.-Y.; Kim, N.-H. Inhibitory effect of ginsenoside Rb1 and compound K on NO and prostaglandin E2 biosyntheses of RAW264.7 cells induced by lipopolysaccharide. *Boil. Pharm. Bull.* **2005**, *28*, 652–656. [CrossRef]
85. Lin, T.-J.; Wu, C.-Y.; Tsai, P.-Y.; Hsu, W.-H.; Hua, K.-F.; Chu, C.-L.; Lee, Y.-C.; Chen, A.; Lee, S.-L.; Lin, Y.-J.; et al. Accelerated and Severe Lupus Nephritis Benefits From M1, an Active Metabolite of Ginsenoside, by Regulating NLRP3 Inflammasome and T Cell Functions in Mice. *Front. Immunol.* **2019**, *10*, 1951. [CrossRef] [PubMed]
86. Ren, S.; Liu, R.; Wang, Y.; Ding, N.; Li, Y. Synthesis and biological evaluation of Ginsenoside Compound K analogues as a novel class of anti-asthmatic agents. *Bioorganic Med. Chem. Lett.* **2019**, *29*, 51–55. [CrossRef] [PubMed]
87. Shin, Y.-W.; Kim, D.-H. Antipruritic effect of ginsenoside rb1 and compound k in scratching behavior mouse models. *J. Pharmacol. Sci.* **2005**, *99*, 83–88. [CrossRef]
88. Kim, J.R.; Choi, J.; Kim, J.; Kim, H.; Kang, H.; Kim, E.H.; Chang, J.-H.; Kim, Y.-E.; Choi, Y.J.; Lee, K.; et al. 20-O-β-d-glucopyranosyl-20(S)-protopanaxadiol-fortified ginseng extract attenuates the development of atopic dermatitis-like symptoms in NC/Nga mice. *J. Ethnopharmacol.* **2014**, *151*, 365–371. [CrossRef]
89. Jie, Z.; Chun-Yan, L.; Jing-Ping, L.; Ren, G.; Hui, W.; Juan, P.; Sheng-Lan, L. Immunoregulation on Mice of Low Immunity and Effects on Five Kinds of Human Cancer Cells of Panax japonicus Polysaccharide. *Evidence-Based Complement. Altern. Med.* **2015**, *2015*, 839697. [CrossRef]
90. Song, J.; Han, S.-K.; Bae, K.-G.; Lim, D.-S.; Son, S.-J.; Jung, I.-S.; Yi, S.-Y.; Yun, Y.-S. Radioprotective effects of ginsan, an immunomodulator. *Radiat. Res.* **2003**, *159*, 768–774. [CrossRef]
91. Lim, Y.-J.; Na, H.-S.; Yun, Y.-S.; Choi, I.S.; Oh, J.-S.; Rhee, J.H.; Cho, B.-H.; Lee, H.C. Suppressive Effects of Ginsan on the Development of Allergic Reaction in Murine Asthmatic Model. *Int. Arch. Allergy Immunol.* **2009**, *150*, 32–42. [CrossRef] [PubMed]
92. Jung, I.D.; Kim, H.; Park, J.W.; Lee, C.-M.; Noh, K.-T.; Kang, H.-K.; Heo, D.-R.; Lee, S.-J.; Son, K.-H.; Park, H.-J.; et al. RG-II from Panax ginseng C.A. Meyer suppresses asthmatic reaction. *BMB Rep.* **2012**, *45*, 79–84. [CrossRef] [PubMed]
93. Ebeling, C.; Wu, Y.; Skappak, C.; Gordon, J.; Ilarraza, R.; Adamko, D. Compound CVT-E002 attenuates allergen-induced airway inflammation and airway hyperresponsiveness, in vivo. *Mol. Nutr. Food Res.* **2011**, *55*, 1905–1908. [CrossRef] [PubMed]
94. Lee, J.-Y.; Jin, H.J.; Park, J.-W.; Jung, S.K.; Jang, J.-Y.; Park, H.-S. A Case of Korean Ginseng-Induced Anaphylaxis Confirmed by Open Oral Challenge and Basophil Activation Test. *Allergy Asthma Immunol. Res.* **2011**, *4*, 110–111. [CrossRef] [PubMed]
95. Hon, K.L.; Leung, T.F. Neonatal urticaria due to American ginseng or not? *Clin. Exp. Dermatol.* **2010**, *35*, 103–104. [PubMed]
96. Erdle, S.C.; Chan, E.S.; Yang, H.; Vallance, B.A.; Mill, C.; Wong, T. First-reported pediatric cases of American ginseng anaphylaxis and allergy. *Allergy, Asthma Clin. Immunol.* **2018**, *14*, 79. [CrossRef]
97. Jang, S.-E.; Jung, I.-H.; Joh, E.-H.; Han, M.J.; Kim, D.-H. Antibiotics attenuate anti-scratching behavioral effect of ginsenoside Re in mice. *J. Ethnopharmacol.* **2012**, *142*, 105–112. [CrossRef]
98. Joh, E.-H.; Lee, I.-A.; Jung, I.-H.; Kim, D.-H. Ginsenoside Rb1 and its metabolite compound K inhibit IRAK-1 activation—The key step of inflammation. *Biochem. Pharmacol.* **2011**, *82*, 278–286. [CrossRef]

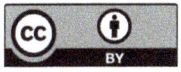

© 2020 by the authors. Licensee MDPI, Basel, Switzerland. This article is an open access article distributed under the terms and conditions of the Creative Commons Attribution (CC BY) license (http://creativecommons.org/licenses/by/4.0/).

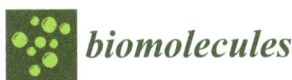

Review

Biotechnological Interventions for Ginsenosides Production

Saikat Gantait [1,†], Monisha Mitra [2,†] and Jen-Tsung Chen [3,*]

[1] Crop Research Unit (Genetics and Plant Breeding), Bidhan Chandra Krishi Viswavidyalaya, Mohanpur, Nadia, West Bengal 741252, India; saikatgantait@yahoo.com
[2] Department of Agricultural Biotechnology, Faculty of Agriculture, Bidhan Chandra Krishi Viswavidyalaya, Mohanpur, Nadia, West Bengal 741252, India; monisha25.mitra@gmail.com
[3] Department of Life Sciences, National University of Kaohsiung, Kaohsiung 811, Taiwan
* Correspondence: jentsung@nuk.edu.tw
† These authors contributed equally to the manuscript.

Received: 3 March 2020; Accepted: 1 April 2020; Published: 2 April 2020

Abstract: Ginsenosides are secondary metabolites that belong to the triterpenoid or saponin group. These occupy a unique place in the pharmaceutical sector, associated with the manufacturing of medicines and dietary supplements. These valuable secondary metabolites are predominantly used for the treatment of nervous and cardiac ailments. The conventional approaches for ginsenoside extraction are time-consuming and not feasible, and thus it has paved the way for the development of various biotechnological approaches, which would ameliorate the production and extraction process. This review delineates the biotechnological tools, such as conventional tissue culture, cell suspension culture, protoplast culture, polyploidy, in vitro mutagenesis, hairy root culture, that have been largely implemented for the enhanced production of ginsenosides. The use of bioreactors to scale up ginsenoside yield is also presented. The main aim of this review is to address the unexplored aspects and limitations of these biotechnological tools, so that a platform for the utilization of novel approaches can be established to further increase the production of ginsenosides in the near future.

Keywords: bioreactor; cell suspension; hairy root; polyploidy; protoplast

1. Introduction

Ginsenosides, commonly called triterpenoids or ginseng saponins, are secondary metabolites bearing immense medicinal importance, especially in the pharmaceutical sector. These secondary metabolites have multifaceted pharmacological properties, owing to their resemblance to steroidal hormones. The amphiphilic nature of ginsenosides allows them to cross the plasma membrane, subsequently inducing signaling cascades that comprise major pathways, e.g., the adenosine-monophosphate–activated protein kinase pathway (which activates B cells). Ginsenosides also trigger receptors, including the glucocorticoid, estrogen, and N-methyl-D-aspartate receptors [1]. Ginsenosides are synthesized mainly by *Panax* species that belong to the family Araliaceae. The plants belonging to the *Panax* genus grow in the Northern hemisphere, and their cultivation is confined to North America. On a commercial basis, ginsenosides have been regarded as profitable drugs that can be utilized for medicinal purposes and have a good stand in the global market. The total revenue achieved in the sales of these metabolites is about 2,000 million US dollars. The major countries where ginsenoside production is commercially exploited are the United States of America, Canada, China, and South Korea. In European countries, ginsenoside production is primarily aimed at manufacturing pharmaceutical drugs, whereas in America, ginsenosides are used to manufacture retail products [2]. The chemical annotation of ginsenoside is 'Rx', wherein 'R' signifies root, and 'x' indicates the chromatographic polarity arranged in alphabetical order. The chemical structure of ginsenosides is common to all the compounds reported till date. The structure consists of 1,2-cyclopentanoperhydrophenanthrene. Ginsenoside compounds can be distinguished from each other on the basis of the number of moieties of sugar attached, the type of sugar, and the linkage position. Ginsenosides are further classified into two categories (Figure 1) based on stereochemistry structure, namely, 20(S)-protopanaxadiol (PPD) (Rb1, Rb2, Rb3, Rc, Rd, Rg3, Rh2, Rs1), wherein an extra carbonyl group is present in PPDs, at the C_6 position, and 20(S)-protopanaxatriol (PPT) (Re, Rf, Rg1, Rg2, Rh1) [3]. The PPD group of ginsenosides is abundantly found in *Panax quinquefolium*, whereas the PPT group of ginsenosides is commonly found in *Panax ginseng*. There are other types of ginsenoside also available, which are pentacyclic oleane saponin Ro and ocotillol saponin F11. The ocotillol ginsenosides are found mainly in *P. quinquefolium*, whereas the oleane ginsenosides are major constituents of *P. ginseng* [4]. Ginsenosides are further divided into two categories, namely, acidic ginsenosides (consisting of four ginsenosides, viz., Rb1, Rb2, Rc, and Rd, which are malonyl derivatives) and neutral ginsenosides, which are actually in fact esterified derivatives. The malonyl ginsenosides are more abundant in *Panax notoginseng* than in *P. ginseng*. The ginsenoside content of a plant is dependent on distinctive factors, like growing conditions, age of the root, root size (which is further dependent on primary roots, secondary roots, and adventitious-root hair). Ginsenoside accumulation is maximum in roots, but new ginsenosides have been isolated from the aerial parts of plant as well, for instance, the floral ginsenosides A–P, derived from the floral buds of *P. ginseng*, and the floral ginsenosides A–E, derived from the floral buds of *P. quinquefolium*. *Gynostemma pentaphyllum* is the only species that does not belong to the Araliaceae family and is a rich source of dammarane triterpene ginsenosides. The conventional approaches of ginsenoside extraction are time-consuming; since the conventional propagation of plants requires approximately six years and is not convenient. Moreover, the conventional method of metabolite extraction requires a long time and the use of methanol, which poses health hazards. The conventional method of extraction involves the basic steps of heating, boiling, and refluxing that can cause the loss of active phytochemicals due to temperature fluctuations and chemical changes induced by reactions such as hydrolysis and oxidation [5]. Thus, to address the shortcomings of the conventional mode of metabolite extraction, cutting-edge biotechnological approaches like tissue culture-mediated mass regeneration technologies, *Agrobacterium*-mediated genetic transformation, and cell suspension culture coupled with elicitation have been implemented in the past three decades to enhance the production efficiency of ginsenosides in a much refined way. These approaches are highlighted in this review.

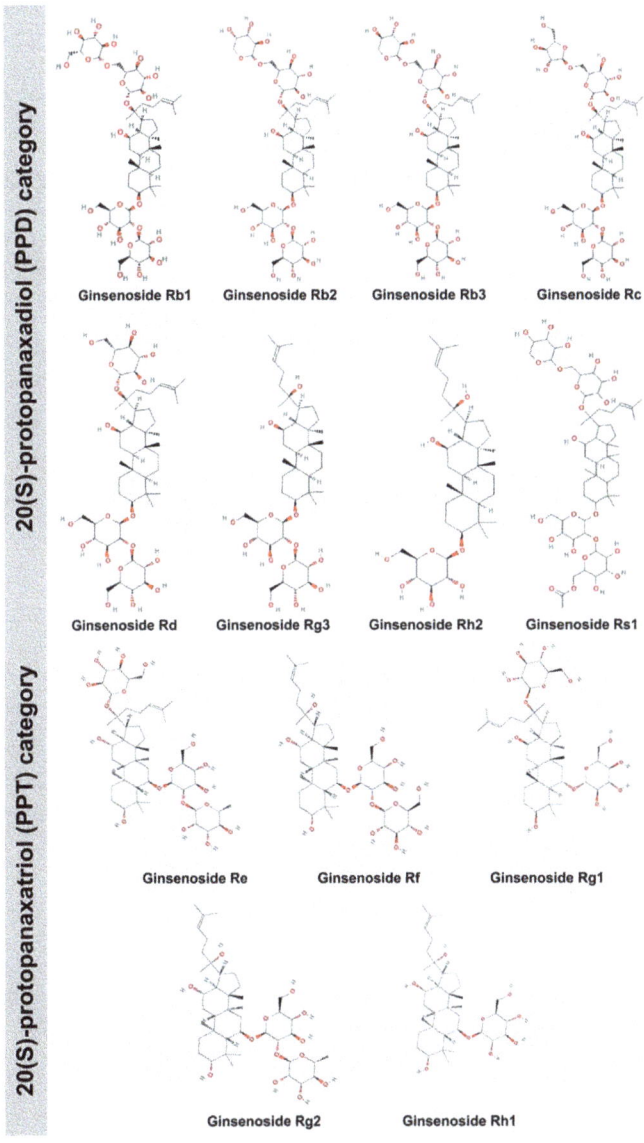

Figure 1. Major structures of ginsenosides belonging to the 20(S)-protopanaxadiol (PPD) and 20(S)-protopanaxatriol (PPT) categories (Structure source: PubChem https://pubchem.ncbi.nlm.nih.gov) (Source: unpublished photograph of Saikat Gantait).

2. Medicinal Uses

Ginsenosides have a broad-spectrum curing capability against several ailments, which is reason enough for them to hold a unique place in the pharmaceutical sector. Ginsenosides possess anti-microbial and anti-fungal properties. They serve as anti-cancerous agents since they restrict metastasis and growth of tumor through a direct cytotoxic action, induce apoptosis, thus preventing tumor invasion, and further restrict chromosome aberrations, which is a prime reason for metastasis [6].

The Rh2 ginsenoside has better anti-cancerous properties than the other ginsenosides. Intravenous application of ginsenoside Rb2 resulted in a decrease of metastasis in the lungs. It possesses immunomodulatory properties that help in the activation of macrophages and lymphocytes, and this provides protection from many infectious diseases. The major ginsenosides with immunomodulatory properties are Rg1, Rg2, Rb1, Re, and Rc. The Rb1 ginsenoside was shown to promote a significant increase of humoral and cell-mediated immunity as a result of the increase of T cells and helper T cells [7]. Anti-inflammatory properties are exhibited by ginsenoside Rg1 in microglial cells of the central nervous system [8]. The anti-inflammatory effects of ginsenosides have even proven to be better than those of the popular drug disodium cromoglycate, which is a commercial anti-allergic drug. Ginsenosides also exhibit anti-allergic properties since they inhibit histamine secretion from mast cells. They also possess membrane-stabilizing properties that restrict membrane disturbances, which is a major mechanism of their anti-allergic properties [9]. Ginsenosides play a major role in the treatment of cardiac ailments by suppressing thrombin production and reducing the activity of sympathetic nerves, thus directly lowering vascular activity and, as a consequence, blood pressure [10]. Ginsenosides release NO that leads to the production of cyclic GMP, which minimizes vascular activity. They also act as regulators of total cholesterol and high-density cholesterol levels, thus preventing chronic diseases like atherosclerosis and other cardiac diseases. The ginsenosides Rg2 and Rg3 are responsible for the inhibition of platelet aggregation via regulating the levels of cyclic GMP and cyclic AMP and suppressing the conversion of fibrinogen to fibrin [11]. They also help in the reduction of hypertension by promoting vasorelaxation. The ginsenosides Rb3 and Rb1 regulate the levels of polyamines that are responsible for cellular growth and regeneration of neural cells [12]. Polyamines are also called stress-based stimuli markers. Rb3 and Rb1 are responsible for blocking the enzyme ornithine carboxylase, which is further responsible for generating polyamines. Ginsenosides play an important role in the treatment of neurological disorders like Alzheimer's and Parkinson's diseases. They have also been utilized for the treatment of nervous ailments like amnesia, wherein they enhance cholinergic activity by promoting the uptake of choline, thus improving synaptic transmission [13]. The ginsenoside Rb1 has been shown to increase neural outgrowth, a property that can be utilized for the treatment of dementia. The ginsenosides Rb1 and Rg1 are also responsible for reversing the detrimental effects of cell death and also aid in modulating nerve transmission by further regulating the levels of neurotransmitters [14]. Ginsenosides are also involved in the treatment of several stomach ailments. The ginsenoside Rf has multifold beneficial effects on metabolism, which further contributes to prevent various diseases like lipid disorders, diabetes, and obesity [15].

3. Natural Biosynthesis

Ginsenosides are specialized plant metabolites that share precursors with the primary sterol biosynthesis pathway. The biosynthesis of triterpene ginsenosides takes place inside the cytosol and plastids via the mevalonic acid (MVA) pathway and the methylerythritol (MEP) pathway, respectively (Figure 2). Ginsenosides are synthesized via an isoprenoid pathway form the precursors isopentenyl diphosphate (IPP) and dimethylallyl diphosphate (DMAPP) [16,17]. The enzymes responsible for ginsenoside production in biological systems are squalene synthase (SS), farnesyl diphosphate synthase (FPS), and geranyl diphosphate synthase (GPPS). Ginsenosides biosynthesis involves one molecule of DMAPP that binds with two molecules of IPP to form FPP (farnesyl diphosphate), and the combination of two molecules of FPP produces a linear chain of squalene, which contains 30 carbon atoms [18]. The linear molecule squalene is epoxidized to 2,3-oxidosqualene, which is then cyclized to dammarenediol, the specific precursor of ginsenoside in *Panax* spp. It is from this process that ginsenosides can directly be synthesized via oxidation, mediated by cytochrome P450-dependent monooxygenases [19]. Although ginsenoside biosynthesis can occur via both MVA and MEP pathways, ginsenoside production occurs mainly through the MVA pathway, as shown by Schramek et al. [20] through a pulse-chase experiment in a 6-year-old *P. ginseng* plantlet using carbon isotopes. The MVA pathway is a universal pathway active in both eukaryotic and prokaryotic organisms. Inhibition experiments pointed out that the MEP pathway is activated when there is a limited supply of products from the MVA pathway. The MVA pathway is inhibited by light, whereas the MEP pathway is stimulated by light or enhanced by phytochrome signaling. Ginsenosides accumulate in the root epidermis. Histochemical assays showed that ginsenoside accumulation is found in the oil canals of the outer cortex but is totally absent in xylem cells and pith cells. The genes responsible for ginsenoside biosynthesis are expressed mainly in phloem cells, suggesting that these are the major sites for ginsenoside production [3]. Ginsenoside production was also reported to occur in cell organelles like vacuoles, plastids, and peroxisomes in leaves. The ginsenosides thus produced are transported to the root cortex. The transportation of ginsenosides is regulated by a complex cassette transporter, which involves adenosine triphosphate (ATP) [3].

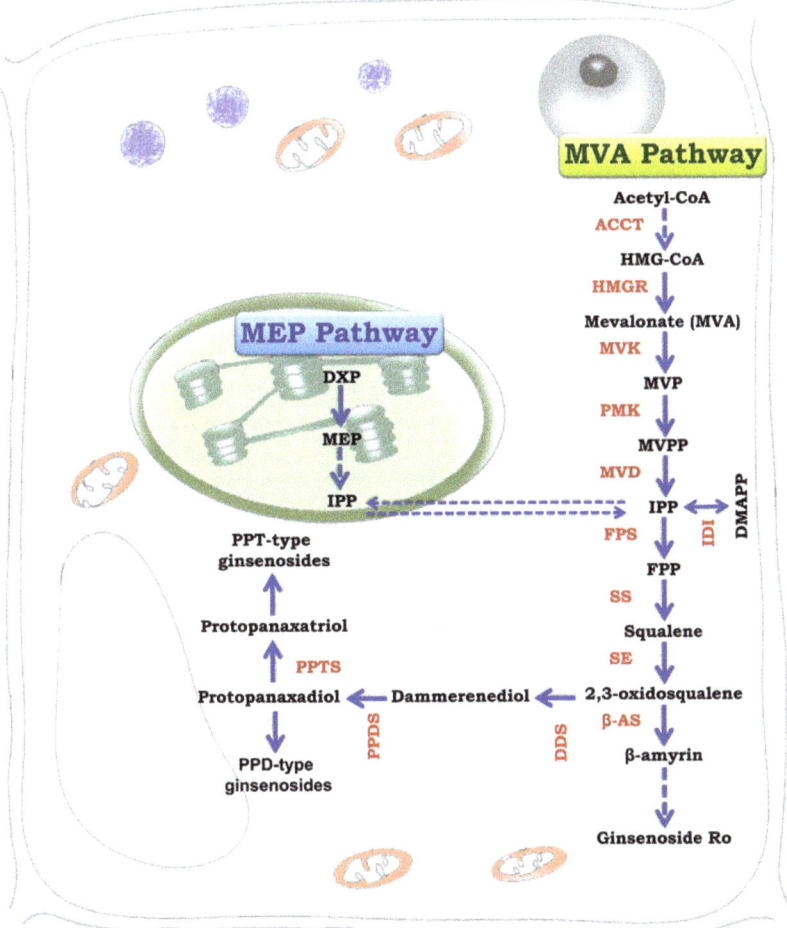

Figure 2. Biosynthesis of ginsenosides via the mevalonic acid (MVA) pathway (inside the cytosol) and the methylerythritol (MEP) pathway (inside plastids) (Concept source: Kim et al. [17]; modified and redrawn by Saikat Gantait).

4. In Vitro Approaches for Secondary Metabolite Production

4.1. Adventitious Shoot Culture

Adventitious shoot culture is a synonymous term for direct organogenesis. Direct organogenesis is defined as the induction of roots and shoots from explants without the formation of an intervening callus. This phenomenon is regulated by the endogenous accumulation of plant growth regulators as well as by their exogenous application [21]. Not many reports on direct organogenesis for ginsenoside estimation are available; the limited few are summarized in Table 1. In addition, there is only a single report on direct organogenesis coupled with ginsenoside estimation in *P. ginseng*, wherein leaves were utilized as explants and inoculated in basal media supplemented with 6-benzyladenine (BA), a cytokinin that promoted the lateral development of shoot buds [22]. Hence, the utilization of a wide array of explants such as shoot tip, nodal segment, hypocotyl, etc., can be employed for the production of ginsenosides in vitro, since this approach is simple and reliable.

4.2. Callus Culture, Somatic Embryogenesis, and Regeneration.

Indirect organogenesis or callogenesis is defined as the phenomenon of regeneration of plantlets from a mass of unorganized cells termed callus. Callus is categorized into two groups, namely, friable callus and compact callus, which are employed for suspension culture and regeneration experiments, respectively [21]. There are extensive reports on callus induction and estimation of ginsenosides in the callus cells, which are summarized in Table 2. The utilization of leaves as explants has been adopted owing to their larger surface area. The utilization of auxins in the basal medium leads to the formation of friable calli. The process of regeneration of plantlets from callus is effectuated by the addition of gibberellic acid (GA_3) and 6-benzylaminopurine (BAP) in the basal medium [23,24]. Compounds like picloram or dicamba can also be used to induce callus from an array of explants, since they possess auxin-mimicking activity.

Somatic embryogenesis is defined as the phenomenon via which somatic embryos are induced from a group of cells that are somatic in origin. The induction of a somatic embryo from callus is regulated by the type and dosage of plant growth regulators used in the growth medium [25]. For ginsenoside production in vitro, there are ample reports available on somatic embryogenesis, which are listed in Table 1. There is also a single instance wherein somatic embryos underwent the process of acclimatization following germination [26].

Table 1. Factors involved in and their influence on ginsenoside production during indirect organogenesis.

Panax sp.	Explant	Surface Sterilization	Basal Medium	Carbon Source	PGRs (mg/L or μM*)	Other Media Additives (mg/L or g/L*)	Culture Condition [Temp; PP; LI lux or PPTD#; RH]	Response	Acclimatization [Substrate Used (v/v); % Survival]	Ginsenoside Yield	Reference
P. ginseng	Leaf	70% EtOH 30 sec → 0.625% NaOCl 1 min	MS	3% sucrose	10* NAA + 9* 2,4-D	NM	NM; 12 h; 24#; NM	Somatic embryo	NM	NM	[23]
					3* GA3 + 5* BAP			Shoot regeneration and rooting			
P. ginseng	Anther	70% EtOH 30s → 2% NaOCl 1 min with drops of Tween 20	MS	9% sucrose	4.53* 2,4-D	NM	25 ± 1 °C; NM; NM; NM	Callus induction	NM	NM	[24]
					28.9* GA3			Shoot regeneration			
P. pseudoginseng	Rhizome	70% EtOH 30s → 2% NaOCl 1 min with drops of Tween 20 → 0.1% HgCl2	MS	3% sucrose	2.5 2,4-D + 2.5 BAP	NM	NM	Somatic embryo	Black garden soil + compost+ leaf litter (1:1:1); 70%	NM	[26]
					1 GA3			Somatic embryo generation			
P. ginseng	Cotyledon	70% EtOH → 1% NaOCl	MS	3% sucrose	NM	40 mM NH4NO3	22 ± 2 °C; 16 h; 24#; NM	Callus induction	NM	4.39 mg/g	[27]
P. quinquefolium	Root	NM	MS	3% sucrose	2.5 2,4-D	NM	NM	Callus induction	NM	NM	[28]
P. ginseng	Root	70% EtOH 30s → 1% NaOCl 1 min	SH	3% sucrose	1 2,4-D + 0.1 KIN	NM	25 ± 2 °C; NM; NM; NM	Callus induction	NM	83.37 mg/L	[29]
P. ginseng	Root	70% EtOH 30 sec → 20% NaOCl 1 min with drops of Tween 20	MS	3% sucrose	2 2,4-D	0.1%(w/v) myo inositol	25 °C; NM; NM; NM	Callus induction	NM	NM	[30]
P. ginseng	Root	75% EtOH	MS	3% sucrose	2 2,4-D + 0.5 KIN	NM	23 ± 2 °C; NM; NM; NM	Callus induction	NM	132.9 mg/L	[31]
P. ginseng	Root	NM	MS	5% sucrose	25* IBA	NM	22 ± 1 °C; NM; NM; NM	Callus induction	NM	7.3 mg/L	[32]
P. ginseng	Leaf	70% EtOH 30 sec → 0.1% HgCl2 for 1 min	MS	3% sucrose	4 BAP	NM	25 ± 2 °C; 16 h; 24#; 80	Shoot induction	NM	NM	[33]
P. quinquefolium	Root	70% EtOH 30 sec	MS	3% sucrose	1 2,4-D + 0.25 KIN	NM	23 ± 2 °C; NM; NM; NM	Callus induction	NM	NM	[34]

Abbreviations: 2,4-D, 2,4-dichlorophenoxyacetic acid; BAP, 6-benzylaminopurine; MS, Murashige and Skoog [35]; NAA, α-naphthalene acetic acid; IAA, indole acetic acid; KIN, kinetin; LI, light intensity; RH, relative humidity; PP, photoperiod; IBA, indole butyric acid; NA, not applicable; NM, not mentioned; PGR, plant growth regulator; PP, photoperiod; SH Schenk and Hildebrandt [36].

4.3. Cell Suspension Culture

Cell suspension culture is regarded as a convenient approach for the production of secondary metabolites, since it is not season-dependent, and harvesting of cells devoid of biotic contaminants is much easier [37]. Multiple reports on ginsenoside production, based on cell suspension culture in *Panax* spp., are available and are summarized in Table 2. Generally, the induction of callus is initiated with the help of plant growth regulators, mainly auxins, to obtain friable calli [38]. Elicitors are low-molecular-weight compounds that induce secondary metabolite formation in plants by inducing stress-like conditions and have a direct effect on the biosynthetic pathway [39]. Elicitors are also employed for further enhancement of ginsenoside production. Yu et al. [40] used the fungal strain *Alternaria panax*, which acted as a biotic elicitor; the exudates from the fungal cell wall, which contained oligosaccharides along with chitin, aided in the enhancement of ginsenoside accumulation. The utilization of jasmonate compounds also elevated ginsenoside accumulation in the cell cultures, since jasmonates induce oxidative stress in the culture and downregulate many genes, which leads to the augmentation of secondary metabolite levels. Generally, the elicitors aid in stimulating ginsenoside accumulation by activating phenylalanine amino lyase. This enzyme, in turn, helps in the synthesis of defense compounds, which indirectly affects the ginsenoside biosynthetic pathway [41–43].

Table 2. Factors involved in and their influence on ginsenoside production in cell suspension culture.

Panax sp.	Basal Media	Carbon Source	PGR (mg/L or *µM)	Elicitor (µM/*mg/L)	Culture Conditions (Temp, PP, RH, LI, rpm)	Yield	References
P. ginseng	MS	3% sucrose	0.1 KIN + 1 2,4-D	NM	25 °C, dark, NM, NA, NM	54 mg/g	[30]
P. ginseng	MS	4% sucrose	1 2,4-D	NM	24 ± 1 °C, dark, NM, NA, NM	3.08 mg/g	[38]
P. ginseng	MS	3% sucrose	0.25 KIN	6* *Alternaria panax*	25 °C, dark, NM, NA, NM (30 days)	276 mg/L	[40]
P. ginseng	MS (no NH$_4$NO$_3$)	5% sucrose	2 NAA	150 MJ	22 °C, dark, NM, NA, 110 rpm (40 days)	48 mg/g	[41]
P. notoginseng	MS	NM	NM	100 2-hydroxyethyl jasmonate	NM, NM, NM, NM, NM	32.7 mg/L	[42]
P. ginseng	MS	3% sucrose	2 IBA + 0.1 KIN	2* JA	NM, dark, NM, NA, 100 rpm	255 mg/L	[43]
P. quinquefolium	MS	3% sucrose	0.25 KIN + 1 2,4-D	NM	23 ± 2 °C, dark, NA, 120 rpm (90 days)	3.36 mg/g	[44]
P. vietnamensis	MS	3% sucrose	0.1 KIN + 3 2,4-D	NM	25 °C, dark, NM, NA, 105 rpm	5.7 mg/g	[45]
P. ginseng	MS	3% sucrose	25* IBA	NM	25 °C, dark, NM, NA, 100 rpm	5.4 mg/g	[46]
P. ginseng	MS	3% sucrose	0.5 BAP + 2 2,4-D	500* CH	25 °C, dark, NM, NA, 100 rpm	NM	[47]
P. quinquefolium	MS	3% sucrose	0.002 TDZ + 0.2 2,4-D	NM	26 ± 2 °C, 90%, NM, 40 µE/m^2/s, 100 rpm (40 days)	29.11 mg/g	[48]

Abbreviations: MJ, methyl jasmonate; JA, jasmonic acid; CH, casein hydrolysate; NM, not mentioned; NA, not applicable; TDZ, thidiazuron.

4.4. Protoplast Culture

Protoplast culture is regarded as a promising tool for the development of interspecific hybrids of those species that are incompatible when crossed conventionally. In protoplast culture, protoplasts are isolated from the counter parents and are fused to form a hybrid in vitro [21]. There is a sole report available on enhanced ginsenoside production based on protoplast fusion between carrot and American ginseng (*P. quinquefolius*). The hybrid obtained was subjected to high-performance liquid chromatography (HPLC) analysis, and ginsenoside accumulation in the hybrid calli (seven in number) was observed; introgression among these lines enhanced the ginsenoside concentration [49].

4.5. Bioreactor: Large-Scale Propagation

Bioreactors are now emerging implements in bioprocessing industries, wherein the optimum environmental conditions are maintained to achieve the required biological products on a large scale. The advantages of bioreactors include a better rate of product multiplication, lesser time for multiplication, and minimum cost [50]. Ginsenoside production in various bioreactors, under different culture conditions, is presented in Table 3. There are various kinds of bioreactors. Stirred-tank bioreactors are the most commonly used (they were utilized by Wang et al. [44] and Kochan et al. [51]), since they allow easier accumulation of cells at various stages due to their large capacities and for their capability to scale up nutrients [52]. The airlift and balloon-type airlift bioreactors are also utilized for ginsenoside production. This type of bioreactors have the additional advantage of better oxygen transfer efficiency with better prediction of flow patterns thus reducing cell shearing [53]. In sprinkle bioreactors, homogeneous culture conditions are usually maintained, and therefore, monitoring becomes much easier [54]. Overall, in all the reports, a pH ranging between 5 to 7 was maintained. Owing to the breakdown of substrate, release of ammonia occurred, which in turn resulted in a decrease of pH; therefore, pH monitoring was a priority [55]. The temperature maintained in the bioreactors was above 20 °C, which is the most favorable temperature for enhanced root biomass and ginsenoside accumulation. Increased aeration rate in bioreactors resulted in an increase in the volume of roots and further metabolite accumulation. The impact of atmospheric gases also determined ginsenoside accumulation, whereby a higher concentration of ethylene and carbon dioxide led to a decrease in ginsenoside production. The increase in ginsenoside accumulation was made possible by the accumulation of nitrate ions and the decrease in ammonia ions. There is a report on the utilization of squalene as an elicitor in bioreactors, wherein squalene resulted in the accumulation of protopanaxatriol groups (the building blocks of ginsenosides) [56].

Table 3. Factors involved in and their influence on ginsenoside production during regeneration via bioreactors.

Species	Type of Bioreactor	Basal Media	PGR (mg/L)	Elicitor/Additives	Culture Condition (Temp, PP, Other)	Ginsenoside Yield	References
P.quinquefolius	Balloon type airlift	MS	5 IBA	4 mg/L *Alternaria panax*	26 °C, dark, 100 vvm	276 mg/L	[40]
P.quinquefolium	Stirred tank	MS	0.25 KIN + 1 2,4-D	100 mg/L Lactoalbumin hydrolysate	23 ± 2 °C, 1 vvm	31.52 mg/L	[44]
P.quinquefolium	Stirred tank	MS	0.1 KIN + 1 2,4-D	NM	26 °C, 100 vvm	9 mg/g	[51]
P.quinquefolium	Nutrient sprinkle	B5	NM	NM	26 ± 2 °C	32.25 mg/g	[54]
P. ginseng	Airlift	MS	NM	10 mM Copper sulphate	0.1 vvm, 23 ± 1 °C	12.42 mg/g	[56]
P. notoginseng	Airlift	MS	NM	1 mM copper, 3.75 mM phosphate	Aeration rate: 0.8 vvm	1.75 g/L	[57]
P. ginseng	NM	MS	NM	18.5 mH NO_3^-	NM	9.9 mg/g	[58]
P. ginseng	Balloon type bubble	MS	7 IBA + 0.5 KIN	200 µM MJ	25 °C, dark	8.82 mg/g	[59]
P. ginseng	Balloon type airlift	MS	7 IBA + 0.5 KIN	20 ppm Ethylene	NM	NM	[60]
P. ginseng	Balloon type airlift	MS	5 IBA + 0.5 KIN	200 µM MJ and salicylic acid	NM	NM	[61]
P. ginseng	NM	MS	24.6 µM IBA	NM	0.1 vvm	1.91 mg/g	[62]
P.quinquefolium	Nutrient sprinkle	B5	NM	NM	26 °C, dark	12.45 mg/g	[63]
P.quinquefolium	Nutrient sprinkle	B5	NM	250 µM MJ	26 °C	24.77 mg/g	[64]

4.6. In Vitro Mutagenesis

Ginsenosides production from in vitro cultures is a popular approach to enhance their production rate. Although somaclonal variants during in vitro cultures are detected at a lower frequency, they are desirable to augment the synthesis of ginsenosides [65]. In vitro mutagenesis incorporates a genotypic change in a culture, and the derived population can be maintained via rigorous subculturing. Cotyledonary explants were inoculated in callus induction medium supplemented with 1 mg/L 2,4-D and 0.1 mg/L kinetin. The induced calli were then exposed to gamma radiations ranging from 10 to 100 Gy (Gray). A dosage of 30 Gy was selected as the adequate dose, and via HPLC analysis, it was confirmed that there was an increase in ginsenoside production in the mutant lines [66]. Similarly, Kim et al. [2] conducted an experiment wherein the in vitro grown calli were exposed to gamma radiations in the 50 Gy range and then cultured in MS media supplemented with 3 mg/L indole butyric acid (IBA). An increase in the concentration of primary ginsenosides in the mutant lines was confirmed subsequently by thin-layer chromatography (TLC) and HPLC analysis. The same was further validated with gene expression studies using RT-PCR, whereby the expression of squalene epoxidase, dammarenediol synthase, and phytosterol synthase genes were enhanced in the mutant lines. There are also reports wherein spontaneous mutation resulted in the overexpression of the *DDS* gene, which is responsible for ginsenoside accumulation. Recently, Le et al. [67] conducted an experiment to determine the sensitivity of mutagens, wherein somatic embryos were exposed to gamma radiation ranging from 20 to 400 Gy, and the optimal radiation dose was standardized at 80 Gy. The gamma-irradiated somatic embryos were germinated in MS medium supplemented with gibberellic acid.

4.7. Induction of Polyploidization

The induction of polyploidy or artificial chromosome doubling with the help of anti-mitotic agents is mainly implemented for enhancing the biomass of a plant and, thus consequently amplifying the metabolite profile as well [68]. In *P. ginseng*, in vitro adventitious roots were excised, treated with 100 mg/L colchicine over 60 h and inoculated in MS medium supplemented with 50 mg/L sucrose and 2 mg/L α-naphthalene acetic acid (NAA). After 40 days, the treated roots were subjected to HPLC analysis, whereby the accumulation of ginsenosides was observed in the resultant regenerated octaploid plantlets, suggesting that chromosome doubling can enhance biomass and ginsenoside accumulation, simultaneously [69]. Hence, based on these studies, it is evident that polyploidization can be a viable approach to increase ginsenosides yield. The utilization of anti-mitotic agents like oryzalin or trifluralin can ensure a successful polyploidization. In addition, flow cytometry analysis can also be used to confirm the polyploidy level in anti-mitotic agent-treated explants, in addition to the conventional chromosome counting method.

4.8. Hairy Root Culture

Genetic transformation with the help of *Agrobacterium rhizogenes* gives rise to transformed hairy roots. The induced hairy roots often exhibit a comparable or higher biosynthetic capacity for secondary metabolite production with respect to non-transformed roots, owing to the presence of auxin-responsive genes and overexpression of *rol* genes that can further lead to an increase in biomass [70]. This observation gave rise to the development of a new direction associated with the use of hairy roots for the production of these secondary metabolites. Hairy root culture has innumerable advantages. For instance, the growth phase of the culture remains stable throughout, and the culture possesses high genetic stability and negative geotropism. Even under control conditions, hairy roots grow at a higher rate than normal adventitious roots. The most positive aspect of hairy roots is that they exhibit a higher biosynthetic rate than the mother plant [71]. There are extensive reports on ginsenoside production using this technique, some of which are listed in Table 4. The leaf is the explant of choice in most cases, since it possesses a large surface area and allows a more effective adhesion of the bacterial suspension, resulting in better chances of transformation [72]. As for the maintenance medium, MS is prevalently employed due to the presence of a high amount of ammonia and nitrate ions [73]. Cefotaxime is recurrently used in all the experiments for genetic transformation due to its broad-spectrum activities against Gram-positive and Gram-negative bacteria [74]. Molecular confirmation of gene integration was carried out via PCR amplification of *rol* genes, which are responsible for the positive regulation of metabolite production [54,75]. Kim et al. [66] performed transcriptional profiling of putative genes for ginsenosides production, viz., *PgSS* (squalene synthase), *PgSE* (squalene epoxidase), and *PNA* (dammarenediol synthase-II) genes. In genetically transformed hairy roots, the presence of ocotillol ginsenosides was detected at a considerable concentration when compared to the roots collected from conventionally grown ex vitro plants.

Table 4. Factors involved in and their influence on ginsenoside production during hairy root culture.

Species	Explant	Strain	Basal Media (for induction)	Antibiotics (mg/L)	Elicitors (mg/L)	Basal Media (for maintenance)	Ginsenoside Yield	Reference
P. ginseng	Root	A4	NM	NM	NM	MS + 3% sucrose	3.62 mg/g	[76]
P. ginseng	Root	A4	NM	NM	MJ	SH	NM	[77]
P. ginseng	Cotyledon	R1000	NM	800 cefotaxime	NM	½ MS	NM	[78]
P. ginseng	Rhizome	A4	YEB	500 cefotaxime	NM	SH	72.9 mg/L	[79]
P. ginseng	NM	A4	NM	NM	NM	NM	17.12 mg/g	[80]
P. ginseng	Root	KCTC 2703	Nutrient broth	300 cefotaxime	2 JA	½ MS	2 mg/L	[81]
P. ginseng	Root	NM	NM	NM	0.1 mM MJ	½ MS	6.83 mg/g	[82]
P. quinquefolium	Leaf	ATCC 15834	NM	NM	NM	B5	3 mg/g	[83]
P. quinquefolium	Leaf	ATCC 15834	NM	500 ampicillin	NM	B5	9 mg/g	[84]
P. vietnamensis	Shoot tip	ATCC 15834	NM	250 cefotaxime	NM	½ SH	10 g/L	[85]

Abbreviations: B5, Gamborg et al. [86].

5. Conclusions and Future Prospect

The most recent biotechnological advances regarding ginsenoside production under in vitro conditions have been highlighted (Figure 3) and described extensively in this review. There are only a handful of reports available on direct and indirect organogenesis experiments, wherein tissue culture-mediated technologies like direct organogenesis, indirect organogenesis, and somatic embryogenesis have not been extensively investigated for the purpose of ginsenoside production, and the quantitative estimation of ginsenosides via HPLC or high-performance thin-layer chromatography (HPTLC) has not been attempted as well. The utilization of additives, elicitors, or precursors in organogenesis experiments and somatic embryogenesis experiments needs to be addressed properly, since these are compounds that can interfere with the signaling pathways that directly or indirectly affect ginsenoside biosynthesis and can enhance their production. There are ample reports on cell suspension cultures and bioreactors, yet the use of elicitors needs to be explored more extensively, since these compounds may greatly contribute to ginsenoside amelioration. These methods have been mainly implemented to increase plant biomass and to further promote metabolite production in a much shorter period of time and are not season-dependent. There are several reports on hairy root culture and the use of other approaches of genetic transformation like direct methods that employ gene guns, particle bombardment, etc., or the use of *Agrobacterium tumifaciens*. On the other hand, few reports on polyploidy that are available till date and this technique needs to be studied furthermore with the extensive applications of antimitotic agents like oryzalin or trifluralin in variable concentrations at different exposure times to enhance the production of ginsenosides. In vitro mutagenesis is the most innovative approach that has gained recognition only recently and needs to be analyzed furthermore to explore its beneficial effects for the increased production of ginsenosides. In conclusion, this review provides an overview of the current biotechnological advancements for ginsenoside production in vitro and also highlights the main unexplored research areas that need to be addressed in the near future.

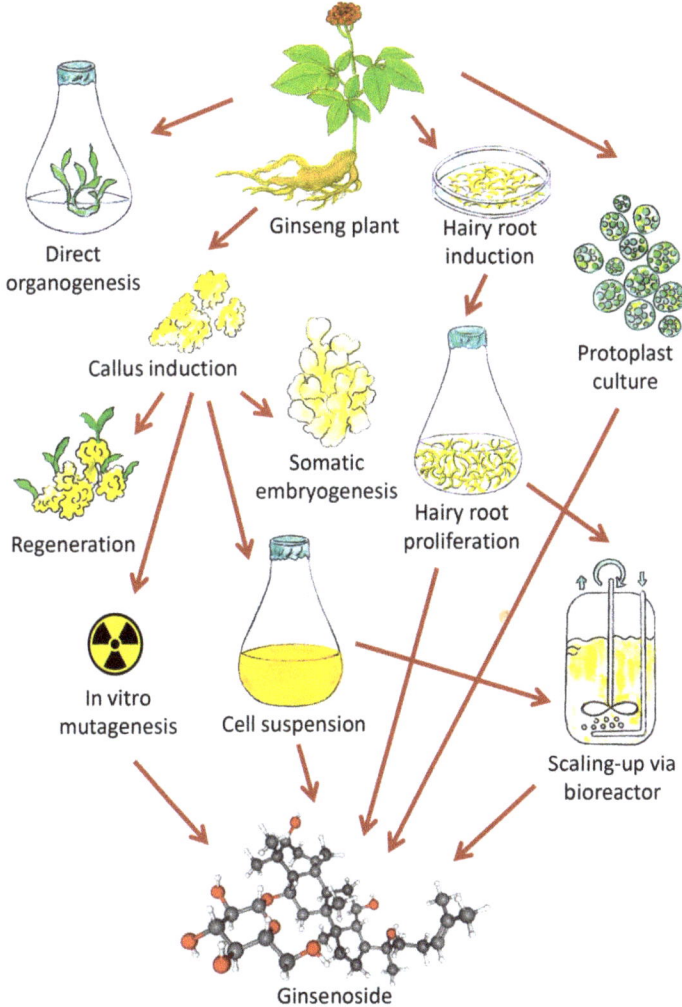

Figure 3. Diagram showing the enhanced production of ginsenosides through various in vitro biotechnological approaches (Source: unpublished photograph of Saikat Gantait).

Author Contributions: S.G. and M.M.—designed and wrote the manuscript. J.-T.C.—comprehensively revised and improved the quality of the manuscript. All authors have read and agreed to the published version of the manuscript.

Funding: This research received no external funding.

Acknowledgments: The authors acknowledge e-library assistance from the Bidhan Chandra Krishi Viswavidyalaya, West Bengal, India. We are further thankful to the anonymous reviewers, the editor of this article for their critical comments and suggestions on the manuscript, and Hsun-Fang Liang for the modification and improvement of Figure 3.

Conflicts of Interest: The authors declare no conflict of interest.

Ethical approval: This article does not contain any studies with human participants or animals performed by any of the authors.

References

1. Mohanan, P.; Subramaniyam, S.; Mathiyalagan, R.; Yang, D.C. Molecular signaling of ginsenosides Rb1, Rg1, and Rg3 and their mode of actions. *J. Ginseng Res.* **2018**, *42*, 123–132. [CrossRef] [PubMed]
2. Kim, D.S.; Song, M.; Kim, S.H.; Jang, D.S.; Kim, J.B.; Ha, B.K.; Kim, S.H.; Lee, K.J.; Kang, S.Y.; Jeong, I.Y. The improvement of ginsenoside accumulation in *Panax ginseng* as a result of γ-irradiation. *J. Ginseng Res.* **2013**, *37*, 332. [CrossRef] [PubMed]
3. Zhao, S.; Wang, L.; Liu, L.; Liang, Y.; Sun, Y.; Wu, J. Both the mevalonate and the non-mevalonate pathways are involved in ginsenoside biosynthesis. *Plant Cell Rep.* **2014**, *33*, 393–400. [CrossRef] [PubMed]
4. Hemmerlin, A.; Harwood, J.L.; Bach, T.J. A raison d'être for two distinct pathways in the early steps of plant isoprenoid biosynthesis? *Progress Lipid Res.* **2012**, *51*, 95–148. [CrossRef] [PubMed]
5. Sasidharan, S.; Jothy, S.L.; Vijayarathna, S.; Kavitha, N.; Oon, C.E.; Chen, Y.; Dharmaraj, S.; Lai, N.S.; Kanwar, J.R. Conventional and non-conventional approach towards the extraction of bioorganic phase. In *Bioorganic Phase in Natural Food: An Overview*; Mohana Roopan, S., Madhumitha, G., Eds.; Springer: Cham, Switzerland, 2018; pp. 41–57.
6. Yue, P.Y.K.; Wong, D.Y.L.; Wu, P.K.; Leung, P.Y.; Mak, N.K.; Yeung, H.W.; Liu, L.; Cai, Z.; Jiang, Z.-H.; Fan, T.P.D. The angiosuppressive effects of 20(R)-ginsenoside Rg3. *Biochem. Pharm.* **2006**, *72*, 437–445. [CrossRef]
7. Lee, C.H.; Kim, J.H. A review on the medicinal potentials of ginseng and ginsenosides on cardiovascular diseases. *J. Ginseng Res.* **2014**, *38*, 161–166. [CrossRef]
8. Radad, K.; Gille, G.; Moldzio, R.; Saito, H.; Ishige, K.; Rausch, W.-D. Ginsenosides Rb1 and Rg1 effects on survival and neurite growth of MPPþ -affected mesencephalic dopaminergic cells. *J. Neural Transm.* **2004**, *111*, 37–45. [CrossRef]
9. Park, E.K.; Choo, M.K.; Kim, E.J.; Han, M.J.; Kim, D.H. Antiallergic activity of ginsenoside Rh2. *Biol. Pharm. Bull.* **2003**, *26*, 1581–1584. [CrossRef]
10. Leung, K.W.; Wong, A.S.T. Pharmacology of ginsenosides: A literature review. *Chin. Med.* **2010**, *5*, 20. [CrossRef]
11. Rhule, A.; Navarro, S.; Smith, J.R.; Shepherd, D.M. *Panax notoginseng* attenuates LPS-induced pro-inflammatory mediators in RAW264.7 cells. *J. Etnopharmacol.* **2006**, *106*, 121–128. [CrossRef]
12. Xue, J.-F.; Liu, Z.-J.; Hu, J.-F.; Chen, H.; Zhang, J.-T.; Chen, N.-H. Ginsenoside Rb1 promotes neurotransmitter release by modulating phosphyrolation of synapsis through a cAMP-dependent protein kinase pathway. *Brain Res.* **2006**, *1106*, 91–98. [CrossRef] [PubMed]
13. Rudakewich, M.; Ba, F.; Benishin, C.G. Neurotrophic and neuroprotective actions of ginsenosides Rb1 and Rg1. *Planta Med.* **2001**, *67*, 533–537. [CrossRef] [PubMed]
14. Joo, S.S.; Won, T.J.; Lee, D.I. Reciprocal activity of ginsenosides in the production of proinflammatory repertoire, and their potential roles in neuroprotection *in vitro*. *Planta Med.* **2005**, *71*, 476–481. [CrossRef] [PubMed]
15. Kaneko, H.; Nakanishi, K. Proof of the mysterious efficacy of ginseng: Basic and clinical trials: Clinical effects of medical ginseng, Korean red ginseng: Specifically, its anti-stress action for prevention of disease. *J. Pharmacol. Sci.* **2004**, *95*, 158–162. [CrossRef] [PubMed]
16. Linsefors, L.; Björk, L.; Mosbach, K. Influence of elicitors and mevalonic acid on the biosynthesis of ginsenosides in tissue cultures of *Panax ginseng*. *Biochem. Physiol. Pflanz.* **1989**, *184*, 413–418. [CrossRef]
17. Kim, Y.-J.; Zhang, D.; Yang, D.-C. Biosynthesis and biotechnological production of ginsenosides. *Biotechnol. Adv.* **2015**, *33*, 717–735. [CrossRef]
18. Lee, M.H.; Jeong, J.H.; Seo, J.W.; Shin, C.G.; Kim, Y.S.; In, J.G.; Yang, D.C.; Yi, J.S.; Choi, Y.E. Enhanced triterpene and phytosterol biosynthesis in *Panax ginseng* overexpressing squalene synthase gene. *Plant Cell Physiol.* **2004**, *45*, 976–984. [CrossRef]

19. Han, J.Y.; Kim, M.J.; Ban, Y.W.; Hwang, H.S.; Choi, Y.E. The involvement of β-amyrin 28-oxidase (CYP716A52v2) in oleanane-type ginsenoside biosynthesis in *Panax ginseng*. *Plant Cell Physiol.* **2013**, *54*, 2034–2046. [CrossRef]
20. Schramek, N.; Huber, C.; Schmidt, S.; Dvorski, S.E.; Knispel, N.; Ostrozhenkova, E.; Eisenreich, W. Biosynthesis of ginsenosides in field-grown *Panax ginseng*. *JSM Biotechnol. Bioeng.* **2014**, *2*, 1033.
21. Gantait, S.; El-Dawayati, M.M.; Panigrahi, J.; Labrooy, C.; Verma, S.K. The retrospect and prospect of the applications of biotechnology in *Phoenix dactylifera* L. *Appl. Microbiol. Biotechnol.* **2018**, *102*, 8229–8259. [CrossRef]
22. Laloue, M.; Pethe, C. Dynamics of cytokinin metabolism in tobacco cells. In *Plant Growth Substances, Proceedings of the 11th International Conference on Plant Growth Substances, Aberystwyth, UK, 12–16th July 1982*; Wareing, P.F., Ed.; Academic Press: New York, NY, USA, 1982; pp. 185–195.
23. Punja, Z.K.; Feeney, M.; Schluter, C.; Tautorus, T. Multiplication and germination of somatic embryos of American ginseng derived from suspension cultures and biochemical and molecular analyses of plantlets. *In Vitro Cell. Dev. Biol.-Plant* **2004**, *40*, 329–338. [CrossRef]
24. Lee, H.Y.; Khorolragchaa, A.; Sun, M.S.; Kim, Y.J.; Kim, Y.J.; Kwon, W.S.; Yang, D.C. Plant regeneration from anther culture of *Panax ginseng*. *Korean J. Plant Resour.* **2013**, *26*, 383–388. [CrossRef]
25. Gantait, S.; Kundu, S. Neoteric trends in tissue culture-mediated biotechnology of Indian ipecac [*Tylophora indica* (Burm. f.) Merrill]. *3 Biotech* **2017**, *7*, 231. [CrossRef] [PubMed]
26. Kharwanlang, L.; Das, M.C.; Kumaria, S.; Tandon, P. High frequency somatic embryos induction from the rhizome explant of *Panax pseudoginseng* Wall. Using thin cell layer section. *Int. J. Appl. Biol. Pharm. Technol.* **2016**, *7*, 31–34.
27. Choi, Y.E.; Jeong, J.H.; Shin, C.K. Hormone-independent embryogenic callus production from ginseng cotyledons using high concentrations of NH_4NO_3 and progress towards bioreactor production. *Plant Cell Tissue Organ Cult.* **2003**, *72*, 229–235. [CrossRef]
28. Mathur, A.; Mathur, A.K.; Sangwan, R.S.; Gangwar, A.; Uniyal, G.C. Differential morphogenetic responses, ginsenoside metabolism and RAPD patterns of three *Panax* species. *Genet. Resour. Crop Evol.* **2003**, *50*, 245–252. [CrossRef]
29. Yu, K.W.; Gao, W.Y.; Hahn, E.J.; Paek, K.Y. Effects of macro elements and nitrogen source on adventitious root growth and ginsenoside production in ginseng (*Panax ginseng* CA Meyer). *J. Plant Biol.* **2001**, *44*, 179–184. [CrossRef]
30. Bonfill, M.; Cusidó, R.M.; Palazón, J.; Piñol, M.T.; Morales, C. Influence of auxins on organogenesis and ginsenoside production in *Panax ginseng* calluses. *Plant Cell Tissue Organ Cult.* **2002**, *68*, 73–78. [CrossRef]
31. Huang, T.; Gao, W.Y.; Wang, J.; Cao, Y.; Zhao, Y.X.; Huang, L.Q.; Liu, C.X. Selection and optimization of a high-producing tissue culture of *Panax ginseng* CA Meyer. *Acta Physiol. Plant.* **2010**, *32*, 765–772. [CrossRef]
32. Kim, Y.S.; Yeung, E.C.; Hahn, E.J.; Paek, K.Y. Combined effects of phytohormone, indole-3-butyric acid, and methyl jasmonate on root growth and ginsenoside production in adventitious root cultures of *Panax ginseng* CA Meyer. *Biotechnol. Lett.* **2007**, *29*, 1789–1792. [CrossRef]
33. Nhut, D.T.; Huy, N.P.; Luan, V.Q.; Van Binh, N.; Nam, N.B.; Thuy, L.N.M.; Cuong, L.K. Shoot regeneration and micropropagation of *Panax vietnamensis* Ha et Grushv. from *ex vitro* leaf derived callus. *African J. Biotechnol.* **2011**, *10*, 19499–19504.
34. Wang, J.; Liu, H.; Gao, W.Y.; Zhang, L. Comparison of ginsenoside composition in native roots and cultured callus cells of *Panax quinquefolium* L. *Acta Physiol. Plant.* **2013**, *35*, 1363–1366. [CrossRef]
35. Murashige, T.; Skoog, F. A Revised Medium for Rapid Growth and Bio Assays with Tobacco Tissue Cultures. *Physiol. Plant.* **1962**, *15*, 473–495. [CrossRef]
36. Schenk, R.U.; Hildebrandt, A.C. Medium and techniques for induction and growth of monocotyledonous and dicotyledonous plant cell cultures. *Can. J. Bot.* **1972**, *50*, 199–204. [CrossRef]
37. Vijaya Sree, N.; Udayasri, P.; Aswani Kumar, V.V.Y.; Ravi, B.B.; Phani, K.Y.; Vijay, V.M. Advancements in the production of secondary metabolites. *J. Nat. Prod.* **2010**, *3*, 112–123.
38. Lee, J.W.; Jo, I.H.; Kim, J.U.; Hong, C.E.; Bang, K.H.; Park, Y.D. Determination of mutagenic sensitivity to gamma rays in ginseng (*Panax ginseng*) dehiscent seeds, roots, and somatic embryos. *Hort. Env. Biotechnol.* **2019**, *60*, 721–731. [CrossRef]
39. Hussain, M.S.; Fareed, S.; Saba Ansari, M.; Rahman, A.; Ahmad, I.Z.; Saeed, M. Current approaches toward production of secondary plant metabolites. *J. Pharm Bioallied Sci.* **2012**, *4*, 10. [CrossRef]

40. Yu, Y.; Zhang, W.B.; Li, X.Y.; Piao, X.C.; Jiang, J.; Lian, M.L. Pathogenic fungal elicitors enhance ginsenoside biosynthesis of adventitious roots in *Panax quinquefolius* during bioreactor culture. *Industrial Crop. Prod.* **2016**, *94*, 729–735. [CrossRef]
41. Kim, Y.S.; Hahn, E.J.; Murthy, H.N.; Paek, K.Y. Effect of polyploidy induction on biomass and ginsenoside accumulations in adventitious roots of ginseng. *J. Plant Biol.* **2004**, *47*, 356–360. [CrossRef]
42. Wang, W.; Zhao, Z.J.; Xu, Y.; Qian, X.; Zhong, J.J. Efficient induction of ginsenoside biosynthesis and alteration of ginsenoside heterogeneity in cell cultures of *Panax notoginseng* by using chemically synthesized 2-hydroxyethyl jasmonate. *Appl. Microbiol. Biotechnol.* **2006**, *70*, 298–307. [CrossRef]
43. Yu, K.W.; Gao, W.; Hahn, E.J.; Paek, K.Y. Jasmonic acid improves ginsenoside accumulation in adventitious root culture of *Panax ginseng* CA Meyer. *Biochem. Engg. J.* **2002**, *11*, 211–215. [CrossRef]
44. Wang, J.; Gao, W.Y.; Zhang, J.; Zuo, B.M.; Zhang, L.M.; Huang, L.Q. Production of ginsenoside and polysaccharide by two-stage cultivation of *Panax quinquefolium* L. cells. *Vitr. Cell. Dev. Biol—Plant* **2012**, *48*, 107–112. [CrossRef]
45. Thanh, N.T.; Anh, H.T.; Yoeup, P.K. Effects of macro elements on biomass and ginsenoside production in cell suspension culture of Ngoc Linh ginseng {*Panax vietnamensis* Ha et Grushv. *Vnu J. Sci. Nat. Sci. Technol.* **2008**, *24*, 248–252.
46. Jeong, C.S.; Murthy, H.N.; Hahn, E.J.; Lee, H.L.; Paek, K.Y. Inoculum size and auxin concentration influence the growth of adventitious roots and accumulation of ginsenosides in suspension cultures of ginseng (*Panax ginseng* CA Meyer). *Acta Physiol. Plant.* **2009**, *31*, 219–222. [CrossRef]
47. Smolenskaya, I.N.; Reshetnyak, O.V.; Smirnova, Y.N.; Chernyak, N.D.; Globa, E.B.; Nosov, A.M.; Nosov, A.V. Opposite effects of synthetic auxins, 2, 4-dichlorophenoxyacetic acid and 1-naphthalene acetic acid on growth of true ginseng cell culture and synthesis of ginsenosides. *Russian J. Plant Physiol.* **2007**, *54*, 215–223. [CrossRef]
48. Kochan, E.; Chmiel, A. Dynamics of ginsenoside biosynthesis in suspension culture of *Panax quinquefolium*. *Acta Physiol. Plant.* **2011**, *33*, 911–915. [CrossRef]
49. Han, L.; Zhou, C.; Shi, J.; Zhi, D.; Xia, G. Ginsenoside Rb1 in asymmetric somatic hybrid calli of *Daucus carota* with *Panax quinquefolius*. *Plant Cell Rep.* **2009**, *28*, 627–638. [CrossRef]
50. Almusawi, A.H.A.; Sayegh, A.J.; Alshanaw, A.M.; Griffis, J.L. Plantform bioreactor for mass micropropagation of date palm. In *Date Palm Biotechnology Protocols*; Vol I. Methods in molecular biology; Al-Khayri, J.M., Jain, S.M., Johnson, D., Eds.; Humana Press: New York, NY, USA, 2017; Volume 1637, pp. 251–265.
51. Kochan, E.; Caban, S.; Szymańska, G.; Szymczyk, P.; Lipert, A.; Kwiatkowski, P.; Sienkiewicz, M. Ginsenoside content in suspension cultures of *Panax quinquefolium* L. cultivated in shake flasksand stirred-tank bioreactor. *Annales Universitatis Mariae Curie-Sklodowska Sectio C–Biol.* **2017**, *72*. [CrossRef]
52. Marks, D.M. Equipment design considerations for large scale cell culture. *Cytotechnology* **2003**, *42*, 21–33. [CrossRef]
53. Chen, N.; Srinivasa, S.; Leavit, R.I.; Coty, V.F.; Kondis, E. Low-pressure airlift fermentor for single cell protein production. *Biotechnol. Bioeng.* **1987**, *29*, 421. [CrossRef]
54. Kochan, E.; Szymczyk, P.; Kuźma, Ł.; Lipert, A.; Szymańska, G. Yeast extract stimulates ginsenoside production in hairy root cultures of American ginseng cultivated in shake flasks and nutrient sprinkle bioreactors. *Molecules* **2017**, *22*, 880. [CrossRef] [PubMed]
55. Elmahdi, I.; Baganz, F.; Dixon, K.; Harrop, T.; Sugden, D.; Lye, G.J. pH control in microwell fermentations of *S. erythraea* CA340: Influence on biomass growth kinetics and erythromycin biosynthesis. *Biochem. Engg. J.* **2003**, *16*, 299–310. [CrossRef]
56. Sivakumar, G.; Yu, K.W.; Paek, K.Y. Production of biomass and ginsenosides from adventitious roots of *Panax ginseng* in bioreactor cultures. *Engg. Life Sci.* **2005**, *5*, 333–342. [CrossRef]
57. Han, J.; Zhong, J.J. Effects of oxygen partial pressure on cell growth and ginsenoside and polysaccharide production in high density cell cultures of *Panax notoginseng*. *Enzyme Microb. Technol.* **2003**, *32*, 498–503. [CrossRef]
58. Yu, K.W.; Hahn, E.J.; Paek, K.Y. Effects of NH_4^+ : NO_3^- ratio and ionic strength on adventitious root growth and ginsenoside production in bioreactor culture of *Panax ginseng* CA Meyer. *Acta Hortic.* **2001**, 259–262. [CrossRef]

59. Thanh, N.T.; Murthy, H.N.; Yu, K.W.; Hahn, E.J.; Paek, K.Y. Methyl jasmonate elicitation enhanced synthesis of ginsenoside by cell suspension cultures of *Panax ginseng* in 5-l balloon type bubble bioreactors. *Appl. Microbiol. Biotechnol.* **2005**, *67*, 197–201. [CrossRef]
60. Thanh, N.T.; Yoeup, P.K. Cultivation of ginseng (*Panax ginseng* CA Meyer) in bioreactor: Role of ethylene on cell growth and ginsenosides production. *Tap Chi Sinh Hoc* **2007**, *29*, 42–48.
61. Ali, M.B.; Yu, K.W.; Hahn, E.J.; Paek, K.Y. Methyl jasmonate and salicylic acid elicitation induces ginsenosides accumulation, enzymatic and non-enzymatic antioxidant in suspension culture *Panax ginseng* roots in bioreactors. *Plant Cell Rep.* **2006**, *25*, 613–620. [CrossRef]
62. Jeong, C.S.; Chakrabarty, D.; Hahn, E.J.; Lee, H.L.; Paek, K.Y. Effects of oxygen, carbon dioxide and ethylene on growth and bioactive compound production in bioreactor culture of ginseng adventitious roots. *Biochem. Eng. J.* **2006**, *27*, 252–263. [CrossRef]
63. Kochan, E.; Szymczyk, P.; Szymańska, G. Nitrogen and phosphorus as the factors affecting ginsenoside production in hairy root cultures of *Panax quinquefolium* cultivated in shake flasks and nutrient sprinkle bioreactor. *Acta Physiol. Plant.* **2016**, *38*, 149. [CrossRef]
64. Kochan, E.; Balcerczak, E.; Lipert, A.; Szymańska, G.; Szymczyk, P. Methyl jasmonate as a control factor of the synthase squalene gene promoter and ginsenoside production in American ginseng hairy root cultured in shake flasks and a nutrient sprinkle bioreactor. *Ind. Crop. Prod.* **2018**, *115*, 182–193. [CrossRef]
65. Yang, H.; Tabei, Y.; Kamada, H.; Kayano, T. Detection of somaclonal variation in cultured rice cells using digoxigenin-based random amplified polymorphic DNA. *Plant Cell Rep.* **1999**, *18*, 520–526. [CrossRef]
66. Kim, D.S.; Kim, S.Y.; Jeong, I.Y.; Kim, J.B.; Lee, G.J.; Kang, S.Y.; Kim, W. Improvement of ginsenoside production by *Panax ginseng* adventitious roots induced by γ-irradiation. *Biol. Plant.* **2009**, *53*, 408. [CrossRef]
67. Le, K.C.; Jeong, C.S.; Lee, H.; Paek, K.Y.; Park, S.Y. Ginsenoside accumulation profiles in long-and short-term cell suspension and adventitious root cultures in *Panax ginseng*. *Hort. Environ. Biotechnol.* **2019**, *60*, 125–134. [CrossRef]
68. Mitra, M.; Gantait, S.; Mandal, N. *Coleus forskohlii*: Advancements and prospects of *in vitro* biotechnology. *Appl. Microbiol. Biotechnol.* **2020**, *104*, 2359–2371. [CrossRef] [PubMed]
69. Kim, Y.S.; Hahn, E.J.; Murthy, H.N.; Paek, K.Y. Adventitious root growth and ginsenoside accumulation in *Panax ginseng* cultures as affected by methyl jasmonate. *Biotechnol. Lett.* **2004**, *26*, 1619–1622. [CrossRef] [PubMed]
70. Chandra, S.; Chandra, R. Engineering secondary metabolite production in hairy roots. *Phytochem. Rev.* **2011**, *10*, 371–395. [CrossRef]
71. Shanks, J.V.; Morgan, J. Plant hairy root culture. *Curr. Opin. Biotechnol.* **1999**, *10*, 151–155. [CrossRef]
72. Wang, Y.M.; Wang, J.B.; Luo, D.; Jia, J.F. Regeneration of plants from callus cultures of roots induced by *Agrobacterium rhizogenes* on *Alhagi pseudoalhagi*. *Cell Res.* **2001**, *11*, 279–284. [CrossRef]
73. Bosela, M.J.; Michler, C.H. Media effects on black walnut (*Juglans nigra* L.) shoot culture growth in vitro: Evaluation of multiple nutrient formulations and cytokinin types. *Vitr. Cell. Dev. Biol.—Plant* **2008**, *44*, 316–329. [CrossRef]
74. Carmine, A.A.; Brogden, R.N.; Heel, R.C.; Speight, T.M.; Avery, G.S. Cefotaxime. *Drugs* **1983**, *25*, 223–289. [CrossRef] [PubMed]
75. Hahn, E.J.; Paek, K.Y.; Yu, K.W. Ginsenoside production by hairy root cultures of Panax ginseng CA Meyer in bioreactors. In *International Conference on Medicinal and Aromatic Plants (Part II)*; ISHS: Budapest, Hungary, 2001; pp. 237–243.
76. Yang, D.C.; Yang, K.J.; Choi, Y.E. Production of red ginseng specific ginsenosides (Rg2, Rg3, Rh1 and Rh2) from Agrobacterium—transformed hairy roots of *Panax ginseng* by heat treatment. *J. Photosci.* **2001**, *8*, 19–22.
77. Palazón, J.; Cusidó, R.M.; Bonfill, M.; Mallol, A.; Moyano, E.; Morales, C.; Piñol, M.T. Elicitation of different *Panax ginseng* transformed root phenotypes for an improved ginsenoside production. *Plant Physiol. Biochem.* **2003**, *41*, 1019–1025. [CrossRef]
78. Chung, H.J.; Cho, I.S.; Kim, J.H.; In, D.S.; Hur, C.G.; Song, J.S.; Woo, S.S.; Choi, D.W.; Liu, J.R. Changes in gene expression during hairy root formation by *Agrobacterium rhizogenes* infection in ginseng. *J. Plant Biol.* **2003**, *346*, 187. [CrossRef]
79. Mallol, A.; Cusidó, R.M.; Palazón, J.; Bonfill, M.; Morales, C.; Piñol, M.T. Ginsenoside production in different phenotypes of *Panax ginseng* transformed roots. *Phytochemistry* **2001**, *57*, 365–371. [CrossRef]

80. Woo, S.S.; Song, J.S.; Lee, J.Y.; In, D.S.; Chung, H.J.; Liu, J.R.; Choi, D.W. Selection of high ginsenoside producing ginseng hairy root lines using targeted metabolic analysis. *Phytochemistry* **2004**, *65*, 2751–2761. [CrossRef]
81. Yu, K.W.; Gao, W.Y.; Son, S.H.; Paek, K.Y. Improvement of ginsenoside production by jasmonic acid and some other elicitors in hairy root culture of ginseng (*Panax ginseng* CA Meyer). *Vitr. Cell. Dev. Biol.—Plant* **2000**, *36*, 424–428. [CrossRef]
82. Kim, O.T.; Bang, K.H.; Kim, Y.C.; Hyun, D.Y.; Kim, M.Y.; Cha, S.W. Upregulation of ginsenoside and gene expression related to triterpene biosynthesis in ginseng hairy root cultures elicited by methyl jasmonate. *Plant Cell Tissue Organ Cult.* **2009**, *98*, 25–33. [CrossRef]
83. Kochan, E.; Szymańska, G.; Szymczyk, P. Effect of sugar concentration on ginsenoside biosynthesis in hairy root cultures of *Panax quinquefolium* cultivated in shake flasks and nutrient sprinkle bioreactor. *Acta Physiol. Plant.* **2014**, *36*, 613–619. [CrossRef]
84. Kochan, E.; Królicka, A.; Chmiel, A. Growth and ginsenoside production in *Panax quinquefolium* hairy roots cultivated in flasks and nutrient sprinkle bioreactor. *Acta Physiol. Plant.* **2012**, *34*, 1513–1518. [CrossRef]
85. Ha, L.T.; Pawlicki-Jullian, N.; Pillon-Lequart, M.; Boitel-Conti, M.; Duong, H.X.; Gontier, E. Hairy root cultures of *Panax vietnamensis*, a promising approach for the production of ocotillol-type ginsenosides. *Plant Cell Tissue Organ Cult.* **2016**, *126*, 93–103. [CrossRef]
86. Gamborg, O.L.; Miller, R.A.; Ojima, K. Nutrient requirements of suspension cultures of soyabean root cells. *Exp. Cell Res.* **1968**, *50*, 151–158. [CrossRef]

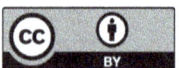 © 2020 by the authors. Licensee MDPI, Basel, Switzerland. This article is an open access article distributed under the terms and conditions of the Creative Commons Attribution (CC BY) license (http://creativecommons.org/licenses/by/4.0/).

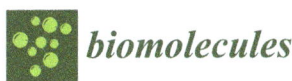

Article

Characterization of a Novel Ginsenoside MT1 Produced by an Enzymatic Transrhamnosylation of Protopanaxatriol-Type Ginsenosides Re

Byeong-Min Jeon [1,†], Jong-In Baek [1,†], Min-Sung Kim [1], Sun-Chang Kim [1,2,3,*] and Chang-hao Cui [2,*]

1   Department of Biological Sciences, Korea Advanced Institute of Science and Technology, 291 Daehak-Ro, Yuseong-Gu, Daejeon 305-701, Korea; jbm0901@kaist.ac.kr (B.-M.J.); baekji@kaist.ac.kr (J.-I.B.); mskim8906@kaist.ac.kr (M.-S.K.)
2   Intelligent Synthetic Biology Center, 291 Daehak-Ro, Yuseong-Gu, Daejeon 305-701, Korea
3   KAIST Institute for Biocentury, Korea Advanced Institute of Science and Technology, 291 Daehak-Ro, Yuseong-Gu, Daejeon 305-701, Korea
*   Correspondence: sunkim@kaist.ac.kr (S.-C.K.); chcui@kaist.ac.kr (C.-h.C.); Tel.: +82-42-3502619 (S.-C.K.); +82-43-2388575 (C.-h.C.)
†   These authors contributed equally to this work.

Received: 26 February 2020; Accepted: 26 March 2020; Published: 31 March 2020

Abstract: Background: Ginsenosides, triterpene saponins of *Panax* species, are considered the main active ingredients responsible for various pharmacological activities. Herein, a new protopanaxatriol-type ginsenoside called "ginsenoside MT1" is described; it was accidentally found among the enzymatic conversion products of ginsenoside Re. Method: We analyzed the conversion mechanism and found that recombinant β-glucosidase (MT619) transglycosylated the outer rhamnopyranoside of Re at the C-6 position to glucopyranoside at C-20. The production of MT1 by trans-rhamnosylation was optimized and pure MT1 was obtained through various chromatographic processes. Results: The structure of MT1 was elucidated based on spectral data: (20S)-3β,6α,12β,20-tetrahydroxydammarene-20-O-[α-L-rhamnopyranosyl(1→2)-β-D-glucopyranoside]. This dammarane-type triterpene saponin was confirmed as a novel compound. Conclusion: Based on the functions of ginsenosides with similar structures, we believe that this ginsenoside MT1 may have great potential in the development of nutraceutical, pharmaceutical or cosmeceutical products.

Keywords: ginsenosides; dammarane-type triterpene saponin; ginsenoside MT1; transglycosylation; biotransformation; biotechnology

---

1. Introduction

Ginsenosides—triterpene saponins composed of a dammarane skeleton with several glycosylation positions—are generally considered the main active components of ginseng, that has been used as a traditional herbal medicine in East Asian countries for thousands of years to stimulate physical and mental activity [1,2]. Ginsenosides can be categorized as protopanaxadiol (PPD) and protopanaxatriol (PPT) saponins based on the structure of their aglycon. More than 100 kinds of ginsenosides have been found [3,4]; their pharmacological effects vary according to their attached sugars and aglycon structures [5–7]. Six major kinds of ginsenoside (Rb_1, Rb_2, Rc, Re, Rd and Rg_1), as shown in Figure S1, constitute >90% of the total ginsenosides in ginseng [2,8]. They are relatively abundant in ginseng and can be converted into minor ginsenosides, which naturally exist in smaller amounts and have higher chemical reactivities [9–11].

Various methods have been reported for preparing minor ginsenosides with high conversion efficiency and few byproducts [12]. Many enzymes have been explored to efficiently convert major ginsenosides into pharmacologically active, rare minor ginsenosides [5,13,14]. Prior to this study, our research group cloned, characterized and applied many efficient glycoside hydrolases for the gram-scale production and purification of minor ginsenosides [15–21].

In our investigation into the enzymatic conversion of major ginsenosides, a new transformation product of ginsenoside Re that is different from the other hydrolyzing products (ginsenoside PPT, F_1, Rg_1 and Rg_2) was accidentally found using a novel recombinant glucosidase (MT619) [15]. This compound was prepared at the gram scale using recombinant MT619 and isolated from the product mixture using chromatographic methods. Finally, the structure of this novel ginsenoside was elucidated based on spectral data.

2. Materials and Methods

2.1. Chemicals and Reagents

The standard forms of various ginsenosides (Rg_1 and Re) used in the present study were purchased from Sigma Co., Ltd. (Louis, MO, USA). F_1, Rg_2(S), Rh_1(S) and PPT were prepared as described in our previous study [22]. The other chemical reagents used were at least extra or better in quality than pure grade. Butanol, ethyl acetate, chloroform, ethanol and pyridine-d5 (Merck KGaA, Darmstadt, Germany) were purchased from Sam Chun Pure Chemical Co. (Pyeongtaek, Korea).

2.2. Biotransformation of Ginsenosides Using Recombinant MT619

Recombinant MT619 was expressed in *Escherichia coli* BL21 as described previously [15]. Briefly, the MT619-harboring pEX vector was inserted into the *E. coli* BL21 strain using heat-shock transformation. The cells grown in LB medium were supplemented with ampicillin at 37 °C until the culture reached an optical density of 600 nm (OD600) of 0.6, at which point protein expression was induced by adding 0.1 mM isopropyl-β-D-thiogalactopyranoside (IPTG). The bacterial cells were incubated further for 24 h at 18 °C and then harvested by centrifugation at 4000 rpm for 15 min. The cells were washed with 50 mM sodium phosphate and then resuspended in 50 mM sodium phosphate and 1% Triton X-100 (pH 7.0). The cells were disrupted by ultrasonication (Vibra-Cell; Sonics & Materials, Danbury, CT, USA). Intact cells and debris were removed by centrifugation at 13,000 rpm for 10 min to obtain a crude cell extract. His-tagged MT619 protein was purified by a HisTrap column (GE Healthcare, Menlo Park, California, USA). The 100 mM imidazole eluted protein was further purified by DEAE-cellulose DE-52 chromatography (Whatman, Maidstone, UK). Purified MT619 was used to examine its MT1 production efficiency by reacting with ginsenoside Re (2.0 mg/mL, pH 7.0) in a shaking incubator at 37 °C for 24 h. The ginsenosides in the samples were extracted with an equal volume of butanol and identified by thin layer chromatography (TLC).

2.3. Optimization of the Substrate Concentration

Ginsenoside MT1 production was evaluated using crude MT619 cell extracts. To determine the optimal concentration of selected substrates for the biotransformation reaction, cells were mixed with an equal volume of a substrate at 3.0–22.5 mg/mL at 37 °C. Samples were then withdrawn at regular intervals and analyzed by TLC.

2.4. Scaled-Up Ginsenoside MT1 Production

Production was scaled up to 1 L and a final concentration of 6.0 mg/mL substrate (ginsenoside Re). The transformation was performed by adding 300 mL of crude cell lysate in a shaking incubator at 200 rpm and 37 °C. After incubating for 24 h, the mixture was centrifuged at $4000 \times g$ for 15 min and the supernatant was loaded into a column packed with HP20 resin (120 g) (Sigma-Aldrich, St Louis, MO, USA). One liter of water was used to remove unbound hydrophilic compounds and free sugar molecules, and the absorbed ginsenosides were eluted using three bed volumes of 95% ethanol. The eluted ethanol was evaporated in vacuo to produce dry powders.

2.5. Purification of MT1 from the Enzymatically Converted Products

Chromatographic pre-purification was performed with an LC-Forte/R system (YMC Korea Co. Ltd., Sungnam, Korea). One gram of the crude MT1 was dissolved in 20 mL of 10% methanol and centrifuged at 4000 × g for 20 min. After filtering with a syringe filter (0.2 µm), the dissolved sample was subjected to liquid chromatography (YMC-C18, 25 µm 120 g, 39 mm × 157 mm) and eluted with methanol-water (300 mL each at 5:5, 6:4, 7:3 and 8:2) to yield 13 fractions. The elution was fractionated every 100 mL, and the fractions containing MT1 were collected for purification.

2.6. Recycling Preparative High-Performance Liquid Chromatography (RPHPLC) Purification of MT1 from Biotransformed Products

The collected MT1 was further purified using RPHPLC (JAI NEXT Recycling Preparative HPLC LC-9210II NEXT, Japan Analytical Industry Co, Tokyo, Japan). RPHPLC was performed using a pre-packed column (JAIGEL-ODS-AP-L, 10 µm, 20 mm i.d. × 500 mm) purchased from Japan Analytical Industry Co. (Japan). The mobile phase was 50% acetonitrile; the flow rate was 7.0 mL/min. The MT1 solution was prepared by dissolving a sufficient quantity of the collected MT1 in 50% acetonitrile to give a final concentration of 35 mg/mL; 10 mL of the MT1 solution was loaded for purification.

2.7. High-Performance Liquid Chromatography (HPLC) Analysis

HPLC analysis of samples in the present study was performed using an Agilent 1260 Infinity HPLC system (Agilent Co., Santa Clara, CA, USA). Ginsenosides were separated on an YMC ODS C18 column (5 µm, 250 × 4.6 mm; YMC, Kyoto, Japan) with a guard column (Eclipse XDB C18, 5 µm, 12.5 × 4.6 mm; Agilent Co., Santa Clara, CA, USA). The gradient elution system consisted of water (A) and acetonitrile (B), and used the following gradient program: 0 → 10 min, 20% B; 10 → 40 min, 20 → 32% B; 40 → 48 min, 32 → 42% B; 48 → 60 min, 42 → 45% B; 60 → 83 min, 45 → 75% B; 83 → 85 min, 75 → 100% B; 85 → 95 min, 100% B; 95 → 95.01 min, 100 → 20% B; 95.01 → 100 min, 20% B. The detection wavelength was set to 203 nm and the flow rate was 1.6 mL/min.

2.8. Nuclear Magnetic Resonance (NMR) and Mass Spectrometry (MS) Analyses

NMR spectra were obtained using a Bruker AVANCE III 700 NMR spectrometer (Bruker, Rheinstetten, Germany) at 700 MHz (^{1}H) and 175 MHz (^{13}C), with chemical shifts given in ppm. Samples were separated with an Acquity UHPLC BEH C18 column (2.1 × 100 mm i.d., 1.7 µm) at room temperature. The mobile phases comprised deionized water containing 0.2% (v/v) formic acid (A) and acetonitrile (B). Quantitative analysis of the novel compound was performed using an LTQ-Orbitrap XL mass spectrometer (Thermo Scientific, Bremen, Germany) equipped with an ESI source (Thermo Electron, Bremen, Germany) in negative ion mode with a mass range of m/z 100–1500 Da. Optimal conditions were employed as follows: capillary voltage 20 V, capillary temperature 350 °C, spray voltage 3.5 kV and tube lens voltage 110 V.

2.9. Acidic Hydrolysis of MT1 and TLC Analysis

The purified compound (10 mg) was heated with 5% HCl mixture for 2 h at 70 °C. The residues from filtration and standard sugars were compared through cellulose TLC (Butanol:Ethanol:H_2O, 50:50:30). TLC was conducted using 60F_{254} silica gel plates (Merck, Darmstadt, Germany) and $CHCl_3$-CH_3OH-H_2O (65:35:10, v/v/v) as the developing solution. The results were visualized with 10% H_2SO_4 by heating at 110 °C for 5 min.

3. Results

3.1. Ginsenoside Re Transformation of MT619

MT619 was purified by Ni column and DEAE column chromatography as described in a previous study [15]. To analyze the transformation pathways, ginsenosides Re and Rg_2 were reacted as substrates with purified MT619 ginsenoside and F_1 and the conversion products were subjected to TLC analysis. The newly produced band (MT1), which had a different Rf value from those of ginsenoside Rg_1 and Rg_2, was identified from Re reaction mixtures (Figure 1). $Rg_2(S)$ was also hydrolyzed by MT619 into PPT, but MT1 was not reported. Interestingly, MT1 was only found in the Rg_2 mixture containing F_1 (Sample 5 in Figure 1), which clearly suggests that F_1 is the recipient in trans-rhamnosyl reactions. No MT1 was formed in the PPT conversion mixture, suggesting that PPT cannot receive rhamnose. Rg_1 and Rh_1 were not found in the Re and Rg_2 conversion mixtures; the existence of rhamnose was inferred by the rapid decomposition of Rg_1 and Rh_1 by MT619 into F_1 and PPT. Released glucose and rhamnose moieties were also identified in the Re and Rg_2 mixtures (Figure S2).

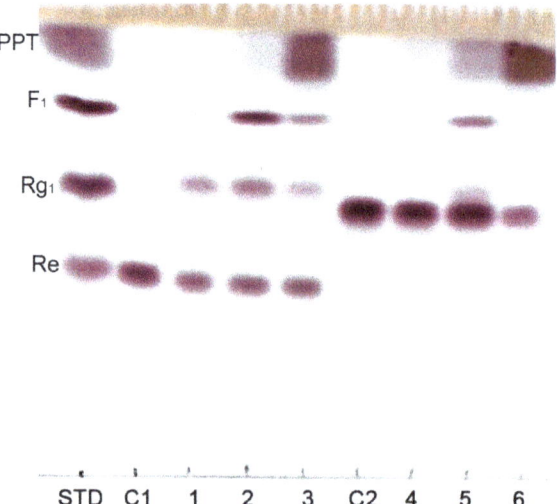

Figure 1. Thin layer chromatography of hydrolyzation products by MT619. C1, Re; 1, Re transformation products; 2, Re transformation products with F1 added; 3, Re transformation products with PPT added; C2, $Rg_2(S)$; 4, $Rg_2(S)$ transformation products; 5, $Rg_2(S)$ transformation products with F1 added; 6, $Rg_2(S)$ transformation products with PPT added.

3.2. Optimization for Ginsenoside MT1 Production

Optimal conditions for the biotransformation of Re into MT1 were determined by examining the substrate concentrations in the reaction mixture. Enzyme reactions were performed using of ginsenoside Re, which is one of the major ginsenosides in ginseng [23,24]. The concentration of MT1 increased in proportion to the substrate concentration (Figure 2A); the maximum concentration of MT1 produced was 8.0 mg/mL with 22.5 mg/mL Re 24 h after reaction. Note that >41.2% of Re remained after 24 h when the Re concentration was >15.0 mg/mL (Figure 2B); however, nearly all the Re was converted when the Re concentration was 6.0 mg/mL. Therefore 6.0 mg/mL Re was used for the scaled-up production of MT1.

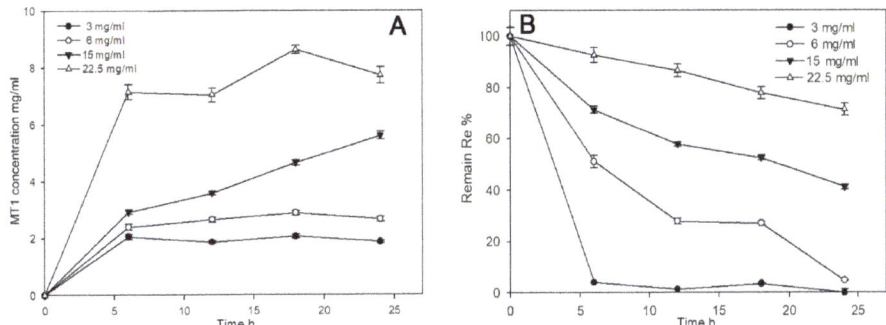

Figure 2. Effects of the substrate Re concentrations (**A**) and remaining Re concentrations (**B**) in the reaction mixture.

3.3. Mass Production of MT1

Six grams of Re in 1.0 L of phosphate buffer (pH 7.0) was reacted with cell lysates containing MT619. Re was completely converted 24 h after adding MT619 (Figure 3; Figure 4B). To remove proteins and impurities, the supernatants of the reaction mixture were applied to a 120 g HP20 macroporous resin. After washing with water, ethanol was used to elute the ginsenosides from the resin. The eluate was then evaporated in vacuo, yielding 3.8 g of mixed dry ginsenosides. In preparation for further purification, 1.0 g MT1 was dissolved in 200 mL of 10% methanol; the undissolved precipitants were separated using an ODS column to yield 13 fractions (Figure S3). MT1 was eluted in the 70% methanol fractions (9 and 10), yielding 655 mg of dry compounds.

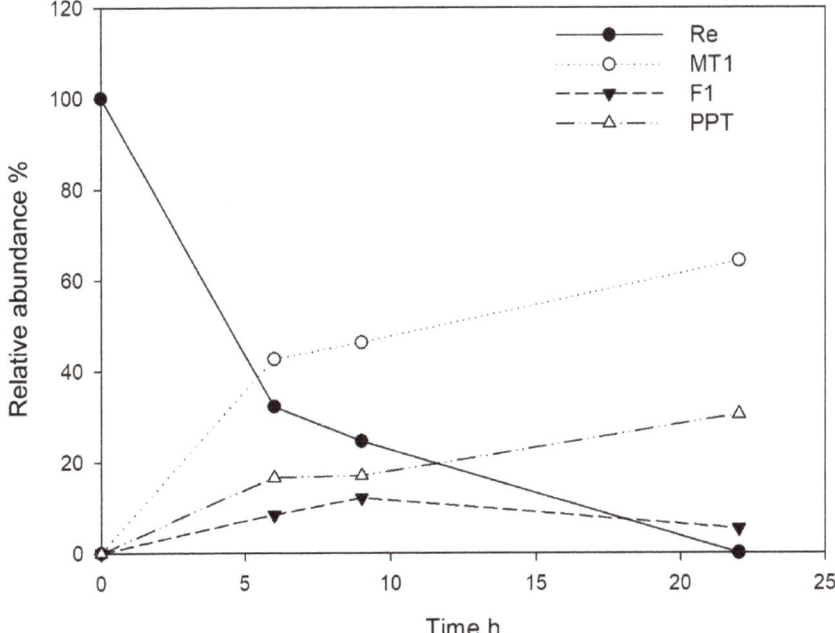

Figure 3. The relative abundance of ginsenosides Re, MT1, F1 and PPT in a scaled-up production reactor over time.

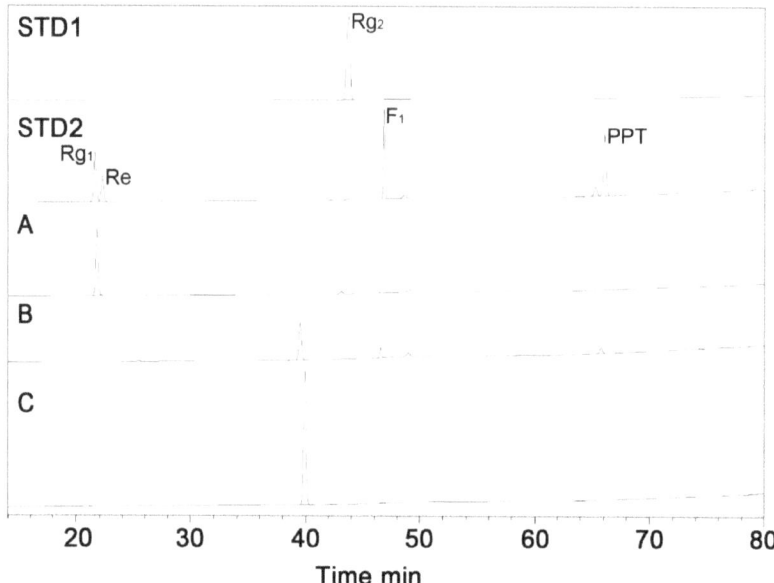

Figure 4. HPLC analysis of purified MT1 from the product mixture. (STD1), ginsenoside Rg$_2$(S) standard; (STD2), standards of ginsenosides Rg$_1$, Re, F$_1$ and PPT; (**A**), substrate ginsenoside Re before purification; (**B**), biotransformed products from the MT619 conversion mixture; (**C**), MT1 isolated using Recycling preparative high-performance liquid chromatography (RPHPLC).

3.4. Purification of MT1 using RPHPLC

Recycling preparative HPLC, which can enhance the separation of compounds by recycling the effluent sample many times over the column without increasing the length of the chromatographic column, was used for further purification. MT1 was purified from the product mixture with a preparative ODS column by RPHPLC. Dry MT1 mixture (300 mg) was loaded onto the RPHPLC column for separation. MT1 was baseline-resolved after three effective columns (Figure S4). The purification process resulted in 214 mg of MT1 with 98.9% chromatographic purity (Figure 4C). The total yield of the production of MT1 from Re was 47.4%.

3.5. Structural Characterization of Ginsenoside MT1

Pure ginsenoside MT1 was obtained as a white powder with a molecular ion peak at m/z 785.5 in the positive LC-MS, which corresponds to the molecular formula C$_{42}$H$_{72}$O$_{13}$ (Figure S5). Acidic hydrolysis of the compound yielded neohesperidose, the signals of which were similar to those of other neohesperidose-containing compounds, such as ginsenoside Rg$_2$(S) and neohesperidin (Figure S6).

Structural characterization was performed by a Bruker AVANCE III 700 NMR spectrometer operating at 700 MHz (^{1}H) and 175 MHz (^{13}C) with chemical shifts given in ppm for atomic force microscopy (AFM) to determine the chemical structure of MT1 (Table 1). The ^{1}H-NMR spectrum showed one olefinic (δH 5.28), two anomeric (δ 5.25 and 6.61) protons and a methyl proton signal (δ 1.83) like in L-rhamnopyranoside. Coupling constants suggested the configuration of the anomeric positions to be α-and-β form for the anomeric proton signals in the ^{1}H-NMR spectrum. The ^{13}C-NMR signals of the sugar were observed as one hemiacetal (δ_C 96.7), four oxygenated methines (δ_C 79.8, 78.4, 76.6 and 71.6) and one oxygenated methylene (δ_C 62.95), indicating that the sugar is b-glucopyranose.

Table 1. ^{1}H- (700 MHz) and ^{13}C-NMR (175 MHz) spectra of MT1.

Aglycon Moiety Position	δ$_H$ mult., (J Hz)	δ$_C$ mult.	Sugar Moiety Position	δ$_H$ mult., (J Hz)	δ$_C$ mult.
1	1.73 m, 1.06 m	39.4 t	Glc-1'	5.25 d (6.3)	96.7 d
2	1.93 m, 1.88 m	28.2 t	Glc-2'	4.29 ^{b}	76.6 d
3	3.56 t-like (5.6)	78.4 d	Glc-3'	4.29 ^{b}	79.8 d
4		40.4 s	Glc-4'	4.09 t (9.1)	71.6 d
5	1.27 d (10.5)	61.8 d	Glc-5'	3.88 m	78.4 d
6	4.40 ^{c}	67.8 d	Glc-6'	4.40 ^{c}, 4.25 m	62.5 t
7	2.04 m, 1.90 m	47.5 t	Rha-1"	6.61 s	101.4 d
8		41.2 s	Rha-2"	4.79 brs	72.5 d
9	1.67 m	49.7 d	Rha-3"	4.64 t (4.9)	72.6 d
10		39.3 s	Rha-4"	4.40 ^{c}	74.2 d
11	2.20 m, 1.55 m	31.1 t	Rha-5"	4.89 dd (9.1, 5.6)	69.4 d
12	4.11 m	70.7 d	Rha-6"	1.83 d (5.6)	19.0 q
13	2.00 m	49.0 d	3'-OH	7.50 brs	
14		51.6 s	4'-OH	7.40 d (4.2)	
15	1.58 m, 1.03 m	30.9 t	6'-OH	5.90 brs	
16	1.95 m, 1.44 m	26.7 t	2"-OH	6.76 d (4.2)	
17	2.77 dd (18.2, 10.5)	53.3 d	3"-OH	6.46 brs	
18	1.12 s	17.4 q	4"-OH	6.81 d (3.5)	
19	1.05 s	17.5 q			
20		84.0 s			
21	1.59 s	22.8 q			
22	2.45 m, 1.98 m	35.9 t			
23	2.29 m	24.0 t			
24	5.28 ^{d}	126.0 d			
25		130.8 s			
26	1.62 s	25.8 q			
27	1.65 s	17.9 q			
28	2.02 s	32.0 q			
29	1.48 s	16.5 q			
30	1.17 s	17.2 q			
3-OH	5.76 d (5.6)				
6-OH	5.28 ^{d}				
12-OH	5.58 s				

^{a} Measured at 700 and 175 MHz; obtained in C5D5N with TMS as an internal standard. The assignments were based on ^{1}H-^{1}HCOSY, HSQC, and HMBC experiments. $^{b–d}$ Overlapped with other signals.

The β-D-glucopyranosyl anomeric proton signals were confirmed to be linked at the C-20 position by long-range heteronuclear multiple bond connectivity (HMBC) correlations between the proton signal at δ 5.25 (H-1") and the carbon signal at δ 84.0 (C-20). A large downfield shift in the C-2" (δ 76.6) was observed for the inner β-D-glucopyranosyl moiety at C-20 of the aglycone, which showed that the C-1"' (δ 6.61) in the terminal α-L-rhamnopyranosyl moiety is linked to the inner β-D-glucopyranosyl moiety at C-20 [25]. In summary, these results indicate that the metabolite of MT619 is (20S)-3β,6α,12β,20-tetrahydroxydammarene-20-O-[α-L-rhamnopyranosyl(1→2)-β-D-glucopyranoside] (Figure 5) or ginsenoside MT1.

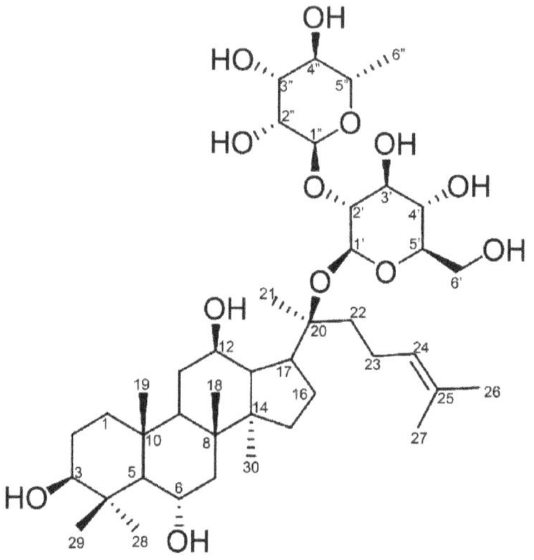

Figure 5. The structure ginsenoside MT1 based on the spectral data.

Based on the above experimental results, the conversion pathways were deduced as shown in Figure 6. In the conversion of Re, the rhamnopyranoside moieties were released from the substrates and transformed into the C-20 outer glucopyranoside of ginsenoside F_1. When MT619 reacted with Rg_2, the rhamnosyl transformation could only occur with the existence of the attached glucopyranoside at C-20 positions such as F_1. The mechanisms of rhamnose transformation by MT619 warrant further exploration.

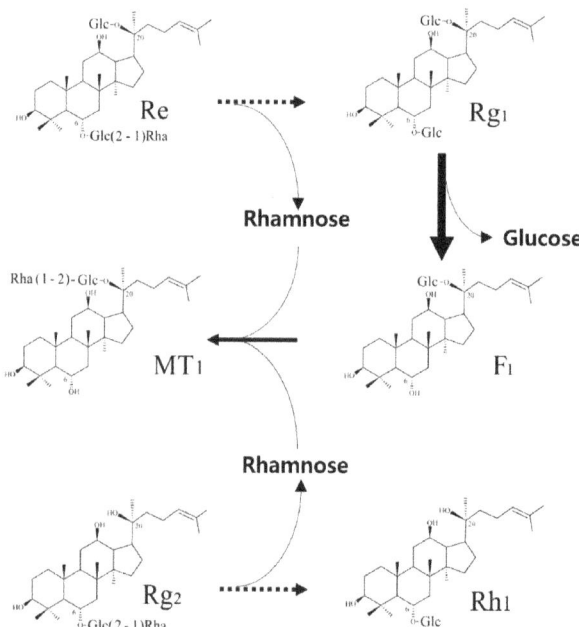

Figure 6. Conversion pathways of ginsenosides Re and $Rg_2(S)$ by MT619.

4. Discussion

Many glycoside hydrolases have been shown to possess transglycosylation capabilities in addition to hydrolytic activity [26]. In substrate transglycosylation of glycoside hydrolases, the glycosyl part of the substrate is transferred to a hydroxyl-containing compound instead of water moieties [27]. Some GH family 3 enzymes also show transglycosylation capabilities from various substrates. A GH3 cellobiase from *Phanerochaete chrysosporium* can hydrolyze and transglycosylate glucopyranoside from laminarioligosaccharides [28]. β-glucosidase from *Aspergiluus niger* strain ASKU28 also showed transglucosidase activity against various substrates [29]. MT619 has been classified into GH family 3 according to the Carbohydrate-Active enZymes (CAZy). To the best of our knowledge, this is the only transrhamnosylation activity reported in glycoside hydrolase family 3 to date. Further studies are needed to reveal its sequence-activity relevance.

Some glycosylated ginsenoside derivatives from various natural ginsenosides have been synthesized using enzymatic methods. A novel α-glycosylated ginsenoside F_1((20S)-3β,6α,12β-trihydroxydammar-24ene-(20-O-β-D-glucopyranosyl-(1→2)-α-D-glucopyranoside)) was synthesized using a cyclodextrin glucanotransferase [30]; ginsenoside Ia((20S)-3b,6a,12b,20-tetrahydroxydammar-24-ene-20-O-b-D-glucopyranosyl-3-O-b-D-glucopyranoside) was synthesized using UDP- glycosyl transferase (BSGT1) from ginsenoside F_1 [31]. In addition, various Rg_1 a-glycosylated ginsenosides (α-1,3-, α-1,4- or α-1,6-glucosidic linkage in β-glucose moieties) linked at C-6 and C-20 positions of aglycones have been synthesized using rice seed a-glucosidases [32], although no trans-rhamnosyl activity has been found using ginsenosides as rhamnose receptors.

A similar ginsenoside—ginsenoside Rg_{18} (Figure S1), which differs from MT1 in that it is linked to an additional glucose moiety at the C-6 position—was recently found, isolated and characterized from *Panax ginseng* roots [33]. Rg_{18} has been shown to have various important pharmacological effects, such as anticancer [34] and neuroprotective effects [35]. However, the content of Rg_{18} in ginseng is <36.0 µg/g of ginseng, which means that its application is limited by its scarcity in plants. Fortunately, MT1 can be produced efficiently from the relatively abundant ginsenoside Re using the recombinant MT619 with high recovery, which can make it industrially applicable. Furthermore, the deglycosylated ginsenosides generally have shown enhanced pharmacological effects and absorbances than the original ginsenosides [36–38]. Our group is drawing on the properties of MT1 to conduct experiments on compounds with higher anticancer, anti-inflammatory, anti-oxidation and anti-aging.

5. Conclusions

In summary, this paper describes characterization and mass production of a new dammarane-type triterpene saponin from enzymatic converted products. The trans-rhamnosyl activity of MT619 against ginsenoside Re to F_1 resulted in the new ginsenoside MT1, a PPT-type ginsenoside containing one neohesperidose moiety at the C-20 position (confirmed based on spectral data). This unknown compound can be efficiently produced from abundant ginsenoside Re using MT619. Various studies are on-going by our group to investigate its pharmacological effects. We expect potential commercial uses of MT1 in nutraceutical, pharmaceutical or cosmeceutical areas.

Supplementary Materials: The following are available online at http://www.mdpi.com/2218-273X/10/4/525/s1, Figure S1: Chemical structures of ginsenosides; Figure S2. Released glucose (orange arrow) and rhamnose (blue arrow)s in the supernatant of the reaction products of Re and Rg_2(S); Figure S3. Thin layer analysis of the fractions for the purification of MT1 using the ODS column; Figure S4. RPHPLC chromatogram showing the resolution of the Rb3 and Rd; Figure S5. Positive-ion mode HPLC-ESI-MS/MS of the molecular ion (sodium adduct) of MT1; Figure S6. TLC analysis of acidic hydrolysis products from neohesperidose-moiety harboring substrates by hydrogen chloride.

Author Contributions: Conceptualization, C.-h.C., S.-C.K. and B.-M.J.; methodology, C.-h.C., B.-M.J., S.-C.K. and J.-I.B.; software, C.-h.C., B.-M.J., S.-C.K. and J.-I.B.; validation, C.-h.C., J.-I.B., S.-C.K. and B.-M.J. formal analysis, B.-M.J. and J.-I.B.; investigation, C.-h.C., J.-I.B., M.K. and S.-C.K.; resources, C.-h.C., B.-M.J. and J.-I.B.; data curation, C.-h.C., J.-I.B., S.-C.K. and B.-M.J.; writing — original draft preparation, C.-h.C. and J.-I.B.; writing — review & editing, J.-I.B., M.-S.K., S.-C.K. and B.-M.J.; Visualization, C.-h.C. and J.-I.B.; supervision, S.-C.K.;

project administration, S.-C.K. and C.-h.C.; funding acquisition, S.-C.K.. All authors have read and agreed to the published version of the manuscript.

Funding: This work was supported by the Intelligent Synthetic Biology Center of The Global Frontier Project (2011-0031955), funded by the Ministry of Education, Science and Technology, Republic of Korea.

Conflicts of Interest: The authors declare no conflict of interest.

References

1. Chung, H.S.; Lee, Y.C.; Rhee, Y.K.; Lee, S.Y. Consumer acceptance of ginseng food products. *J. Food Sci.* **2011**, *76*, S516–S522. [CrossRef]
2. Shi, Y.; Sun, C.J.; Zheng, B.; Gao, B.; Sun, A.M. Simultaneous Determination of Ten Ginsenosides in American Ginseng Functional Foods and Ginseng Raw Plant Materials by Liquid Chromatography Tandem Mass Spectrometry. *Food Anal. Methods* **2013**, *6*, 112–122. [CrossRef]
3. Jia, L.; Zhao, Y.Q. Current Evaluation of the Millennium Phytomedicine-Ginseng (I): Etymology, Pharmacognosy, Phytochemistry, Market and Regulations. *Curr. Med. Chem.* **2009**, *16*, 2475–2484. [CrossRef]
4. Leung, K.W.; Leung, F.P.; Mak, N.K.; Tombran-Tink, J.; Huang, Y.; Wong, R.N. Protopanaxadiol and protopanaxatriol bind to glucocorticoid and oestrogen receptors in endothelial cells. *Brit. J. Pharmacol.* **2009**, *156*, 626–637. [CrossRef]
5. Wong, A.S.T.; Che, C.M.; Leung, K.W. Recent advances in ginseng as cancer therapeutics: A functional and mechanistic overview. *Nat. Prod. Rep.* **2015**, *32*, 256–272. [CrossRef]
6. Biswas, T.; Mathur, A.K.; Mathur, A. A literature update elucidating production of Panax ginsenosides with a special focus on strategies enriching the anti-neoplastic minor ginsenosides in ginseng preparations. *Appl. Microbiol. Biot.* **2017**, *101*, 4009–4032. [CrossRef]
7. Hao, H.P.; Zheng, X.; Wang, G.J. Insights into drug discovery from natural medicines using reverse pharmacokinetics. *Trends Pharmacol. Sci.* **2014**, *35*, 168–177. [CrossRef]
8. Zhou, S.S.; Xu, J.D.; Zhu, H.; Shen, H.; Xu, J.; Mao, Q.; Li, S.L.; Yan, R. Simultaneous determination of original, degraded ginsenosides and aglycones by ultra high performance liquid chromatography coupled with quadrupole time-of-flight mass spectrometry for quantitative evaluation of Du-Shen-Tang, the decoction of ginseng. *Molecules* **2014**, *19*, 4083–4104. [CrossRef]
9. Kim, W.Y.; Kim, J.M.; Han, S.B.; Lee, S.K.; Kim, N.D.; Park, M.K.; Kim, C.K.; Park, J.H. Steaming of ginseng at high temperature enhances biological activity. *J. Nat. Prod.* **2000**, *63*, 1702–1704. [CrossRef]
10. Bae, E.A.; Han, M.J.; Kim, E.J.; Kim, D.H. Transformation of ginseng saponins to ginsenoside Rh2 by acids and human intestinal bacteria and biological activities of their transformants. *Arch. Pharm. Res.* **2004**, *27*, 61–67. [CrossRef]
11. Yun, T.K.; Lee, Y.S.; Lee, Y.H.; Kim, S.I.; Yun, H.Y. Anticarcinogenic effect of Panax ginseng CA Meyer and identification of active compounds. *J. Korean Med. Sci.* **2001**, *16*, S6–S18. [CrossRef] [PubMed]
12. Cui, C.H.; Kim, S.C.; Im, W.T. Characterization of the ginsenoside-transforming recombinant beta-glucosidase from Actinosynnema mirum and bioconversion of major ginsenosides into minor ginsenosides. *Appl. Microbiol. Biot.* **2013**, *97*, 649–659. [CrossRef] [PubMed]
13. Shin, K.-C.; Oh, D.-K. Classification of glycosidases that hydrolyze the specific positions and types of sugar moieties in ginsenosides. *Crit. Rev. Biotechnol.* **2016**, *36*, 1036–1049. [CrossRef] [PubMed]
14. Park, C.S.; Yoo, M.H.; Noh, K.H.; Oh, D.K. Biotransformation of ginsenosides by hydrolyzing the sugar moieties of ginsenosides using microbial glycosidases. *Appl. Microbiol. Biotechnol.* **2010**, *87*, 9–19. [CrossRef] [PubMed]
15. Cui, C.-h.; Jeon, B.-M.; Fu, Y.; Im, W.-T.; Kim, S.-C. High-density immobilization of a ginsenoside-transforming β-glucosidase for enhanced food-grade production of minor ginsenosides. *Appl. Microbiol. Biotechnol.* **2019**, *103*, 7003–7015. [CrossRef] [PubMed]
16. An, D.-S.; Cui, C.-H.; Siddiqi, M.Z.; Yu, H.S.; Jin, F.-X.; Kim, S.-G.; Im, W.-T. Gram-Scale Production of Ginsenoside F1 Using a Recombinant Bacterial β-Glucosidase. *Appl. Microbiol. Biotechnol.* **2017**, *27*, 1559–1565. [CrossRef] [PubMed]
17. Cui, C.-H.; Fu, Y.; Jeon, B.-M.; Kim, S.-C.; Im, W.-T. Novel enzymatic elimination method for the chromatographic purification of ginsenoside Rb3 in an isomeric mixture. *J. ginseng Res.* **2019**. [CrossRef]

18. Siddiqi, M.Z.; Cui, C.H.; Park, S.K.; Han, N.S.; Kim, S.C.; Im, W.T. Comparative analysis of the expression level of recombinant ginsenoside-transforming beta-glucosidase in GRAS hosts and mass production of the ginsenoside Rh2-Mix. *PLoS ONE* **2017**, *12*, e0176098. [CrossRef]
19. Cui, C.H.; Kim, J.K.; Kim, S.C.; Im, W.T. Characterization of a ginsenoside-transforming beta-glucosidase from Paenibacillus mucilaginosus and its application for enhanced production of minor ginsenoside F(2). *PLoS ONE* **2014**, *9*, e85727.
20. Park, M.K.; Cui, C.H.; Park, S.C.; Park, S.K.; Kim, J.K.; Jung, M.S.; Jung, S.C.; Kim, S.C.; Im, W.T. Characterization of recombinant beta-glucosidase from Arthrobacter chlorophenolicus and biotransformation of ginsenosides Rb1, Rb 2, Rc, and Rd. *J. Microbiol.* **2014**, *52*, 399–406. [CrossRef]
21. Du, J.; Cui, C.H.; Park, S.C.; Kim, J.K.; Yu, H.S.; Jin, F.X.; Sun, C.; Kim, S.C.; Im, W.T. Identification and characterization of a ginsenoside-transforming beta-glucosidase from Pseudonocardia sp. Gsoil 1536 and its application for enhanced production of minor ginsenoside Rg2(S). *PLoS ONE* **2014**, *9*, e96914. [CrossRef]
22. Cui, C.H.; Liu, Q.M.; Kim, J.K.; Sung, B.H.; Kim, S.G.; Kim, S.C.; Im, W.T. Identification and characterization of a Mucilaginibacter sp. strain QM49 beta-glucosidase and its use in the production of the pharmaceutically active minor ginsenosides (S)-Rh1 and (S)-Rg2. *Appl. Environ. Microbiol.* **2013**, *79*, 5788–5798. [CrossRef]
23. Ren, G.; Chen, F. Simultaneous quantification of ginsenosides in American ginseng (Panax quinquefolium) root powder by visible/near-infrared reflectance spectroscopy. *J. Agric. Food Chem.* **1999**, *47*, 2771–2775. [CrossRef] [PubMed]
24. Wang, Y.; Pan, J.Y.; Xiao, X.Y.; Lin, R.C.; Cheng, Y.Y. Simultaneous determination of ginsenosides in Panax ginseng with different growth ages using high-performance liquid chromatography-mass spectrometry. *Phytochem. Anal.* **2006**, *17*, 424–430. [CrossRef] [PubMed]
25. Iwamoto, M.; Fujioka, T.; Okabe, H.; Mihashi, K.; Yamauchi, T. Studies on the Constituents of Actinostemma-Lobatum Maxim.1. Structures of Actinostemmoside-a, Actinostemmoside-B, Actinostemmoside-C, Actinostemmoside-D, Dammarane Triterpene Glycosides Isolated from the Herb. *Chem. Pharm. Bull.* **1987**, *35*, 553–561. [CrossRef]
26. Bissaro, B.; Monsan, P.; Faure, R.; O'Donohue, M.J. Glycosynthesis in a waterworld: New insight into the molecular basis of transglycosylation in retaining glycoside hydrolases. *Biochem. J.* **2015**, *467*, 17–35. [CrossRef] [PubMed]
27. Geronimo, I.; Payne, C.M.; Sandgren, M. Hydrolysis and Transglycosylation Transition States of Glycoside Hydrolase Family 3 beta-Glucosidases Differ in Charge and Puckering Conformation. *J. Phys. Chem. B* **2018**, *122*, 9452–9459. [CrossRef]
28. Kawai, R.; Igarashi, K.; Kitaoka, M.; Ishii, T.; Samejima, M. Kinetics of substrate transglycosylation by glycoside hydrolase family 3 glucan (1 -> 3)-beta-glucosidase from the white-rot fungus Planerochaete chrysosporium. *Carbohyd. Res.* **2004**, *339*, 2851–2857. [CrossRef]
29. Thongpoo, P.; McKee, L.S.; Araujo, A.C.; Kongsaeree, P.T.; Brumer, H. Identification of the acid/base catalyst of a glycoside hydrolase family 3 (GH3) beta-glucosidase from Aspergillus niger ASKU28. *Bba-Gen. Subjects* **2013**, *1830*, 2739–2749. [CrossRef]
30. Moon, S.S.; Lee, H.J.; Mathiyalagan, R.; Kim, Y.J.; Yang, D.U.; Lee, D.Y.; Min, J.W.; Jimenez, Z.; Yang, D.C. Synthesis of a Novel alpha-Glucosyl Ginsenoside F1 by Cyclodextrin Glucanotransferase and Its In Vitro Cosmetic Applications. *Biomolecules* **2018**, *8*, 142. [CrossRef]
31. Wang, D.D.; Jin, Y.; Wang, C.; Kim, Y.J.; Perez, Z.E.J.; Baek, N.I.; Mathiyalagan, R.; Markus, J.; Yang, D.C. Rare ginsenoside Ia synthesized from F1 by cloning and overexpression of the UDP-glycosyltransferase gene from Bacillus subtilis: Synthesis, characterization, and in vitro melanogenesis inhibition activity in BL6B16 cells. *J. Ginseng. Res.* **2018**, *42*, 42–49. [CrossRef] [PubMed]
32. Kim, M.J.; Kim, Y.H.; Song, G.S.; Suzuki, Y.; Kim, M.K. Enzymatic transglycosylation of ginsenoside Rg1 by rice seed alpha-glucosidase. *Biosci. Biotech. Bioch.* **2016**, *80*, 318–328. [CrossRef] [PubMed]
33. Lee, D.G.; Quilantang, N.G.; Lee, J.S.; Geraldino, P.J.L.; Kim, H.Y.; Lee, S.H. Quantitative Analysis of Dammarane-type Ginsenosides in Different Ginseng Products. *Nat. Prod. Sci.* **2018**, *24*, 229–234. [CrossRef]
34. Leem, D.G.; Shin, J.S.; Kim, K.T.; Choi, S.Y.; Lee, M.H.; Lee, K.T. Dammarane-type triterpene ginsenoside-Rg18 inhibits human non-small cell lung cancer A549 cell proliferation via G1 phase arrest. *Oncol. Lett.* **2018**, *15*, 6043–6049. [CrossRef]

35. Kim, M.; Choi, S.Y.; Kim, K.T.; Rhee, Y.K.; Hur, J. Ginsenoside Rg18 suppresses lipopolysaccharide-induced neuroinflammation in BV2 microglia and amyloid-beta-induced oxidative stress in SH-SY5Y neurons via nuclear factor erythroid 2-related factor 2/heme oxygenase-1 induction. *J. Funct. Foods* **2017**, *31*, 71–78. [CrossRef]
36. Wang, C.Z.; Zhang, B.; Song, W.X.; Wang, A.; Ni, M.; Luo, X.; Aung, H.H.; Xie, J.T.; Tong, R.; He, T.C.; et al. Steamed American ginseng berry: Ginsenoside analyses and anticancer activities. *J. Agric. Food Chem.* **2006**, *54*, 9936–9942. [CrossRef]
37. Wang, J.R.; Yau, L.F.; Zhang, R.; Xia, Y.; Ma, J.; Ho, H.M.; Hu, P.; Hu, M.; Liu, L.; Jiang, Z.H. Transformation of ginsenosides from notoginseng by artificial gastric juice can increase cytotoxicity toward cancer cells. *J. Agric. Food Chem.* **2014**, *62*, 2558–2573. [CrossRef]
38. Qu, Y.; Liu, H.-Y.; Guo, X.-X.; Luo, Y.; Wang, C.-X.; He, J.-H.; Xu, T.-R.; Yang, Y.; Cui, X.-M. Converting ginsenosides from stems and leaves of Panax notoginseng by microwave processing and improving their anticoagulant and anticancer activities. *RSC Adv.* **2018**, *8*, 40471–40482. [CrossRef]

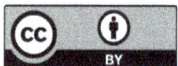

© 2020 by the authors. Licensee MDPI, Basel, Switzerland. This article is an open access article distributed under the terms and conditions of the Creative Commons Attribution (CC BY) license (http://creativecommons.org/licenses/by/4.0/).

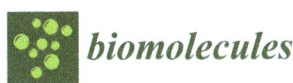

Article

(20S)G-Rh2 Inhibits NF-κB Regulated Epithelial-Mesenchymal Transition by Targeting Annexin A2

Yu-Shi Wang, He Li, Yang Li, Shiyin Zhang and Ying-Hua Jin *

Key Laboratory for Molecular Enzymology and Engineering of the Ministry of Education, School of Life Sciences, Jilin University, Changchun 130012, China; wangyushi0317@hotmail.com (Y.-S.W.); lihe0607@163.com (H.L.); liyang915@jlu.edu.cn (Y.L.); zsyshiyin@163.com (S.Z.)
* Correspondence: yhjin@jlu.edu.cn; Tel.: +86-431-8515-5221

Received: 20 February 2020; Accepted: 30 March 2020; Published: 31 March 2020

Abstract: (1) Background: Epithelial-mesenchymal transition (EMT) is an essential step for cancer metastasis; targeting EMT is an important path for cancer treatment and drug development. NF-κB, an important transcription factor, has been shown to be responsible for cancer metastasis by enhancing the EMT process. Our previous studies showed that (20S)Ginsenoside Rh2 (G-Rh2) inhibits NF-κB activity by targeting Anxa2, but it is still not known whether this targeted inhibition of NF-κB can inhibit the EMT process. (2) Methods: In vivo (20S)G-Rh2-Anxa2 interaction was assessed by cellular thermal shift assay. Protein interaction was determined by immuno-precipitation analysis. NF-κB activity was determined by dual luciferase reporter assay. Gene expression was determined by RT-PCR and immuno-blot. EMT was evaluated by wound healing and Transwell assay and EMT regulating gene expression. (3) Results: Anxa2 interacted with the NF-κB p50 subunit, promoted NF-κB activation, then accelerated mesenchymal-like gene expression and enhanced cell motility; all these cellular processes were inhibited by (20S)G-Rh2. In contrast, these (20S)G-Rh2 effect were completely eliminated by overexpression of Anxa2-K301A, an (20S)G-Rh2-binding-deficient mutant of Anxa2. (4) Conclusion: (20S)G-Rh2 inhibited NF-κB activation and related EMT by targeting Anxa2 in MDA-MB-231 cells.

Keywords: Anxa2; epithelial-mesenchymal transition; NF-κB; (20S)G-Rh2

1. Introduction

Playing key roles in embryonic development, epithelial-mesenchymal transition (EMT) facilitates body formation and tissue differentiation [1–4]. EMT is triggered by a genetic phenotype shift from epithelial-like to mesenchymal-like in response to pleiotropic signal; cells acquire the migratory and invasive properties by modifying adhesion molecules [3–5]. During this process, EMT specific transcription factors (EMT-TFs), in company with other regulatory factors like histone modifier and non-coding RNA, modify the gene expression through different states along EMT [6–11]. With the transcriptional activation of EMT-TFs, the expression of adherent junction components and tight junction components are negative-regulated, followed by the alteration in cadherin intermediate filament composition and cellular adhesion status [1,3,8,9]. EMT is also implicated in other physiological and pathological processes including would healing, tissue repair, fibrosis and cancer [1–6,11,12]. Tumor metastasis is the leading cause for cancer associated mortality; EMT is the main impetus and the essential access within this duration [11,12]. Despite the enhanced migration capability and invasiveness, EMT protects cancer cells from senescence, apoptosis and immuno-response by enhancing stem-cell properties and triggers the metastasis and dissemination to long distance through circulatory systems [13,14]. Focusing on the diverse regulated molecules, multiple drugs have shown their potential as EMT inhibitors by targeting the tumor microenvironment, corresponding extracellular receptors, intracellular kinases and EMT inducing transcription factors [15]. As its well-described clinical signature of EMT in cancer development, therapeutic strategies and targeted drugs towards EMT have been involved in cancer treatment [16–18].

NF-κB is an important transcription factor involved in multiple biologic processes as immune response, stress response, apoptosis, cell proliferation and cell metastasis [18]. The abnormal activation of NF-κB has been regarded as a hallmark of cancer, which promotes both tumorigenesis and tumor development [19–21]. NF-κB has been shown responsible for the expression of EMT-TFs including SNAIL, TWIST1, SLUG, SIP1 and ZEB1 and promotes EMT progression upon diverse signaling and stimuli, especially in cytokine and chemokine-induced cell growth and migration [22,23]. In the meanwhile, EMT promotes mesenchymal and stem-like phenotype of cancer cells and alters tumor microenvironment via autocrine and paracrine signaling, resulting in a constitutive activation of NF-κB in a ligand-receptor manner rather than genetic alteration [24]. Therefore, inhibition of NF-κB seems to be an important way to inhibit the progression of EMT and related tumors [25–27].

In our previous study, (20S)G-Rh2 has been identified as an NF-κB inhibitor targeting Anxa2, a NF-κB p50 subunit binding protein [28]. Here, we investigated the Anxa2 regulation on NF-κB and EMT. We further studied detailed molecular mechanisms for (20S)G-Rh2-induced NF-κB inhibition and the following EMT inhibition in invasive breast cancer cells. The results provide new evidences for the anticancer activity of ginsenosides.

2. Materials and Methods

2.1. Cell lines and Culture

Human breast cancer cell line MDA-MB-231 (ATCC, HTB-26), MCF-7 (ATCC, HTB-26) and HEK-293-T (ATCC, CRL-11268) were cultured in DMEM high-glucose medium (Gibco) supplemented with 10% fetal bovine serum (Biological Industries, BI), 100 units/mL penicillin and 100 μg/mL streptomycin, in a humidified 5% CO_2 atmosphere at 37 °C.

2.2. Chemicals, Antibodies and Plasmids

(20S)G-Rh2, etoposide, phorbol 12-myristate 13-acetate (PMA) were purchased from Sigma-Aldrich.

Antibodies for Twist (25465-1-AP), SIP1 (21672-1-AP), Slug (12129-1-AP), Snail 1 (13099-1-AP), MMP-2 (10373-2-AP), MMP-9 (10375-2-AP), Anxa2 (11256-1-AP), β-actin (66009-1-lg) and myc-tag (16286-1-AP, 60003-2-lg) were purchased from Proteintech (Proteintech Group, Inc.). Antibodies for E-cadherin (sc-8426), N-cadherin (sc-59987), NF-κB p50 subunit (sc-7178), Anxa2 (sc-47696) and IgG (sc-2025) were purchased from Santa Cruz Biotechnology. HRP-conjugated goat anti-rabbit IgG (H + L) secondary antibody (31460) and HRP-conjugated goat anti-mouse IgG (H+L) secondary antibody (31430) were purchased from Invitrogen.

Plasmids for over-expression of wild-type Anxa2 (pcs4-Anxa2-WT-myc) and Anxa2 K031A mutant (pcs4-Anxa2-K301A-myc) were shown as described [28]. A truncation with 1–33 deletion of Anxa2 was amplified by polymerase chain reaction (PCR), followed by a recombination into pcs4-myc vector for over-expression of Anxa2-delta N-terminus (pcs4-Anxa2-dN-myc). For lentivirus package, pLVX-TetOne-Puro (Clontech, 631849), pMD2.G (Addgene plasmid # 12259) and psPAX2 (Addgene plasmid # 12260) were gifts from Professor Zhihua Zou (Collage of Life Sciences, Jilin University). C-terminus-Myc-tagged Anxa2 full-length protein as well as K301A mutant and delta-N truncation were amplified from pcs4 vector and recombined into pLVX-TetOne-Pure vector for myc-tagged Anxa2 over-expression with lentivirus. The primers used within were shown in Table 1. Dual luciferase reporter assay were performed with pNF-κB-TA-luc (Beyotime, Shanghai, China) and pRL-CMV (Promega, WI, USA).

Table 1. Primers for vector construction.

Primer Description	Sequence
pcs4-Anxa2-dN-F	5'- TTGGATCCATGGATGCTGAGCGGGATGCTTTG -3'
pcs4-Anxa2-dN-R	5'- CCGCTCGAGTCATCTCCACCACACAGGTACAG -3'
pLVX-Anxa2-dN-F	5'- GCGTATACATGGATGCTGAGCGGGATGCTTTG -3'
pLVX-Anxa2-F	5'- GCGTATACATGTCTACTGTTCACGAAATCCT -3'
pLVX-Anxa2-R	5'- GCGGATCCTAGCTATCTAGAGGCTCGAGAGG -3'

2.3. Transfection

Lipo3000 (Invitrogen) was used for lentivirus package, transient transfection in MCF-7 cells and dual luciferase reporter assay according to the reagent protocol.

For lentivirus transfection, pLVX, pMD2.G and psPAX2 were co-transfected into HEK-293-T cells and supernatant for 24 h and 48 h was collected then added into MDA-MB-231 cells.

2.4. Immuno-Precipitation

50 µL of Protein A/G Magnetic Beads (MCE, K0202) was washed with 400 µL of IP lysis buffer (Pierce) for 3 times. 5 µg of antibody for immune-precipitation was diluted with 500 µL of IP lysis buffer, then added to the prepared beads, followed by a rotation for 2 h at 4 °C. MDA-MB-231 cells and MCF-7 cells were collected and lysed with IP lysis buffer supplemented with Protease Inhibitor Cocktail (Roche, 04693124001) and 1-mM phenylmethanesulfonyl fluoride (PMSF). Cell lysis was centrifuged with $12,000\times g$ for 20 min at 4 °C and the supernatant was collected. The antibody bonded beads were then collected and combined with cell lysis containing 500 µg of protein with a final volume of 400 µL, followed by another rotation for 2 h at 4 °C. The beads were then washed with IP lysis buffer for 3 times and collected for immuno-blot analysis.

2.5. Cellular Thermal Shift Assay

MDA-MB-231 cells and MCF-7 cells were cultured in 100-mm culture plates until the confluence reached 90%. The culture medium was then replaced with new medium supplemented with 15-µM (20S)G-Rh2 (~10 µg/mL) followed by an incubation for 1 h in a humidified 5% CO_2 atmosphere at 37 °C. After digested with trypsin (0.25%, w/v in PBS) and counted, cells were collected with centrifugation at $400\times g$ for 5 min and re-suspended with PBS containing 1-mM PMSF to a final cell density of 2×10^7 cells/mL. Each 100 µL of cell suspension was added to a 200-µL tube and heated at indicated temperature for 3 min and incubated at 4 °C for another 2 min. After 2-time rapid freeze-thawing from −80 °C to 25 °C, cell suspension was centrifuged with $20,000\times g$ for 20 min at 4 °C, the supernatant was collected for immune-blot analysis.

2.6. Dual Luciferase Reporter Assay

pNF-κB-TA-luc and pRL-CMV (10:1, w:w) were co-transfected into MDA-MB-231 cells and MCF-7 cells with Lipo3000 and cultured for 24 h before chemical treatment. The activity of luciferase was determined with Dual-Luciferase®Reporter Assay System (Promega, E1910) according to the manufacture's protocol. Luminescence generated by luciferase was collected via Infinite F200 Pro (TECAN).

2.7. Real-Time Polymerase Chain Reaction

Whole-cell RNA was isolated with TRIzol (Invitrogen). 2 µg of whole-cell RNA was proceeded with High Capacity cDNA Reverse Transcription Kit (Applied Biosystems, 4368814) for cDNA synthesis followed by real-time PCR analysis via PowerUp SYBR Green Master Mix (Applied Biosystems, A25742) and 7500 Real-Time PCR System (Applied Biosystems). The primers used were shown in Table 2. Gene expression was normalized to that of GAPDH and visualized in histogram format.

Table 2. Primers for RT-PCR.

Gene Name	Sequence
SNAIL-F	5'- TGCCCTCAAGATGCACATCCGA -3'
SNAIL-R	5'- GGGACAGGAGAAGGGCTTCTC -3'
SLUG-F	5'- ATCTGCGGCAAGGCGTTTTCCA -3'
SLUG-R	5'- GAGCCCTCAGATTTGACCTGTC -3'
SIP1-F	5'- GAGTTGATGCCTCGGCTATTGC -3'
SIP1-R	5'- CTGGACATTGAGCTGCTTCGATC -3'
TWIST1-F	5'- GCCAGGTACATCGACTTCCTCT -3'
TWIST1-R	5'- TCCATCCTCCAGACCGAGAAGG -3'
MMP2-F	5'- AGCGAGTGGATGCCGCCTTTAA -3'
MMP2-R	5'- CATTCCAGGCATCTGCGATGAG -3'
MMP9-F	5'- GCCACTACTGTGCCTTTGAGTC -3'
MMP9-R	5'- CCCTCAGAGAATCGCCAGTACT -3'
CDH1-F	5'- GCCTCCTGAAAAGAGAGTGGAAG -3'
CDH1-R	5'- TGGCAGTGTCTCTCCAAATCCG -3'
CDH2-F	5'- CCTCCAGAGTTTACTGCCATGAC -3'
CDH2-R	5'- GTAGGATCTCCGCCACTGATTC -3'
GAPDH-F	5'- GTCTCCTCTGACTTCAACAGCG -3'
GAPDH-R	5'- ACCACCCTGTTGCTGTAGCCAA -3'

2.8. Cell Migration Analysis

A culture-insert 2 well (Ibidi, 81176) was utilized for would healing assay to determine the migration capability of MDA-MB-231 cells. MDA-MB-231 cells were digested and re-suspended to a final density of 5×10^5 cells/mL. Cell suspension was added into chambers as well as outer area and cultured for 24 h for cell adhesion before the inserts were removed. Then the culture medium was replaced with new medium supplemented with indicated chemicals. Then the wound healing status was recorded by microscopy at 12 h, 24 h and 48 h after culture medium alteration.

2.9. Cell Invasion Analysis

A Matrigel Transwell invasion assay was performed to determine the invasiveness of MDA-MB-231 cells. A total of 10^4 cells in serum-free DMEM medium were seeded into upper chamber (8-μm pore, Corning, 3464) pre-coated with 1 mg/mL Matrigel Matrix (Corning, 354234) and DMEM medium containing 20% FBS was added into 24-well plate. After incubation for 24 h in a humidified 5% CO_2 atmosphere at 37 °C, cells were fixed with pre-cooled methanol for 30 min and stained with 0.1% crystal violet (w/v) in PBS for 10 min. Images were collected by microscopy to determine the cells passing through Matrigel basement.

2.10. Statistical Analysis

All data were obtained from independent triple-replicated experiments and presented as the mean ± standard deviation (SD). Significance was determined by a two-tail Student's t-test via GraphPad Prism v.6 (GraphPad Inc., USA) and data with *p*-value < 0.05 were considered of statistical significance.

3. Results

3.1. Anxa2 Bound to NF-κB p50 Subunit in MDA-MB-231 Cells and MCF-7 Cells

It has been well-established that Anxa2 binds to p50 to promote NF-κB activation and cell survival in hepatocellular carcinoma and pancreatic cancer cell lines [28,29]. In order to tell the activity of Anxa2 in NF-κB associated EMT in breast cancer, we first assessed the interaction of Anxa2 with NF-κB p50 subunit in breast cancer MDA-MB-231 and MCF-7 cells by coIP analysis (Figure 1A). As the N-terminus of Anxa2 is responsible for its interaction with p50 [29], we transiently transfected C-terminus myc-tagged full-length Anxa2 and an N-terminus deleted truncated version of Anxa2

(Anxa2-dN). Precipitated by anti-myc antibody, Anxa2-dN failed to interact with p50, demonstrating Anxa2 bound to p50 via its N-terminus in breast cancer cells as does in Hepatoma cells (Figure 1B).

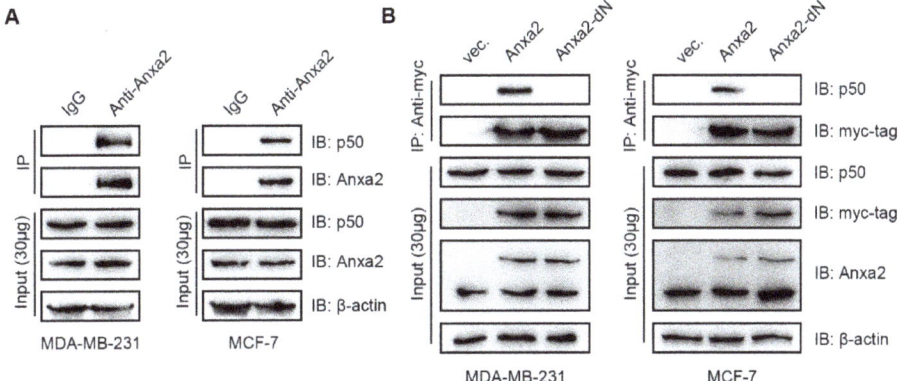

Figure 1. Anxa2 interacts with p50 in breast cancer cell lines. (**A**) An immuno-precipitation was performed with anti-Anxa2 antibody in protein extract from MDA-MB-231 cells and MCF-7 cells and immuno-precipitation with IgG was used as a negative control. (**B**) An immuno-precipitation was performed with anti-myc-tag antibody in protein extract from MDA-MB-231 cells and MCF-7 cells transfected with empty vector (vec.), Anxa2 and Anxa2-dN. A total of 30 μg of whole-cell protein extract was loaded as input. All experiments were repeated for three times.

3.2. Anxa2 Promoted NF-κB Activation and Associated EMT in Invasive Breast Cancer Cells

We co-transfected cells with Anxa2 and dual luciferase reporter system for NF-κB activity analysis, the transfection of full-length Anxa2 enhanced NF-κB activity whereas that of Anxa2-dN failed (Figure 2A). We then analyzed the NF-κB associated EMT-TFs including SNAIL, SLUG, SIP1 and TWIST1, EMT marker (CDH1, gene encoding E-cadherin; CDH2, gene encoding N-cadherin) and pro-invasion matrix metalloproteinases (MMP2, MMP9). The over-expression of full-length Anxa2 increased the expression of three EMT-TFs such as SLUG, SIP1 and TWIST1 and two MMPs (MMP2, MMP9) in invasive breast cancer MDA-MB-231 cells (Figure 2B, left panel). Up-regulated CDH2 and down-regulated CDH1, presenting the accelerated EMT capability were observed in full-length Anxa2 over-expressing MDA-MB-231 cells (Figure 2B, left panel). Correlated with failed activation of NF-κB, the over-expression of Anxa2-dN caused little expression shift in CDH2 and CDH1 (Figure 2B, left panel). In contrast with MDA-MB-231 cells, less-invasive MCF-7 cells presented no obvious alteration in these migration related gene expression under either full-length Anxa2 or Anxa2-dN truncation over-expression (Figure 2B, right panel). Protein levels of these genes in MDA-MB-231 cells were further determined by immune-blot. The up-regulation of protein levels of E-Cadherin and that of down-regulation of N-cadherin, Twist, slug, SIP1, MMP-2 and MMP-9 were observed in accord with the alteration of mRNA levels (Figure 2C).

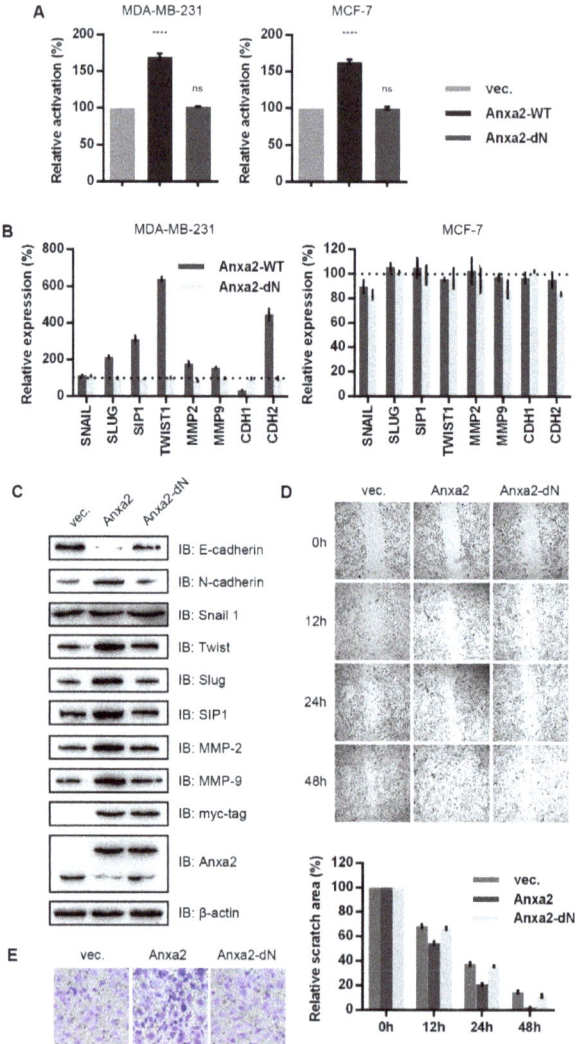

Figure 2. Anxa2 over-expression enhanced NF-κB activation and related cell migration and invasion. (**A**) NF-κB activity was determined via a dual luciferase reporter assay in MDA-MB-231 cells and MCF-7 cells transfected with empty vector, Anxa2 and Anxa2-dN. (**B**) mRNA levels of indicated genes were determined by RT-PCR with RNA extract from MDA-MB-231 cells and MCF-7 cells transfected with Anxa2 and Anxa2-dN t, the dot line at 100% presents mRNA levels in cells transfected with empty vector. (**C**) The protein levels of indicated genes were determined by immuno-blot in MDA-MB-231 cells transfected with empty vector (vec.), Anxa2 and Anxa2-dN. A total of 30 μg of whole-cell protein extract was loaded for immuno-blotting assay. (**D**) A wound healing assay was performed with MDA-MB-231 cells transfected with empty vector (vec.), Anxa2 and Anxa2-dN. Relative scratch area was shown below the microscopy images. (**E**) A Transwell invasion assay was performed with MDA-MB-231 cells transfected with empty vector (vec.), Anxa2 and Anxa2-dN. All experiments were repeated for three times and all data are shown as mean ± SD, with **** presenting $p < 0.0001$, *** presenting $p < 0.001$, ** $p < 0.01$, * presenting $p < 0.05$ and ns presenting $p > 0.05$.

Wound healing assay and Transwell invasion assays were then performed with Anxa2-over-expressing MDA-MB-231 cells. Full-length Anxa2 over-expression enhanced the wound healing efficiency and invasiveness through Matrigel basement whereas Anxa2-dN truncation over-expression showed no facilitation (Figure 2D,E).

3.3. (20S)G-Rh2 Inhibited NF-κB Activation Targeting Anxa2

(20S)G-Rh2 was proven as a natural small-molecule ligand for Anxa2 and inhibited NF-κB activation by interfering Anxa2-p50 interaction in HepG2 cells [28]. For the purpose of investigating the inhibitory effect toward NF-κB of (20S)G-Rh2 in breast cancer cells, a cellular thermal shift assay was performed with MDA-MB-231 cells and MCF-7 cells; (20S)G-Rh2 increased the thermal stability of Anxa2 in both cell lines (Figure 3A), indicating (20S)G-Rh2 bound to Anxa2 in MDA-MB-231 cells and MCF-7 cells. A following immune-precipitation showed (20S)G-Rh2 inhibited Anxa2-p50 interaction at resting state or under co-treatment with NF-κB activator etoposide or PMA in either MDA-MB-231 cells or MCF-7 cells (Figure 3B). NF-κB activity was determined via a dual luciferase reporter assay; (20S)G-Rh2 inhibited NF-κB activity at resting state and co-treated with etoposide or PMA in both MDA-MB-231 cells and MCF-7 cells (Figure 3C).

3.4. (20S)G-Rh2 Inhibited the Migration and Invasion of MDA-MB-231 in a Dose-Dependent Manner

MDA-MB-231 cells and MCF-7 cells were treated with increasing concentration of (20S)G-Rh2 and the result showed that NF-κB activity was down-regulated in a dose-dependent manner upon (20S)G-Rh2 treatment (Figure 4A). A dose-dependent alteration was also appeared in the gene expression analysis of TWIST1, MMP2, MMP9, CDH1 and CDH2, the expression of SLUG and SIP1 presented stable by (20S)G-Rh2 in MDA-MB-231 cells; only Snail1 presented an unexpected increase (Figure 4B, left panel). No regulated shift was seen in MCF-7 cells under (20S)G-Rh2 treatment (Figure 4B right panel). The protein levels of EMT-TFs, MMPs and N-cadherin were down-regulated and that of E-cadherin was up-regulated in a (20S)G-Rh2-dose-dependent manner in MDA-MB-231 cells (Figure 4C). Wound healing assay and Transwell invasion assay were performed MDA-MB-231 cells upon various concentration of (20S)G-Rh2 treatment. (20S)G-Rh2 inhibited the migration and invasion of MDA-MB-231 cells in a dose-dependent manner (Figure 4D,E).

3.5. (20S)G-Rh2 Binding-Deficient Mutant of Anxa2 Protected MDA-MB-231 Cells from (20S)G-Rh2 Induced NF-κB Inhibition

To provide further evidence for the (20S)G-Rh2 effect on Anxa2 function, we over-expressed the (20S)G-Rh2-binding-deficient mutant, Anxa2-K301A, in MDA-MB-231 cells. A cellular thermal shift assay showed that Anxa2-K301A failed to interact with (20S)G-Rh2 (Figure 5A). (20S)G-Rh2 failed to interfere the interaction between Anxa2-K301A and p50; it even enhanced it (Figure 5B). (20S)G-Rh2 induced NF-κB inhibition and downstream gene expression shift were also unchanged or reversed in Anxa2-K301A over-expressing cells (Figure 5C,D). Cell migration capability and invasiveness were unaltered with Anxa2-K301A overexpression under (20S)G-Rh2 treatment (Figure 5E,F).

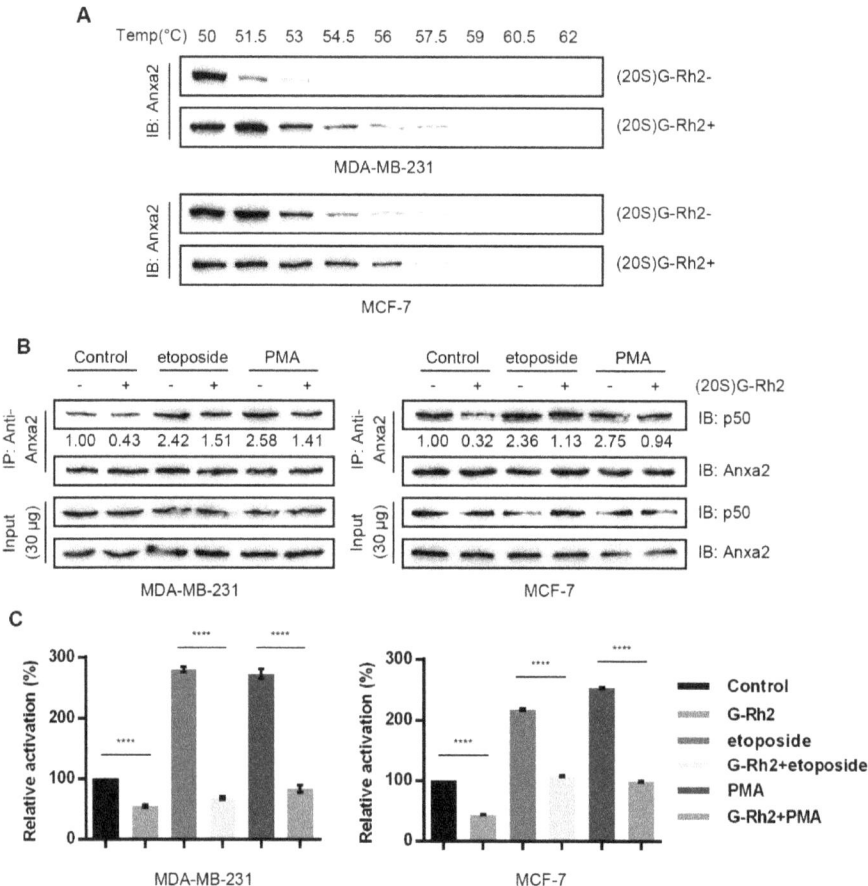

Figure 3. (20S)G-Rh2 inhibits NF-κB activation by binding to Anxa2. (**A**) A cellular thermal shift was performed in MDA-MB-231 cells and MCF-7 cells under 10-μM-(20S)G-Rh2 treatment or not. (**B**) An immuno-precipitation was performed with anti-Anxa2 antibody in protein extract from MDA-MB-231 cells and MCF-7 cells under treatment or 6-μM (20S)G-Rh2, 25 μg/mL etoposide,100 ng/mL PMA and combined chemicals for 12 h. (**C**) NF-κB activity was determined via a dual luciferase reporter assay in MDA-MB-231 cells and MCF-7 cells under treatment or 6-μM (20S)G-Rh2, 25 μg/mL etoposide,100 ng/mL PMA and combined chemicals for 12 h. A total of 30 μg of whole-cell protein extract was loaded as input. All experiments were repeated for three times and all data are shown as mean ± SD, with **** presenting $p < 0.0001$, *** presenting $p < 0.001$, ** $p < 0.01$, * presenting $p < 0.05$ and ns presenting $p > 0.05$.

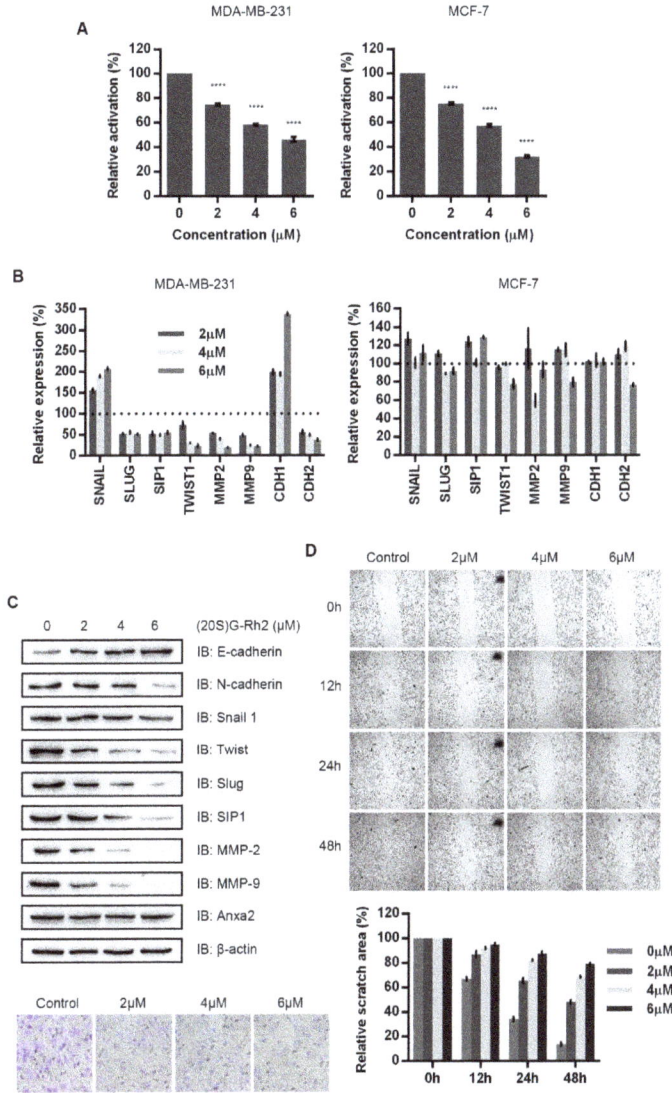

Figure 4. (20S)G-Rh2 inhibits NF-κB related cell migration and invasion. (**A**) NF-κB activity was determined via a dual luciferase reporter assay in MDA-MB-231 cells and MCF-7 cells under (20S)G-Rh2 treatment for 12 h. (**B**) mRNA levels of indicated genes were determined by RT-PCR with RNA extract from MDA-MB-231 cells under (20S)G-Rh2 treatment for 12 h. (**C**) The protein levels of indicated genes were determined by immuno-blot in MDA-MB-231 cells under (20S)G-Rh2 treatment for 12 h. A total of 30 μg of whole-cell protein extract was loaded for immuno-blotting assay. (**D**) A wound healing assay was performed with MDA-MB-231 cells under (20S)G-Rh2 treatment for 12 h. Relative scratch area was shown below the microscopy images. (**E**) A Transwell invasion assay was performed with MDA-MB-231 cells t under (20S)G-Rh2 treatment for 12 h. All experiments were repeated for three times and all data are shown as mean ± SD, with **** presenting $p < 0.0001$, *** presenting $p < 0.001$, ** $p < 0.01$, * presenting $p < 0.05$ and ns presenting $p > 0.05$.

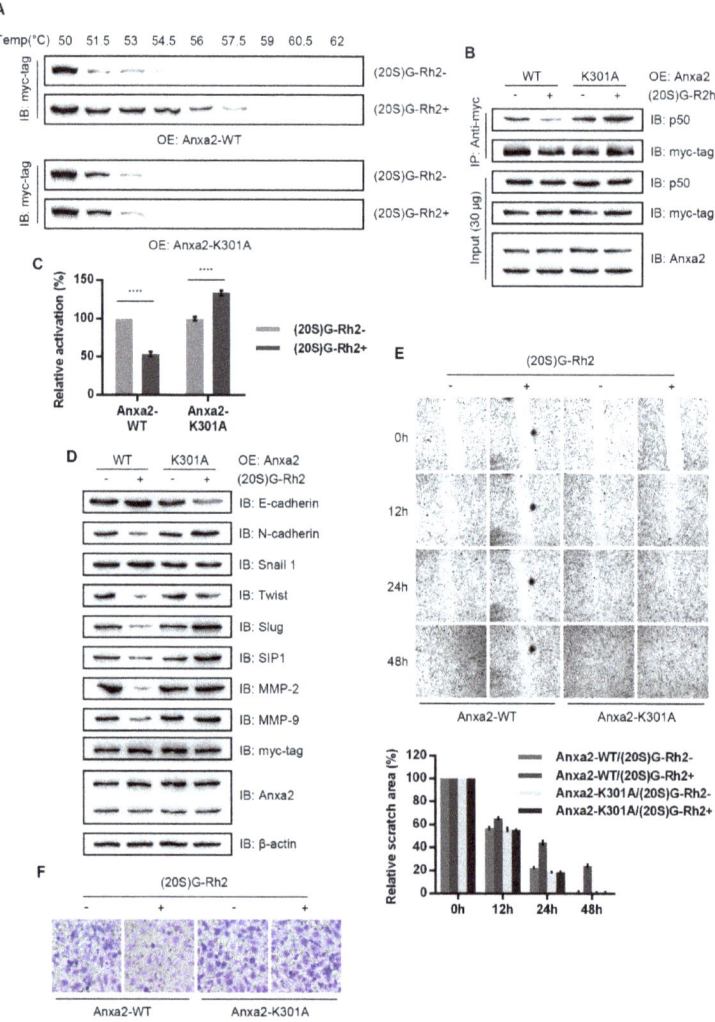

Figure 5. Anxa2-K301A protects MDA-MB-231 cells from (20S)G-Rh2-induced NF-κB inhibition. (**A**) A cellular thermal shift was performed in MDA-MB-231 cells transfected with Anxa2-WT and Anxa2-K301A under 10-μM-(20S)G-Rh2 treatment or not. (**B**) An immuno-precipitation was performed with anti-myc-tag antibody in protein extract from MDA-MB-231 cells transfected with Anxa2-WT and Anxa2-K301A under 6-μM-(20S)G-Rh2 treatment or not. A total of 30 μg of whole-cell protein extract was loaded as input. (**C**) NF-κB activity was determined via a dual luciferase reporter assay in MDA-MB-231 cells transfected with Anxa2-WT and Anxa2-K301A under 6-μM-(20S)G-Rh2 treatment for 12 h or not. (**D**) The protein levels of indicated genes were determined by immuno-blot in MDA-MB-231 cells transfected with Anxa2-WT and Anxa2-K301A under 6-μM-(20S)G-Rh2 treatment or not. A total of 30 μg of whole-cell protein extract was loaded for immuno-blotting assay. (**E**) A wound healing assay was performed with MDA-MB-231 cells transfected with Anxa2-WT and Anxa2-K301A under 6-μM-(20S)G-Rh2 treatment or not. Relative scratch area was shown below the microscopy images. (**F**) A Transwell invasion assay was performed with MDA-MB-231 cells transfected with Anxa2-WT and Anxa2-K301A under 6-μM-(20S)G-Rh2 treatment or not. All experiments were repeated for three times and all data are shown as mean ± SD, with **** presenting $p < 0.0001$, *** presenting $p < 0.001$, ** $p < 0.01$, * presenting $p < 0.05$ and ns presenting $p > 0.05$.

4. Discussion

Cancer metastasis present responsibility for over 90% cancer mortality. EMT—one of the main generators for cancer metastasis—has become an assignable factor in both cancer research and treatment [1,11]. Derived by EMT promoting genes, epithelial-like cancer cells re-program gene expression phenotype, lose epithelial feature, dissociate from primary tumor tissue and spread with circulatory system [2,4–6]. A variety of gene transcriptional regulation was involved in this program, among which EMT-TFs and up-stream transcriptional factors like NF-κB and STAT3, directly alter the expression of key effector molecules [22,23,30,31].

Among them, multi-functional protein Anxa2 behaves as an implicated promoter for EMT and related cellular event. Anxa2 was first associated with cell migration for its heterotetramer with S100A10 [32,33], which promotes extracellular matrix degradation by activating plasmin and following researches indicate Anxa2 is responsible for membrane dynamics in invasive cells by binding to other S100 protein like S100A4 [34], S100A6 [35] and S100A11 [36,37]. Implicated in signaling transduction, phosphorylated Anxa2 at Tyr23 binds to STAT3 and promotes its phosphorylation at Tyr705 as well as following dimerization and nuclear translocation, resulting in up-regulated MMPs and enhanced EMT [38,39]. In addition, couple of researches have demonstrated Anxa2 content is correlated to cell migration capability [40–43].

It has been well-established that NF-κB bound to the promoter region of ZEB-1/2, SNAIL, SLUG, SIP1 and TWIST1 and the transcription of ZEB-1/2, SLUG, SIP1 and TWIST1 accords with NF-κB activation [22,23]. Anxa2, acting as an NF-κB co-activator in hepatocellular carcinoma and pancreatic cancer [28,29], was first identified bound to p50 subunit of NF-κB in breast cancer cells (Figure 1A,B). Over-expression of Anxa2 in invasive breast cancer MDA-MB-231 cells accelerated NF-κB activation (Figure 2A) and the expression EMT-TFs including SLUG, SIP1 and TWIST1 (Figure 2B,C), followed by the down-regulation of E-cadherin and up-regulation of N-cadherin (Figure 2B,C). Though containing NF-κB binding site, SNAIL somehow failed to follow NF-κB regulation, presenting differential variation trend as other EMT-TFs (Figures 2B and 4B) [23]. MMPs responsible for the degradation of extracellular matrix and promote cell motility appeared to be up-regulated in according with EMT phenotype in Anxa2-over-expressing cells (Figure 2B,C). These gene expression alteration resulted in the enhanced migratory properties and invasiveness (Figure 2D,E). In contrast, no altered expression of EMT-TFs was observed in company with the activation of NF-κB in less aggressive MCF-7 cells (Figure 2A,B), indicating EMT-TFs expression requires additional regulatory mechanism, which is necessary to perform further investigation in the future study.

(20S)G-Rh2 is one of the most famous ginsenosides from ginseng extract for its remarkable anti-cancer activity. (20S)G-Rh2 has been proven efficiently inducing growth arrest and apoptosis [44–47]. Moreover, in-vivo study indicates that (20S)G-Rh2 inhibits tumor growth by inhibiting tumor associated angiogenesis and enhancing anti-tumor immunological response [48–50]. In addition, couples of studies have indicated (20S)G-Rh2 presents inhibitory effect towards EMT. Based on our previous research on (20S)G-Rh2-Anxa2 interaction, we supposed that (20S)G-Rh2 inhibited EMT by targeting Anxa2. A cellular thermal shift assay verified the intracellular interaction between Anxa2 and (20S)G-Rh2 (Figure 3A): an immuno-precipitation as well as NF-κB luciferase reporter assay confirmed the inhibitory impact on NF-κB by (20S)G-Rh2 (Figure 3B,C and Figure 4A) in breast cancer cell line MDA-MB-231 and MCF-7. As a result, down-stream pro-EMT genes were down-regulated with epithelial phenotype marker E-cadherin accelerated in MDA-MB-231 cells under (20S)G-Rh2 treatment (Figure 4B,C); cell migration and invasion were also apparently inhibited (Figure 4D,E).

In our previous work, we have identified the Lys301 residue responsible for (20S)G-Rh2 binding; Anxa2-K301A has been shown to be a (20S)G-Rh2 binding deficiency mutant [28]. In addition, Anxa2-K301A mutants maintained p50 binding capacity and promoted NF-κB under (20S)G-Rh2 treatment [28]. Anxa2a-WT and K301A mutants were transfected with MDA-MB-231 cells to examine the targeted inhibition of NF-κB and related EMTs. (20S)G-Rh2 failed to interact with Anxa2-K301A (Figure 5A); p50-Anxa2-K301A interaction and NF-κB activation were surprisingly enhanced under

(20S)G-Rh2 treatment (Figure 5B,C). Functioning as a multi-targeted chemical, (20S)G-Rh2 induced various cellular stress and NF-κB stayed inactive under the targeted inhibition [28,44–50]. This status was reversed when Anxa2 mutant maintained the activation property regardless of (20S)G-Rh2 and stress related NF-κB activation was generated. Under the constitutive NF-κB activation by Anxa2-K301A over-expression presented higher mesenchymal-like phenotype (Figure 5D) and equivalent migratory and invasive properties (Figure 5E,F).

5. Conclusions

Our data suggest that Anxa2 is an important co-activator of NF-κB in breast cancer cells. Over-expression of Anxa2 promoted NF-κB activation and pro-EMT gene expression. With the up-regulation of EMT-TFs and MMPs, MDA-MB-231 cells presented a mesenchymal-like phenotype and achieved enhanced migratory properties as well as invasiveness. (20S)G-Rh2 induced NF-κB inhibition by targeting Anxa2 and led to the suppression in pro-EMT gene expression, resulting in the EMT arrest at the epithelial state. Over expression of Anxa2-K301A maintained NF-κB activation and the mesenchymal-like phenotype under (20S)G-Rh2 treatment in MDA-MB-231 cells. Taken together, (20S)G-Rh2 targets Anxa2 in invasive breast cancer cells, inhibits NF-κB activity and EMT and may be a potent candidate for breast cancer treatment and related research.

Author Contributions: Conceptualization, Y.-S.W. and Y.-H.J.; methodology, Y.-S.W., H.L. and S.Z.; software, Y.-S.W.; formal analysis, Y.-S.W. and H.L.; investigation, Y.-S.W. and Y.L.; resources, Y.S.W. and Y.-H.J.; data curation, Y.-S.W.; writing—original draft preparation, Y.-S.W.; writing—review and editing, Y.-H.J.; visualization, Y.-S.W.; supervision, Y.-H.J.; project administration, Y.-H.J.; funding acquisition, Y.-H.J. All authors have read and agreed to the published version of the manuscript.

Funding: This study was funded by Special Project for Province & University Construction Plan of Jilin Province (SXGJXX2017-13) and Science and Technology Development Program of Jilin Province (20191102059YY).

Conflicts of Interest: All authors declare no conflict of interest.

References

1. Thiery, J.P.; Acloque, H.; Huang, R.Y.J.; Nieto, M.A. Epithelial-mesenchymal transitions in development and disease. *Cell* **2009**, *139*, 871–890. [CrossRef] [PubMed]
2. Nieto, M.A.; Huang, R.Y.J.; Jackson, R.A.; Thiery, J.P. EMT: 2016. *Cell* **2016**, *166*, 21–45. [CrossRef] [PubMed]
3. Lamouille, S.; Xu, J.; Derynck, R. Molecular mechanisms of epithelial-mesenchymal transition. *Nat. Rev. Mol. Cell Biol.* **2014**, *15*, 178–196. [CrossRef]
4. Nieto, M.A. Epithelial plasticity: A common theme in embryonic and cancer cells. *Science* **2013**, *342*, 1234850. [CrossRef] [PubMed]
5. Pastushenko, I.; Brisebarre, A.; Sifrim, A.; Fioramonti, M.; Revenco, T.; Boumahdi, S.; Van Keymeulen, A.; Brown, D.; Moers, V.; Lemaire, S.; et al. Identification of the tumour transition states occurring during EMT. *Nature* **2018**, *556*, 463–468. [CrossRef] [PubMed]
6. Beck, B.; Lapouge, G.; Rorive, S.; Drogat, B.; Desaedelaere, K.; Delafaille, S.; Dubois, C.; Salmon, I.; Willekens, K.; Marine, J.C.; et al. Different levels of Twist1 regulate skin tumor initiation, stemness, and progression. *Cell Stem Cell* **2015**, *16*, 67–79. [CrossRef]
7. Derynck, R.; Weinberg, R.A. EMT and cancer: More than meets the eye. *Dev. Cell* **2019**, *49*, 313–316. [CrossRef]
8. Aiello, N.M.; Maddipati, R.; Norgard, R.J.; Balli, D.; Li, J.; Yuan, S.; Yamazoe, T.; Black, T.; Sahmoud, A.; Furth, E.E.; et al. EMT subtype influences epithelial plasticity and mode of cell migration. *Dev. Cell* **2018**, *45*, 681–695. [CrossRef]
9. Meyer-Schaller, N.; Cardner, M.; Diepenbruck, M.; Saxena, M.; Tiede, S.; Lüönd, F.; Ivanek, R.; Beerenwinkel, N.; Christofori, G. A hierarchical regulatory landscape during the multiple stages of EMT. *Dev. Cell* **2019**, *48*, 539–553. [CrossRef]
10. Yousefi, H.; Maheronnaghsh, M.; Molaer, F.; Mashouri, L.; Reza Aref, A.; Momeny, M.; Alashari, S.K. Long noncoding RNAs and exosomal lncRNAs: Classification, and mechanisms in breast cancer metastasis and drug resistance. *Oncogene* **2020**, *39*, 953–974. [CrossRef]

11. Brabletz, T. EMT and MET in metastasis: Where are the cancer stem cells? *Cancer Cell* **2012**, *22*, 699–701. [CrossRef] [PubMed]
12. Pastushenko, I.; Blanpain, C. EMT transition states during tumor progression and metastasis. *Trends Cell Biol.* **2019**, *29*, 212–226. [CrossRef] [PubMed]
13. Puram, S.V.; Tirosh, I.; Parikh, A.S.; Patel, A.P.; Yizhak, K.; Gillespie, S.; Rodman, C.; Luo, C.L.; Mroz, E.A.; Emerick, K.S.; et al. Single-cell transcriptomic analysis of primary and metastatic tumor ecosystems in head and neck cancer. *Cell* **2017**, *171*, 1611–1624. [CrossRef] [PubMed]
14. Schliekelman, M.J.; Taguchi, A.; Zhu, J.; Dai, X.; Rodriguez, J.; Celiktas, M.; Zhang, Q.; Chin, A.; Wong, C.H.; Wang, H.; et al. Molecular portraits of epithelial, mesenchymal, and hybrid states in lung adenocarcinoma and their relevance to survival. *Cancer Res.* **2015**, *75*, 1789–1800. [CrossRef]
15. Marcucci, F.; Stassi, G.; De Maria, R. Epithelial-mesenchymal transition: A new target in anticancer drug discovery. *Nat. Rev. Drug Discov.* **2016**, *15*, 311–325. [CrossRef]
16. Lo, H.C.; Zhang, X.H. EMT in metastasis: Finding the right balance. *Dev. Cell* **2018**, *45*, 663–665. [CrossRef]
17. Acharyya, S.; Oskarsson, T.; Vanharanta, S.; Madlladi, S.; Kim, J.; Morris, P.G.; Manova-Todorova, K.; Leversha, M.; Hogg, N.; Seshan, V.E.L.; et al. A CXCL1 paracrine network links cancer chemoresistance and metastasis. *Cell* **2012**, *150*, 165–178. [CrossRef]
18. Yang, Y.R.; Kim, D.H.; Seo, Y.K.; Park, D.; Jang, H.J.; Choi, S.Y.; Lee, Y.H.; Lee, G.H.; Nakajima, K.; Taniguchi, N.; et al. Elevated O-GlcNAcylation promotes colonic inflammation and tumorigenesis by modulating NF-κB signaling. *Oncotarget* **2015**, *6*, 12529–12542. [CrossRef]
19. Hanahan, D.; Weinberg, R.A. The hallmarks of cancer. *Cell* **2000**, *100*, 57–70. [CrossRef]
20. AlQathama, A.; Prieto, J.M. Natural products with therapeutic potential in melanoma metastasis. *Nat. Prod. Rep.* **2015**, *32*, 1170–1182. [CrossRef]
21. Karin, M. Nuclear factor-kappaB in cancer development and progression. *Nature* **2006**, *441*, 431–436. [CrossRef] [PubMed]
22. Chua, H.L.; Bhar-Nakshatri, P.; Clare, S.E.; Morumiya, A.; Badve, S.; Nakshatri, H. NF-κB represses E-cadherin expression and enhances epithelial to mesenchymal transition of mammary epithelial cells: Potential involvement of ZEB-1 and ZEB-2. *Oncogene* **2007**, *26*, 711–724. [CrossRef] [PubMed]
23. Pires, B.R.; Mencalha, A.L.; Ferreira, G.M.; de Souza, W.F.; Morgado-Díaz, J.A.; Maia, A.M.; Corrêa, S.; Abdelhay, E.S. NF-KappaB is involved in the regulation of EMT genes in breast cancer cells. *PLoS ONE* **2017**, *12*, e0169622. [CrossRef] [PubMed]
24. Liu, J.; Wu, Z.; Han, D.; Wei, C.; Liang, Y.; Jiang, T.; Chen, L.; Sha, M.; Cao, Y.; Huang, F.; et al. Mesencephalic astrocyte-derived neurotrophic factor inhibits liver cancer through small ubiquitin-related modifier (SUMO)ylation-related suppression of NF-κB/Snail signaling pathway and epithelial-mesenchymal transition. *Hepatology* **2020**. [CrossRef]
25. Shin, S.R.; Sanchez-Velar, N.; Sherr, D.H.; Sonenshein, G.E. 7,12-dimethylbenz(a)anthracene treatment of a c-rel mouse mammary tumor cell line induces epithelial to mesenchymal transition via activation of nuclear factor-κB. *Cancer Res.* **2006**, *66*, 2570–2575. [CrossRef]
26. Liu, P.; Yang, P.; Zhang, Z.; Liu, M.; Hu, S. Ezrin/NF-κB pathway regulates EGF-induced epithelial-mesenchymal transition (EMT), metastasis, and progression of osteosarcoma. *Med. Sci. Monit.* **2018**, *24*, 2098–2108. [CrossRef]
27. Fang, H.; Wu, Y.; Huang, X.; Wang, W.; Ang, B.; Cao, X.; Wan, T. Toll-like receptor 4 (TLR4) is essential for Hsp70-like protein 1 (HSP70L1) to activate dendritic cells and induce Th1 response. *J. Biol. Chem.* **2011**, *286*, 30393–30400. [CrossRef]
28. Wang, Y.S.; Lin, Y.; Li, Y.; Song, Z.; Jin, Y.H. The identification of molecular target of (20S)Ginsenoside Rh2 for its anti-cancer activity. *Sci. Rep.* **2017**, *7*, 12408. [CrossRef]
29. Jung, H.; Kim, J.S.; Kim, W.K.; Oh, K.J.; Lee, H.J.; Han, B.S.; Kim, D.S.; Seo, Y.S.; Lee, S.C.; Park, S.G.; et al. Intracellular annexin A2 regulates NF-κB signaling by binding to the p50 subunit implications for gemcitabbine resistance in pancreatic. *Cell Death Dis.* **2015**, *6*, e1606. [CrossRef]
30. Chung, S.S.; Giehl, N.; Wu, Y.; Vadgama, J.V. STAT3 activation in HER2-overexpressing breast cancer promotes epithelial–mesenchymal transition and cancer stem cell traits. *Int. J. Oncol.* **2014**, *44*, 403–411. [CrossRef]

31. Xiong, H.; Hong, J.; Du, W.; Lin, Y.W.; Ren, L.L.; Wang, Y.C.; Su, W.Y.; Wang, J.L.; Cui, Y.; Wang, Z.H.; et al. Roles of STAT3 and ZEB1 proteins in E-cadherin down-regulation and human colorectal cancer epithelial−mesenchymal transition. *J. Biol. Chem.* **2012**, *287*, 5819–5832. [CrossRef]
32. Bydoun, M.; Waisman, D.M. On the contribution of S100A10 and annexin A2 to plasminogen activation and ongogenesis: An enduring ambiguity. *Future Oncol.* **2014**, *10*, 2469–2479. [CrossRef]
33. Myrvang, H.K.; Guo, X.; Li, C.; Dekker, L.V. Protein interactions between surface annexin A2 and S100A10 mediate adhesion of breast cancer cells to microvascular endothelial cells. *Febs Lett.* **2013**, *587*, 3210–3215. [CrossRef]
34. Semo, A.; Moreno, M.J.; Onichtchenko, A.; Abulrob, A.; Ball, M.; Ekiel, I.; Pietrzynski, G.; Stanimirovic, D.; Alakhov, V. Metastasis-associated protein S100A4 induces angiogenesis through interaction with Annexin II and accelerated plasmin formation. *J. Biol. Chem.* **2005**, *280*, 20833–20841. [CrossRef] [PubMed]
35. Nedjadi, T.; Kitteringham, N.; Campbell, F.; Jenkins, R.E.; Park, B.K.; Navarro, P.; Ashcroft, F.; Tepikin, A.; Neoptolemos, J.P.; Costello, E. S100A6 binds to annexin 2 in pancreatic cancer cells and promotes pancreatic cancer cell motility. *Br. J. Cancer* **2009**, *101*, 1145–1154. [CrossRef] [PubMed]
36. Jaiswal, J.K.; Nylandsted, J. S100 and annexin proteins identify cell membrane damage as the Achilles heel of metastatic cancer cells. *Cell Cycle* **2015**, *14*, 502–509. [CrossRef] [PubMed]
37. Jaiswal, J.K.; Lauritzen, S.P.; Scheffer, L.; Sakaguchi, M.; Bunkenborg, J.; Simon, S.M.; Kallunki, T.; Jäättelä, M.; Nylandsted, J. S100A11 is required for efficient plasma membrane repair and survival of invasive cancer cells. *Nat. Commun.* **2014**, *5*, 3795. [CrossRef] [PubMed]
38. Yuan, J.; Yang, Y.; Gao, Z.; Wang, Z.; Ji, W.; Song, W.; Zhang, F.; Niu, R. Tyr23 phosphorylation of Anxa2 enhances STAT3 activation and promotes proliferation and invasion of breast cancer cells. *Breast Cancer Res. Treat.* **2017**, *164*, 327–340. [CrossRef]
39. Wang, T.; Yuan, J.; Zhang, J.; Tian, R.; Ji, W.; Zhou, Y.; Yang, Y.; Song, W.; Zhang, F.; Niu, R. Anxa2 binds to STAT3 and promotes epithelial to mesenchymal transition in breast cancer cells. *Oncotarget* **2015**, *6*, 30975–30992. [CrossRef]
40. Yan, X.; Zhang, D.; Wu, W.; Wu, S.; Qian, J.; Hao, Y.; Yan, F.; Zhu, P.; Wu, J.; Huang, G.; et al. Mesenchymal Stem Cells Promote Hepatocarcinogenesis via lncRNA-MUF Interaction with ANXA2 and miR-34a. *Cancer Res.* **2017**, *77*, 6704–6716. [CrossRef]
41. Wu, M.; Sun, Y.; Xu, F.; Liang, Y.; Liu, H.; Yi, Y. Annexin A2 Silencing Inhibits Proliferation and Epithelial-to-mesenchymal Transition through p53-Dependent Pathway in NSCLCs. *J. Cancer* **2019**, *10*, 1077–1085. [CrossRef] [PubMed]
42. Liu, Y.; Li, H.; Ban, Z.; Nai, M.; Yang, L.; Chen, Y.; Xu, Y. Annexin A2 inhibition suppresses ovarian cancer progression via regulating β-catenin/EMT. *Oncol. Rep.* **2017**, *37*, 3643–3650. [CrossRef] [PubMed]
43. Cui, L.; Song, J.; Wu, L.; Cheng, L.; Chen, A.; Wang, Y.; Huang, Y.; Huang, L. Role of Annexin A2 in the EGF-induced epithelial-mesenchymal transition in human CaSki cells. *Oncol. Lett.* **2017**, *13*, 377–383. [CrossRef] [PubMed]
44. Guo, X.X.; Guo, Q.; Li, Y.; Lee, S.K.; Wei, X.N.; Jin, Y.H. Ginsenoside Rh2 induces human hepatoma cell apoptosis via bax/bak triggered cytochrome C release and caspase-9/ caspase-8 activation. *Int. J. Mol. Sci.* **2012**, *13*, 15523–15535. [CrossRef] [PubMed]
45. Lee, H.; Lee, S.; Jeong, D.; Kim, S.J. Ginsenoside Rh2 epigenetically regulates cell-mediated immune pathway to inhibit proliferation of MCF-7 breast cancer cells. *J. Ginseng Res.* **2018**, *42*. [CrossRef] [PubMed]
46. Mathiyalagan, R.; Wang, C.; Kim, Y.J.; Castro-Aceituno, V.; Ahn, S.; Subramaniyam, S.; Simu, S.Y.; Jiménez-Pérez, Z.E.; Yang, D.C.; Jung, S.K. Preparation of polyethylene glycol-ginsenoside Rh1 and Rh2 conjugates and their efficacy against lung cancer and inflammation. *Molecules* **2019**, *24*, 4367. [CrossRef]
47. Hou, J.G.; Jeon, B.M.; Yun, Y.J.; Cui, C.H.; Kim, S.C. Ginsenoside Rh2 ameliorates doxorubicin-induced senescence bystander effect in breast carcinoma cell MDA-MB-231 and nomal epithelial cell MCF-10A. *Int. J. Mol. Sci.* **2019**, *20*, 1244. [CrossRef]
48. Qi, Z.; Chen, L.; Li, Z.; Shao, Z.; Qi, Y.; Gao, K.; Liu, S.; Sun, Y.; Li, P.; Liu, J. Immunomodulatory Effects of (24R)-Pseudo-Ginsenoside HQ and (24S)-Pseudo-Ginsenoside HQ on Cyclophosphamide-Induced Immunosuppression and Their Anti-Tumor Effects Study. *Int. J. Mol. Sci.* **2019**, *20*, 836. [CrossRef]

49. Wang, M.; Yan, S.J.; Zhang, H.T.; Li, N.; Liu, T.; Zhang, Y.L.; Li, X.X.; Ma, Q.; Qiu, X.C.; Fan, Q.Y.; et al. Ginsenoside Rh2 enhances the antitumor immunological response of a melanoma mice model. *Onco. Lett.* **2017**, *13*, 681–685. [CrossRef]
50. Huang, Y.; Huang, H.; Han, Z.; Li, W.; Mai, Z.; Yuan, R. Ginsenoside Rh2 Inhibits Angiogenesis in Prostate Cancer by Targeting CNNM1. *J. Nanosci. Nanotechnol.* **2019**, *19*, 1942–1950. [CrossRef]

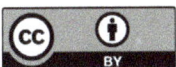 © 2020 by the authors. Licensee MDPI, Basel, Switzerland. This article is an open access article distributed under the terms and conditions of the Creative Commons Attribution (CC BY) license (http://creativecommons.org/licenses/by/4.0/).

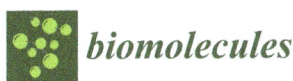

Article

Ginsenoside Compound K Induces Adult Hippocampal Proliferation and Survival of Newly Generated Cells in Young and Elderly Mice

Jung-Mi Oh [1,2,†], Jae Hoon Jeong [1,†], Sun Young Park [1,2] and Sungkun Chun [1,2,*]

1. Department of Physiology, Chonbuk National University Medical School, Jeonju-si, Jeollabuk-do 54907, Korea; biojmi@jbnu.ac.kr (J.-M.O.); jjh8690624@gmail.com (J.H.J.); qirsjm@naver.com (S.Y.P.)
2. Brain Korea 21 Plus Program, Chonbuk National University Medical School, Jeonju-si 54907, Korea
* Correspondence: sungkun.chun@jbnu.ac.kr; Tel.: +82-63-270-4290
† These authors contributed equally.

Received: 29 February 2020; Accepted: 21 March 2020; Published: 23 March 2020

Abstract: Cognitive impairment can be associated with reduced adult hippocampal neurogenesis, and it may contribute to age-associated neurodegenerative diseases such as Alzheimer's (AD). Compound K (CK) is produced from the protopanaxadiol (PPD)-type ginsenosides Rb1, Rb2, and Rc by intestinal microbial conversion. Although CK has been reported as an inducing effector for neuroprotection and improved cognition in hippocampus, its effect on adult neurogenesis has not been explored yet. Here, we investigated the effect of CK on hippocampal neurogenesis in both young (2 months) and elderly (24 months) mice. CK treatment increased the number of cells co-labeled with 5-ethynyl-2'-deoxyuridine (EdU) and proliferating cell nuclear antigen (PCNA); also, Ki67, specific markers for progenitor cells, was more expressed, thus enhancing the generation of new cells and progenitor cells in the dentate gyrus of both young and elderly mice. Moreover, CK treatment increased the number of cells co-labeled with EdU and NeuN, a specific marker for mature neuron in the dentate gyrus, suggesting that newly generated cells survived and differentiated into mature neurons at both ages. These findings demonstrate that CK increases adult hippocampal neurogenesis, which may be beneficial against neurodegenerative disorders such as AD.

Keywords: ginsenoside CK; neurogenesis; cell proliferation; neuroprotection

1. Introduction

Since adult hippocampal neurogenesis in the dentate gyrus [1] has first been reported, it has been considered a main contributor to age-related cognitive impairments [2] and to neurodegenerative diseases such as Alzheimer's disease (AD) [3]. Aging leads to several symptoms, such as inflammation-induced brain metabolic changes, neurovascular defects, memory loss, and increased anxiety level in mice [4]. Furthermore, aging both reduces adult hippocampal neurogenesis [5,6] and increases the risk factors for AD [7–9]. Indeed, age-dependent neurogenesis reduction [5,10,11] leads to decreased learning and memory function [12]. Therefore, any therapy aiming to increase adult hippocampal neurogenesis could be an important strategy to mitigate age-related neurodegenerative diseases such as AD.

Ginsenoside compound K (CK) is conversion from protopanaxadiol (PPD)-type ginsenosides Rb1, Rb2, and Rc by intestinal microbiota [13]. Previous researches reported that CK exhibits beneficial pharmacological effects, including antidiabetic [14], anti-inflammatory [15], anticancer [16], and antiaging [17] activity. Recent evidences suggest that CK has a role in neuroprotection and in cognitive improvement. For instance, CK protects neurons in the stroke mouse model by reducing microglial activation through its anti-inflammatory activity [18]. Also, chemotherapy-induced cognitive impairment was mitigated by CK administration in mice [19]. In vascular dementia rats, CK cleared the beta-amyloid deposition, resulting in the attenuation of both neuronal damage and cognitive deficits [20]. In addition, 10 mg/Kg CK was successfully used in mice to reduce scopolamine-induced memory impairment and negative effects of reactive oxygen species via the induction of Nrf2-mediated antioxidant enzyme [21]. Although previous studies regarding the neuroprotective beneficial effects of CK have been reported, the direct evidence regarding the effect of CK on adult hippocampal neurogenesis is still unknown. Hence, in this study, we investigated the potential of CK to modulate adult hippocampal neurogenesis.

2. Materials and Methods

2.1. Animals

All mouse care and experimental procedures were approved by the Institutional Animal Care and Use Committee of the Chonbuk National University (permit number: CBNU-2018-042, Approval date: 05 June 2018). Two-month-old (-mo) and 24-mo male mice were purchased from Jackson Laboratories (Bar Harbor, ME, USA). Animals were kept grouped in cages at 22 °C with a 12:12-h light–dark cycle and fed a standard chow diet with ad libitum access to water.

2.2. Compound K Administration

Ginsenosides compound K was obtained from the laboratory of Ace EMzyme, Hankyung National University, South Korea. Compound K (CK) was dissolved in 100% dimethyl sulfoxide (DMSO) and then diluted daily in 2-hydroxypropyl-cyclodextrin (cat. no. H5784; Invitrogen). For 3 consecutive days, 2-mo and 24-mo mice were injected intraperitoneally either diluted CK (5, 10, or 15 mg/Kg) or vehicle (0 mg/Kg).

2.3. EdU Administration

To determine the cell proliferation rate induced by CK, on the last CK administration day, all mice received an intraperitoneal injection of phosphate-buffered saline (PBS)-EdU (100 mg/Kg, ab146186, Abcam, Cambridge, Massachusetts, UK). Mice were then sacrificed after 24 h. For neuronal survival analysis, EdU was injected for 3 consecutive days after the last CK injection, and all remaining mice were sacrificed after 4 weeks.

2.4. Perfusion

At the end of the experiment, all mice were perfused with 0.1 M PBS containing heparin (1000 u/mL; cat. no. H3393; Sigma-Aldrich; Merck KGaA, Darmstadt, Germany) and prefixed with 4% paraformaldehyde (PFA) in 0.1 M PBS. All brains were postfixed in a 4% PFA solution for 24 h at 4 °C, dehydrated in a 30% sucrose solution at 4 °C for 72 h, and immediately frozen at −80 °C. Coronal sections (40 μm) were cut with a cryostat (Leica CM 1860, Leica Biosystems Inc., Chicago, IL, USA), and slices were stored in cryoprotectant (25% ethylene glycol and 25% glycerin) in 0.05 M phosphate buffer at −20 °C.

2.5. Immunohistochemistry

Every sixth serial section was tested for cell proliferation with the Click-iT EdU Cell Proliferation Kit for Imaging, Alexa Fluor 488 dye (cat. no. C10337; Invitrogen, Gaisburg, MD, USA) according to the manufacturer's instructions. Briefly, the free-floating sections were washed 3 times in 0.1 M PBS containing 3% bovine serum albumin (BSA), permeabilized with 0.5% Triton-X 100 in PBS for 20 min, and rinsed with 3% BSA in PBS. Then, the sections were incubated with the Click-iT reaction buffer for 30 min at room temperature (RT), washed 3 times in PBS, mounted on a slide-glass using Vectashield antifade mounting medium (cat. no. H-1000; Vector Laboratories, Burlingame, CA, USA), and covered with a coverslip. For EdU and immunohistochemistry double labeling, the sections were incubated in 1 × Target Retrieval Solution (Dako, cat# S1699) at 95 °C for 5 min prior to the EdU staining procedure. After EdU staining, sections were incubated in blocking solution (5% BSA and 0.1% Triton X-100 in PBS) for 2 h at RT and then incubated with anti-proliferating cell nuclear antigen (anti-PCNA) (1:1000; cat. no. 2586; Cell Signaling Technology, Danvers, MA, USA), anti-Ki67 (1:1000; cat. no. ab15580; Abcam), or anti-NeuN (1:1000; cat. no. 24307; Cell Signaling Technology) antibodies for 24 h at 4 °C. Sections were then washed 3 times in PBS and incubated with Alexa 594 anti-mouse IgG (1:1000; cat. no. ab150116; Abcam) or Alexa 594 anti-rabbit IgG (1:1000; cat. no. ab150080; Abcam) for 2 h at RT. Tissues were washed, dried, and mounted with mounting medium. Images were acquired using a Zeiss LSM 880 super resolution confocal microscope.

2.6. Immunoblotting

Radioimmunoprecipitation assay (RIPA) buffer (cat. no. R2002; Biosesang, Seongnam-si, South Korea) containing proteinase inhibitors (cat. no. G652A; Promega, South Korea) was used to obtain total lysates from the hippocampus of 2-mo and 24-mo C57BL/6 mice injected with vehicle or CK. Total lysates (20 μg) were separated on 12% SDS-PAGE gels and transferred to polyvinylidene fluoride (PVDF) membranes and then kept in 5% skim milk blocking buffer for 2 h at RT. Anti-brain-derived neurotrophic factor (anti-BDNF) (1:1000; cat. no. ab108319; Abcam), anti-pAkt (Ser473) (1:1000; cat. no. 4060; Cell Signaling Technology), anti-Akt (1:1000; cat. no. 9272; Cell Signaling Technology), anti-pERK1/2 (1:1000; cat. no. 9101; Cell Signaling Technology), anti-ERK1/2 (1:1000; cat. no. 4696; Cell Signaling Technology), and anti-GAPDH (1:5000; cat. no. AP0066; Bioworld Technology) antibodies diluted in TBST (Tris buffered saline Tween 20) buffer containing 5% BSA, which was used for the membranes' incubation for 24 h at 4 °C. The membranes were then washed in TBST buffer and probed with anti-rabbit IgG, horseradish peroxidase (HRP)-linked or anti-mouse IgG, HRP-linked secondary antibodies (1:3000; cat. no. 7074 and 7076; Cell Signaling Technology) for 2 h at RT. All membranes were washed in TBST buffer and developed using Clarity Western ECL Substrate (cat. no. 1705060; BIO RAD, Hercules, CA, USA).

2.7. Quantitative Reverse Transcription PCR

For qRT-PCR analysis of neurotrophin 3 (NT3) and brain-derived neurotrophic factor (BDNF) genes, total RNA was isolated from hippocampus using the Trizol reagent (Thermo Fisher Scientific, Inc., 15596026) and then first-strand cDNA was synthesized using GoScript Reverse Transcription System (cat. no. A5001; Promega). Real-time qPCR was performed with 7900 HT fast Real-Time PCR System (Applied Biosystems) using SYBR Green I Master Mix (cat. no. RT501M; Enzynomics). Each qPCR reaction was prepared in a final volume of 10 μL, containing 2 μL cDNA and 5 μL of SYBR Green Master mix with a different primer pair (1 μL, 10 pmole/μL). Beta-actin was used as an internal control for the quantification of each sample. The primer pairs employed are F5'-CAAAGGGATCGTTGGAGGTGA-3' and R5'- GTTCGGTCAT TCAGTCTCGC-3' for NT3, F5'-TCATACTTCGGTTGCATGAAGG-3' and R5'-AGACCTCTC GAACCTGCCC-3' for BDNF, and F5'-CCTGACAGACTACCTCATGAAG-3' and R5'- CCATC TCTTGCTCGAAGTCTAG-3' for beta-actin. Relative gene expression was determined using the $^{\Delta\Delta}$Ct method. Relative mRNA expression levels were presented as the fold change compared with the 2-mo mice vehicle group.

2.8. Statistical Analysis

All statistics were performed with GraphPad Prism (version 5.01.) for windows (Graphpad Software, San Diego, CA, USA). Data were expressed as mean ± standard error of the mean (SEM). Statistical significance was assessed using an unpaired t-test. Results with $p < 0.05$ were considered significant.

3. Results

3.1. CK Increases the Number of Newly Born Cells in the Dentate Gyrus

We first purified compound K (>97%, molecular structure in Figure 1A) by acid-heat treatment of PPD-type ginsenoside extracts from Korean ginseng (Panax ginseng). To determine the effect of CK on cell proliferation in young and elderly mice, both mice groups were injected with various concentration of CK (0 mg/Kg, 5 mg/Kg, 10 mg/Kg, and 15 mg/Kg) for 3 consecutive days and then with EdU (Figure 1b). Twenty-four h after EdU injection, all mice were transcardially perfused and the brain was sectioned for histological study using a cryostat (40 μm).

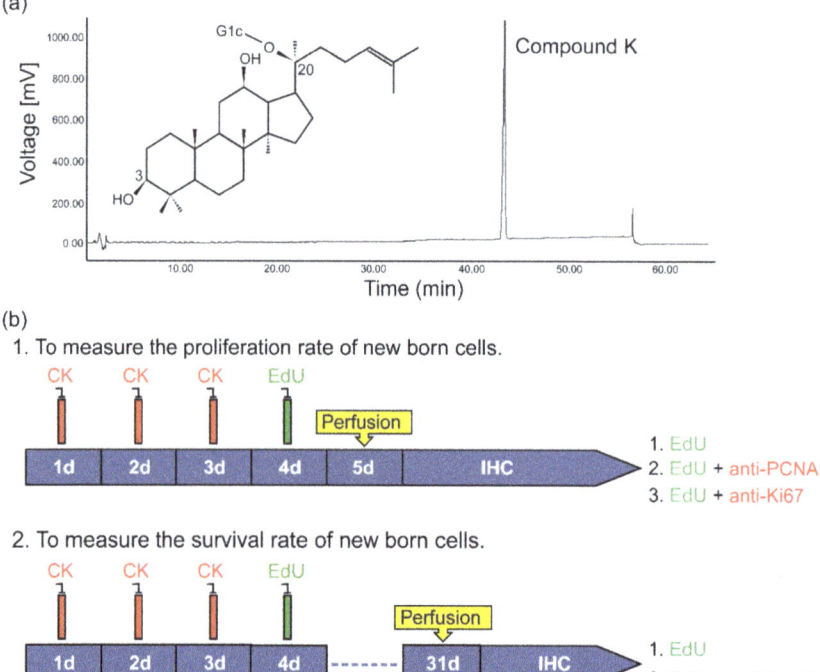

Figure 1. (a) Chemical structure of Compound K (CK) and high-performance liquid chromatography (HPLC) analysis of the transformation of CK: The chromatographic peak was identified by comparison with the reference compounds. (b) Experimental design. In experiment 1: mice were injected with 5-ethynlyl-2'-deoxyuridine (EdU, 100 mg/Kg) once after 3 consecutive CK intraperitoneal injections and sacrificed on day 5 or on day 31 for proliferation or survival studies, respectively. Antibodies for EdU, proliferating cell nuclear antigen (PCNA), and Ki67 were used to measure the proliferation of newly born cells, while antibodies for EdU and NeuN were used to measure the survival rate of newly born cells.

The total number of EdU-incorporated cells was counted in the subgranular zone of the dentate gyrus. The CK dose-dependently increased the number of EdU-incorporated newborn cells in the dentate gyrus of young mice (Figure 2a,c). However, the production of new cells in 24-mo mice was significantly increased only with 15 mg/Kg CK (Figure 2b,c). These results show that the number of new cells does decrease by aging, but this trend could be slowed by treatments with more concentrated ginsenoside CK.

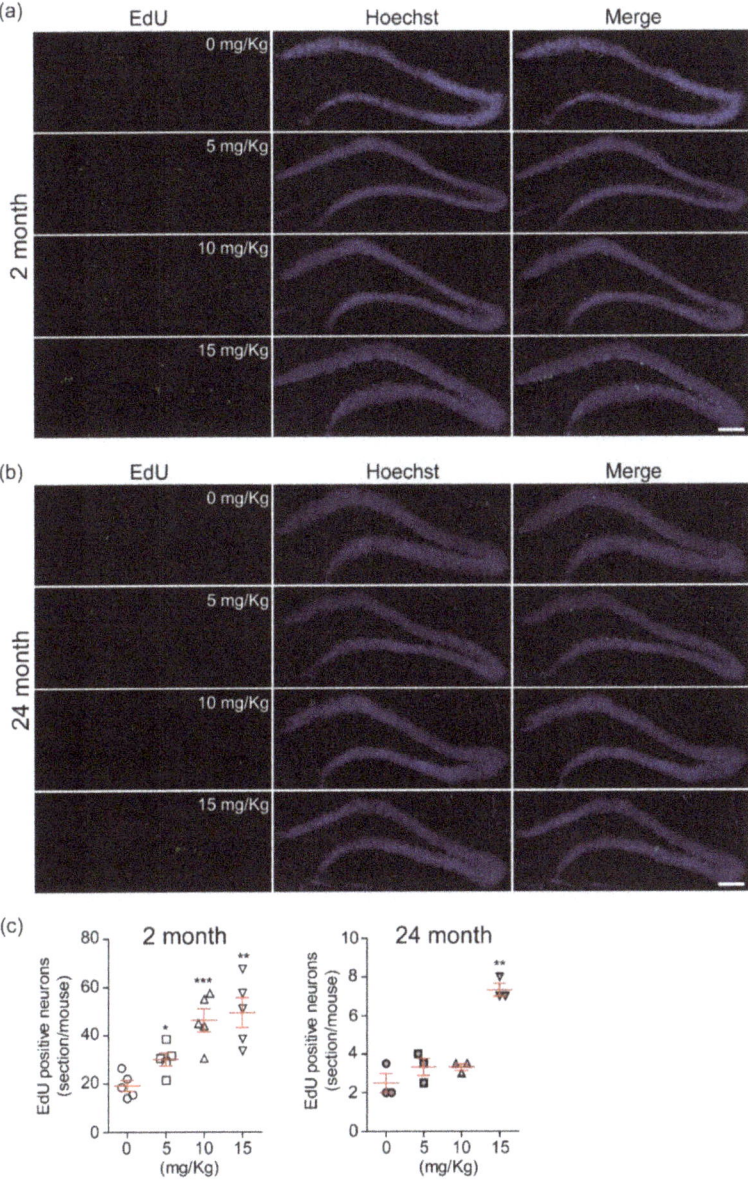

Figure 2. Compound K (CK) induces the production of new cells in the dentate gyrus (DG) of hippocampus: Images of confocal microscopy showing 5-ethynyl-2′-deoxyuridine (EdU)-labeled cells in the dentate gyrus of 2-month-old (-mo) (**a**) and 24-mo mice (**b**). All C57BL/6 mice were intraperitoneally injected with EdU (5 mg/Kg, 10 mg/Kg, and 15 mg/Kg) or vehicle for 3 consecutive days. (**c**) Summary plots showing that CK promotes the generation new cells in a dose-dependent manner ($n = 5$ in 2-mo; $n = 3$ in 24-mo mice, respectively). All data are represented as the mean ± standard error of the mean (SEM). *$p < 0.05$, **$p < 0.01$, and ***$p < 0.001$ vs. vehicle treated groups (unpaired t-test).

3.2. CK Enhances the Proliferation of Newly Born Cells in the Dentate Gyrus

Given that CK showed potent effects on newly born cell production in the dentate gyrus of both age groups, we next investigated its effects using double immunofluorescence staining with the anti-proliferating cell nuclear antigen (PCNA), which is a marker for cell proliferation. We found that 10 mg/Kg CK significantly increased both PCNA-labeled cells and EdU-PCNA double-labeled cells in the dentate gyrus of hippocampus (Figure 3).

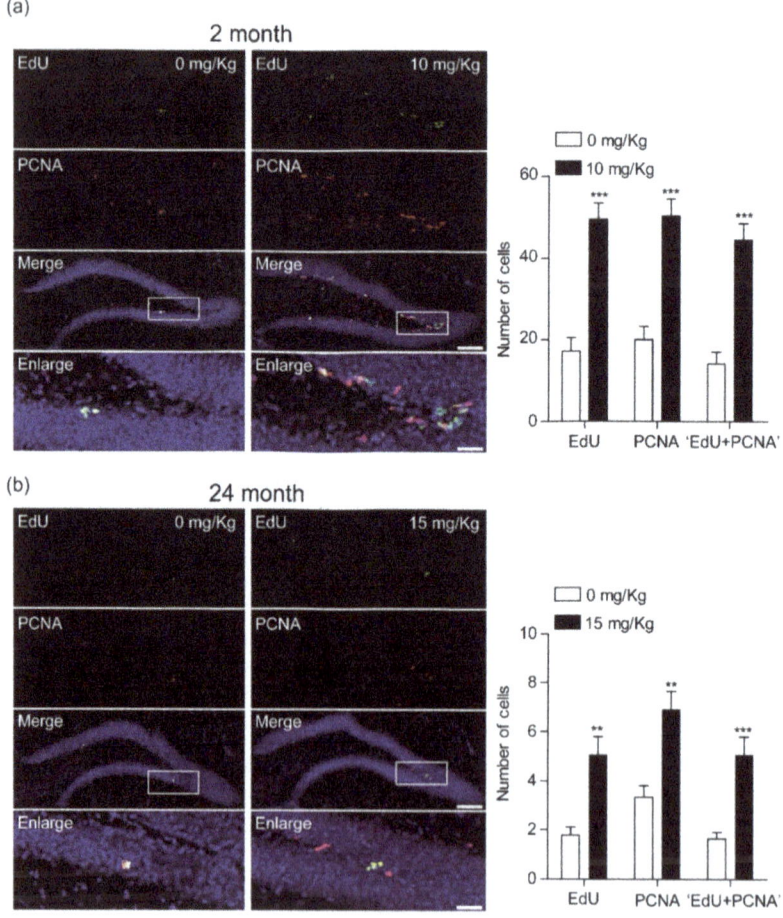

Figure 3. Compound K (CK) increases 5-ethynyl-2′-deoxyuridine (EdU)+/PCNA+ cells as well as PCNA+ cells in the DG of hippocampus. (**a**) Co-expression of PCNA in the EdU-labeled newborn cells in the dentate gyrus (DG) of 2-mo mice (0 mg/Kg, $n = 5$ mice; 10 mg/Kg, $n = 4$ mice; ***$p < 0.001$, unpaired *t*-test). Scale bar = 100 μm (merge) or 20 μm (enlarge). (**b**) Image of confocal microscopy showing expression of PCNA in the EdU-labeled newborn cells of DG of 24-mo mice. Plots showing that CK increases PCNA positive cells in EdU-labeled newborn cells (0 mg/Kg, $n = 7$; 15 mg/Kg, $n = 7$; **$p < 0.01$, ***$p < 0.001$, unpaired *t*-test). Scale bar = 100 μm (merge) or 20 μm (enlarge).

Ki-67 is also a classic marker for cellular proliferation and is preferentially expressed during the late G1, S, G2, and M phases of the cell cycle, whereas resting, non-cycling cells (G0 phase) lack Ki-67 expression. Also, it is reported that the Ki-67 antigen is a more specific marker for cell proliferation than PCNA [22]. We further confirmed the effect of CK on the proliferation of newborn cells in the dentate gyrus of hippocampus. Ten mg/Kg CK significantly enhanced the Ki-67 positive cells in the dentate gyrus of hippocampus as well as Ki-67 and EdU double-positive cells (Figure 4). These results suggest that CK enhances the proliferation rate of newborn cells, resulting in an increase of both PCNA and Ki-67-labeled EdU-positive cells.

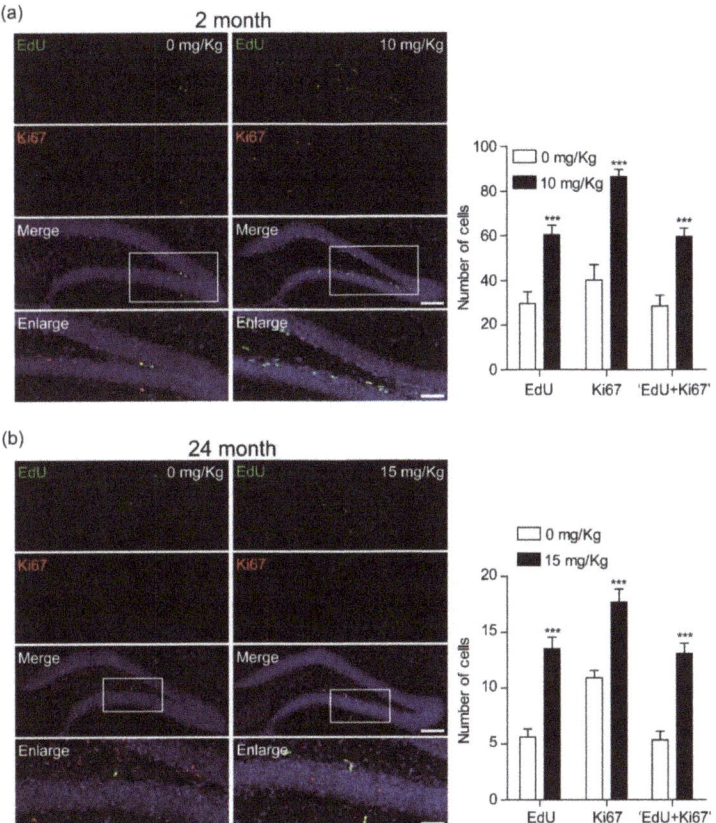

Figure 4. Compound K (CK) induces the number of co-labeled cells with 5-ethynyl-2′-deoxyuridine (EdU) incorporation and anti-Ki67 in the dentate gyrus (DG) of hippocampus. Confocal images showing EdU+/Ki67+ cells in the DG of (**a**) 2-mo (0 mg/Kg, $n = 5$; 10 mg/Kg, $n = 6$) and (**b**) 24-mo mice (0 mg/Kg, $n = 7$; 15 mg/kg, $n = 7$). The summary plots show quantification of positive cells for EdU, Ki67, or EdU/Ki67 in 2-mo or 24-mo mice with CK treatment. All data are represented as the mean ± standard error of the mean (SEM). ***$p < 0.001$ vs. vehicle treated groups (unpaired t-test). Scale bar = 100 μm (merge) or 20 μm (enlarge).

3.3. CK Improves Adult Hippocampal Neurogenesis by Increasing Neuronal Survival

To investigate whether CK induces adult hippocampal neurogenesis through an increasing survival rate of newborn cells in the DG of hippocampus of both 2-mo and 24-mo mice, we performed immunohistochemistry for EdU and mature neuronal marker protein (NeuN) co-labeled neurons.

Both age groups showed a significant increase of EdU cells when treated with CK (Figure 5a,b). Furthermore, CK increased the proportion of EdU-labeled cells that also expressed NeuN in both aged mice (Figure 5a,b), indicating that CK induces not only the survival of newborn cells but also differentiation into neurons. Thus, CK seems to facilitate adult hippocampal neurogenesis.

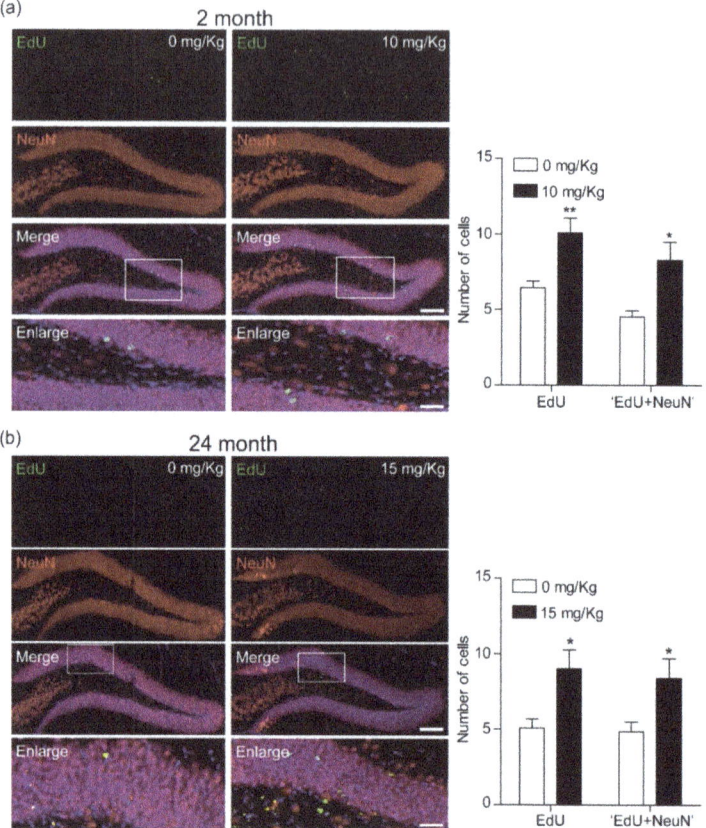

Figure 5. Compound K (CK) enhances the survival of newly generated cells in the dentate gyrus (DG) of hippocampus. Confocal images show that the survival rate of 5-ethynyl-2′-deoxyuridine (EdU)-labeled new born cells were enhanced by CK in the DG of (**a**) 2-mo ($n = 6$ in 0 mg/Kg and 10 mg/Kg, respectively) and (**b**) 24-mo mice ($n = 6$ in 0 mg/Kg; $n = 5$ in 15 mg/Kg). The plots showed a significant induction in co-expression of EdU and NeuN (*$p < 0.05$, **$p < 0.01$, unpaired *t*-test). Scale bar = 100 µm (merge) or 20 µm (enlarge).

3.4. Adult Neurogenesis by CK is Mediated via BDNF Signaling

Neurotrophic factors and growth factors are well known as potent activators of adult hippocampal neurogenesis [23]. We thus examined whether CK-induced neurogenesis is mediated by those factors. Real-time qPCR was performed to determine the expression levels of neurotrophin-3 (NT3) and brain-derived neurotrophic factor (BDNF) in the dentate gyrus of the two age groups treated with CK or with the vehicle. After 3 days of treatment, the NT3 and BDNF mRNA levels in the CK-injected mice were significantly higher than those in the vehicle-injected mice (Figure 6a). In addition, the expression level of NT3 and BDNF was reduced in vehicle-injected 24-mo mice compared with vehicle-injected 2-mo mice, but both gene expression levels after CK administration were higher than those in the vehicle-injected 2-mo mice (Figure 6a). Next, we investigated the effect of CK administration on the influence of the intracellular BDNF signaling pathway over adult hippocampal neurogenesis. The activation of BDNF and its downstream signaling pathway leads neurogenesis through control of neuronal proliferation and survival [24,25]. As observed from our qRT-PCR data, BDNF expression was significantly increased by CK administration in 2-mo mice, while in CK-injected 24-mo mice, it was comparable to that of vehicle-injected 2-mo mice (Figure 6B,C). Furthermore, 10 mg/Kg and 15 mg/Kg CK were sufficient to induce the phosphorylation of Akt and ERK1/2, which are downstream targets of the BDNF signaling pathway in 2-mo and 24-mo mice, respectively (Figure 6b,c). These results indicate that CK-induced adult hippocampal neurogenesis is mediated by the BDNF signaling pathway (Figure 7).

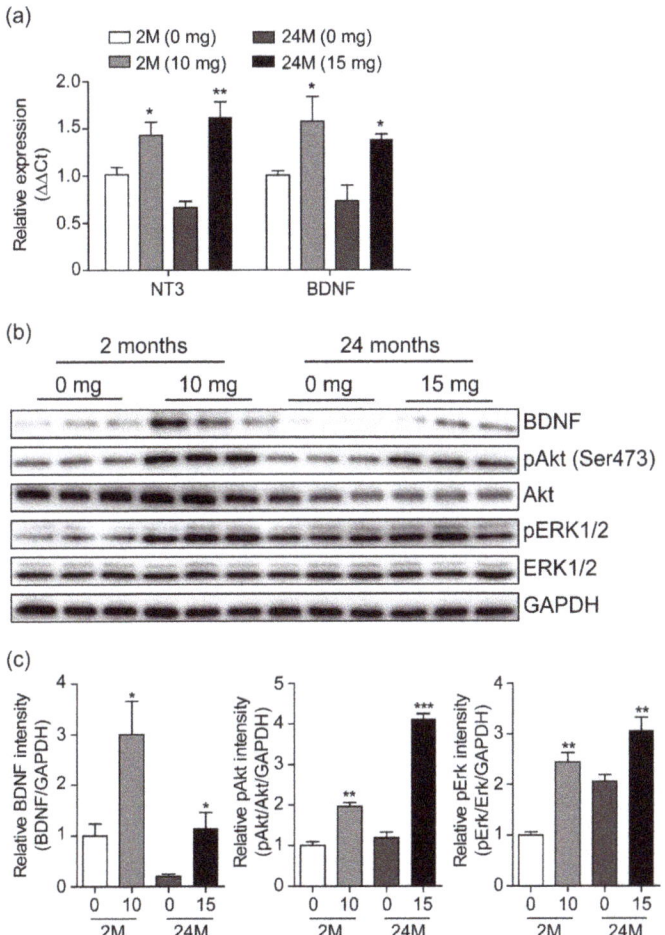

Figure 6. Beneficial effects of Compound K (CK) on adult neurogenesis is mediated via brain-derived neurotrophic factor (BDNF) signaling. (**a**) Summary plots showing neurotrophin-3 (NT3) and brain-derived neurotrophic factor (BDNF) mRNA expression in the dentate gyrus (DG) of hippocampus of 2-mo and 24-mo mice after CK (10 mg/Kg or 15 mg/Kg) or vehicle (0 mg/Kg) injection. Those expressions significantly increased after CK administration ($n = 3$, respectively, $*p < 0.05$, $**p < 0.01$, unpaired t-test). (**b**) Immunoblotting of total lysates from the DG after CK or vehicle treatment of both age groups. BDNF, Akt, and ERK signaling pathways for adult neurogenesis were screened ($n = 3$). (**c**) Summary plots showing the immunoblotting quantification for BDNF expression and its downstream targets: CK was sufficient to increase BDNF expression and the phosphorylation of Akt and ERK1/2, which are downstream targets of BDNF ($*p < 0.05$, $**p < 0.01$, $***p < 0.001$, unpaired t-test).

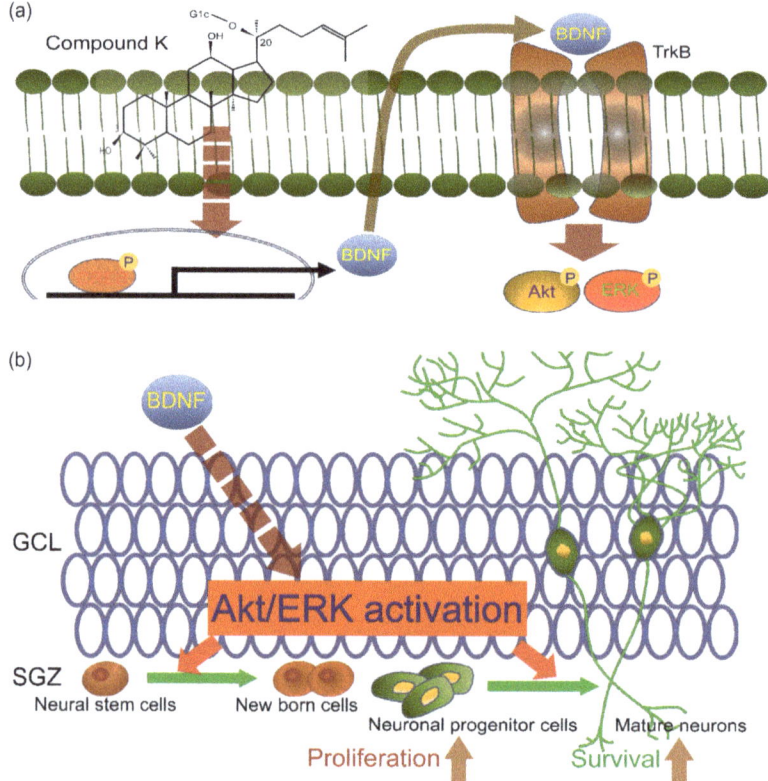

Figure 7. Schematic illustration of the proposed model: Compound K (CK) increases adult neurogenesis in the dentate gyrus (DG) of hippocampus by inducing BDNF signaling cascades. (**a**) CK increases the expression of BDNF and increased BDNF activates Akt and ERK signaling. (**b**) Activated Akt and ERK signals induced the proliferation and differentiation of newly born cells into progenitor cells and mature neurons. GCL, granule cell layer; SGZ, subgranular zone.

4. Discussion

In this study, we provide the first evidence that ginsenoside compound K has the ability to induce the production, proliferation, and survival of newborn cells through the activation of BDNF signaling. Notably, CK administration was sufficient to increase hippocampal neurogenesis even in 24-mo mice, suggesting that CK can contrast age-related cognitive impairment by improving adult neurogenesis.

Compound K is known to have a neuronal protective role following chemotherapy treatment [19]. However, there was no direct evidence for the effect of CK on adult hippocampal neurogenesis so far. The decline of adult hippocampal neurogenesis by aging contributes to cognitive impairment and is associated with age-related neurodegenerative diseases such as AD [26–28]. Furthermore, exercise and dietary energy restriction enhance the adult hippocampal neurogenesis, improve learning and memory, and protect against age-related cognitive decline and AD [26,29,30]. Therefore, the enhancement of neurogenesis by exogenous factors could lead to novel therapeutic strategies for preventing cognitive impairment and AD. We found that CK administration increased newborn cells in the dentate gyrus of 24-mo mice, resulting in more newly generated EdU cells. Also, injections of 10 mg/Kg and 15 mg/Kg CK were sufficient to induce proliferation of newborn cells in 2-mo and 24-mo mice, respectively. In addition, CK significantly enhanced the differentiation of newly generated cells in the dentate gyrus of hippocampus into adult neurons. The rate of neuronal survival in CK-treated 24-mo mice was similar to its rate in 2-mo mice. These results suggest that CK has the ability to facilitate adult hippocampal neurogenesis under declining neurological conditions such as age-related cognitive impairment.

Neurotrophic factors such as BDNF and growth factors including neurotrophin-3 (NT3) are important activators of adult neurogenesis [31–34]. Hence, we examined whether CK-mediated induction of neurogenesis in the dentate gyrus is associated with BDNF and NT3 mRNA levels. Indeed, CK administration significantly increased the mRNA expression of BDNF and NT3 in the dentate gyrus of 2-mo and 24-mo mice. Interestingly, the mRNA levels of BDNF and NT3 in the CK-injected 24-mo mice were higher than 2-mo young mice. Previous studies show that the upregulation of BDNF and NT3 improves cognitive function in AD [35,36], suggesting that CK administration may be able to prevent cognitive impairment. Given that CK administration was sufficient to increase the BDNF mRNA level, we next investigated whether the overexpression of BDNF induced by CK administration could affect the phosphorylation of Akt and ERK1/2, which are downstream targets of the BDNF signaling cascade. In 2-mo and 24-mo mice, CK administration increased BDNF expression, which is consistent with the qRT-PCR results and the phosphorylation of Akt and ERK1/2. In particular, the BDNF protein level in 24-mo mice was lower than those in 2-mo mice (vehicle group) but CK administration was able to restore the BDNF protein up to the young mice level. The BDNF/Trkb signaling pathway has an essential role in the regulation of adult hippocampal neurogenesis [37]. Furthermore, the PI3K-Akt signaling pathway and activation of ERK1/2 signaling play a critical role in neuronal differentiation and in the survival of newly generated cells in the dentate gyrus [38–40], suggesting that CK-mediated activation of BDNF signaling contributes to increase the adult hippocampal neurogenesis in elderly mice (Figure 7).

5. Conclusions

In conclusion, the administration of CK resulted in an enhancement of adult hippocampal neurogenesis in both elderly and young mice. Therefore, ginsenoside compound K can become a therapeutic agent able to prevent age-related cognitive impairments due to reduced adult neurogenesis. Further studies are required to analyze the molecular mechanism by which compound K is able to induce BDNF transcription; promoter assay may help discovering the transcription factors involved in this CK-mediated induction of neurogenesis.

Author Contributions: Conceptualization, J-M.O., J.H.J., and S.C.; methodology, J-M.O., J.H.J., and S.Y.P.; resources, S.Y.P.; validation, J-M.O., J.H.J., S.Y.P., and S.C.; visualization, J-M.O. and S.C.; investigation, J.H.J., J-M.O., S.Y.P., and S.C.; writing—original draft preparation, J.H.J, J-M.O., and S.C.; writing—review and editing, J-M.O. and S.C., funding acquisition, S.C. All authors have read and agreed to the published version of the manuscript.

Funding: This work was supported by research funds from Basic Science Research Program (NRF-2017R1D1A1B03035125) through the National Research Foundation (NRF), which is funded by the Korean government; from Korea Health Technology R&D project through the Korea Health Industry Development Institute (KHIDI), funded by the Ministry of Health & Welfare, Republic of Korea (grant number: HI17C1510); and from Brain Pool Program through the National Research Foundation of Korea (NRF), funded by the Ministry of Science and ICT (NRF-2019H1D3A2A01059349).

Acknowledgments: We would like to thank Wan-Taek Im (Hankyung National University, Anseong, South Korea) for providing the ginsenoside Compound K and thank Editage (www.editage.co.kr) for English language editing.

Conflicts of Interest: The authors declare no conflict of interest.

References

1. Altman, J.; Das, G.D. Autoradiographic and histological evidence of postnatal hippocampal neurogenesis in rats. *J. Comp. Neurol.* **1965**, *124*, 319–335. [CrossRef] [PubMed]
2. Toda, T.; Parylak, S.L.; Linker, S.B.; Gage, F.H. The role of adult hippocampal neurogenesis in brain health and disease. *Mol. Psychiatry* **2019**, *24*, 67–87. [CrossRef] [PubMed]
3. Braskie, M.N.; Thompson, P.M. Understanding cognitive deficits in Alzheimer's disease based on neuroimaging findings. *Trends Cogn. Sci.* **2013**, *17*, 510–516. [CrossRef] [PubMed]

4. Hoffman, J.D.; Parikh, I.; Green, S.J.; Chlipala, G.; Mohney, R.P.; Keaton, M.; Bauer, B.; Hartz, A.M.S.; Lin, A.L. Age Drives Distortion of Brain Metabolic, Vascular and Cognitive Functions, and the Gut Microbiome. *Front. Aging Neurosci.* **2017**, *9*, 298. [CrossRef]
5. Kuhn, H.G.; Dickinson-Anson, H.; Gage, F.H. Neurogenesis in the dentate gyrus of the adult rat: age-related decrease of neuronal progenitor proliferation. *J. Neurosci.* **1996**, *16*, 2027–2033. [CrossRef]
6. Mathews, K.J.; Allen, K.M.; Boerrigter, D.; Ball, H.; Shannon Weickert, C.; Double, K.L. Evidence for reduced neurogenesis in the aging human hippocampus despite stable stem cell markers. *Aging Cell* **2017**, *16*, 1195–1199. [CrossRef]
7. Winner, B.; Kohl, Z.; Gage, F.H. Neurodegenerative disease and adult neurogenesis. *Eur. J. Neurosci.* **2011**, *33*, 1139–1151. [CrossRef]
8. Varela-Nallar, L.; Aranguiz, F.C.; Abbott, A.C.; Slater, P.G.; Inestrosa, N.C. Adult hippocampal neurogenesis in aging and Alzheimer's disease. *Birth Defects Res.* **2010**, *90*, 284–296. [CrossRef]
9. Horgusluoglu, E.; Nudelman, K.; Nho, K.; Saykin, A.J. Adult neurogenesis and neurodegenerative diseases: A systems biology perspective. *Am. J. Med. Genet.* **2017**, *174*, 93–112. [CrossRef]
10. Encinas, J.M.; Michurina, T.V.; Peunova, N.; Park, J.H.; Tordo, J.; Peterson, D.A.; Fishell, G.; Koulakov, A.; Enikolopov, G. Division-coupled astrocytic differentiation and age-related depletion of neural stem cells in the adult hippocampus. *Cell Stem Cell* **2011**, *8*, 566–579. [CrossRef]
11. Gebara, E.; Sultan, S.; Kocher-Braissant, J.; Toni, N. Adult hippocampal neurogenesis inversely correlates with microglia in conditions of voluntary running and aging. *Front. Neurosci* **2013**, *7*, 145. [CrossRef] [PubMed]
12. Gil-Mohapel, J.; Brocardo, P.S.; Choquette, W.; Gothard, R.; Simpson, J.M.; Christie, B.R. Hippocampal neurogenesis levels predict WATERMAZE search strategies in the aging brain. *PLoS ONE* **2013**, *8*, e75125. [CrossRef] [PubMed]
13. Hasegawa, H.; Sung, J.H.; Matsumiya, S.; Uchiyama, M. Main ginseng saponin metabolites formed by intestinal bacteria. *Planta Med.* **1996**, *62*, 453–457. [CrossRef] [PubMed]
14. Yoon, S.H.; Han, E.J.; Sung, J.H.; Chung, S.H. Anti-diabetic effects of compound K versus metformin versus compound K-metformin combination therapy in diabetic db/db mice. *Biol. Pharm. Bull.* **2007**, *30*, 2196–2200. [CrossRef]
15. Chen, J.; Si, M.; Wang, Y.; Liu, L.; Zhang, Y.; Zhou, A.; Wei, W. Ginsenoside metabolite compound K exerts anti-inflammatory and analgesic effects via downregulating COX2. *Inflammopharmacology* **2019**, *27*, 157–166. [CrossRef]
16. Oh, J.M.; Kim, E.; Chun, S. Ginsenoside Compound K Induces Ros-Mediated Apoptosis and Autophagic Inhibition in Human Neuroblastoma Cells In Vitro and In Vivo. *Int J. Mol. Sci.* **2019**, *20*. [CrossRef]
17. Kim, E.; Kim, D.; Yoo, S.; Hong, Y.H.; Han, S.Y.; Jeong, S.; Jeong, D.; Kim, J.H.; Cho, J.Y.; Park, J. The skin protective effects of compound K, a metabolite of ginsenoside Rb1 from Panax ginseng. *J. Ginseng Res.* **2018**, *42*, 218–224. [CrossRef]
18. Park, J.S.; Shin, J.A.; Jung, J.S.; Hyun, J.W.; Van Le, T.K.; Kim, D.H.; Park, E.M.; Kim, H.S. Anti-inflammatory mechanism of compound K in activated microglia and its neuroprotective effect on experimental stroke in mice. *J. Pharmacol. Exp. Ther.* **2012**, *341*, 59–67. [CrossRef]
19. Hou, J.G.; Xue, J.J.; Lee, M.R.; Sun, M.Q.; Zhao, X.H.; Zheng, Y.N.; Sung, C.K. Compound K is able to ameliorate the impaired cognitive function and hippocampal neurogenesis following chemotherapy treatment. *Biochem. Biophys. Res. Commun.* **2013**, *436*, 104–109. [CrossRef]
20. Zong, W.; Zeng, X.; Chen, S.; Chen, L.; Zhou, L.; Wang, X.; Gao, Q.; Zeng, G.; Hu, K.; Ouyang, D. Ginsenoside compound K attenuates cognitive deficits in vascular dementia rats by reducing the Abeta deposition. *J. Pharmacol. Sci.* **2019**, *139*, 223–230. [CrossRef]
21. Seo, J.Y.; Ju, S.H.; Oh, J.; Lee, S.K.; Kim, J.S. Neuroprotective and Cognition-Enhancing Effects of Compound K Isolated from Red Ginseng. *J. Agric. Food Chem.* **2016**, *64*, 2855–2864. [CrossRef] [PubMed]
22. Bologna-Molina, R.; Mosqueda-Taylor, A.; Molina-Frechero, N.; Mori-Estevez, A.D.; Sanchez-Acuna, G. Comparison of the value of PCNA and Ki-67 as markers of cell proliferation in ameloblastic tumors. *Med. Oral Patol. Oral Cir. Bucal.* **2013**, *18*, e174–179. [CrossRef] [PubMed]
23. Shohayeb, B.; Diab, M.; Ahmed, M.; Ng, D.C.H. Factors that influence adult neurogenesis as potential therapy. *Transl. Neurodegener.* **2018**, *7*, 4. [CrossRef] [PubMed]
24. Huang, E.J.; Reichardt, L.F. Neurotrophins: roles in neuronal development and function. *Annu. Rev. Neurosci.* **2001**, *24*, 677–736. [CrossRef] [PubMed]

25. Vilar, M.; Mira, H. Regulation of Neurogenesis by Neurotrophins during Adulthood: Expected and Unexpected Roles. *Front. Neurosci.* **2016**, *10*, 26. [CrossRef]
26. Lazarov, O.; Mattson, M.P.; Peterson, D.A.; Pimplikar, S.W.; van Praag, H. When neurogenesis encounters aging and disease. *Trends Neurosci.* **2010**, *33*, 569–579. [CrossRef]
27. Moreno-Jimenez, E.P.; Flor-Garcia, M.; Terreros-Roncal, J.; Rabano, A.; Cafini, F.; Pallas-Bazarra, N.; Avila, J.; Llorens-Martin, M. Adult hippocampal neurogenesis is abundant in neurologically healthy subjects and drops sharply in patients with Alzheimer's disease. *Nat. Med.* **2019**, *25*, 554–560. [CrossRef]
28. Teixeira, C.M.; Pallas-Bazarra, N.; Bolos, M.; Terreros-Roncal, J.; Avila, J.; Llorens-Martin, M. Untold New Beginnings: Adult Hippocampal Neurogenesis and Alzheimer's Disease. *J. Alzheimers Dis.* **2018**, *64*, S497–S505. [CrossRef]
29. Van Praag, H.; Christie, B.R.; Sejnowski, T.J.; Gage, F.H. Running enhances neurogenesis, learning, and long-term potentiation in mice. *Proc. Natl. Acad. Sci. USA* **1999**, *96*, 13427–13431. [CrossRef]
30. Lee, J.; Seroogy, K.B.; Mattson, M.P. Dietary restriction enhances neurotrophin expression and neurogenesis in the hippocampus of adult mice. *J. Neurochem.* **2002**, *80*, 539–547. [CrossRef]
31. Scharfman, H.; Goodman, J.; Macleod, A.; Phani, S.; Antonelli, C.; Croll, S. Increased neurogenesis and the ectopic granule cells after intrahippocampal BDNF infusion in adult rats. *Exp. Neurol.* **2005**, *192*, 348–356. [CrossRef] [PubMed]
32. Quesseveur, G.; David, D.J.; Gaillard, M.C.; Pla, P.; Wu, M.V.; Nguyen, H.T.; Nicolas, V.; Auregan, G.; David, I.; Dranovsky, A.; et al. BDNF overexpression in mouse hippocampal astrocytes promotes local neurogenesis and elicits anxiolytic-like activities. *Transl. Psychiatry* **2013**, *3*, e253. [CrossRef] [PubMed]
33. Ockel, M.; Lewin, G.R.; Barde, Y.A. In vivo effects of neurotrophin-3 during sensory neurogenesis. *Development* **1996**, *122*, 301–307. [PubMed]
34. Shimazu, K.; Zhao, M.; Sakata, K.; Akbarian, S.; Bates, B.; Jaenisch, R.; Lu, B. NT-3 facilitates hippocampal plasticity and learning and memory by regulating neurogenesis. *Learn. Mem.* **2006**, *13*, 307–315. [CrossRef] [PubMed]
35. Blurton-Jones, M.; Kitazawa, M.; Martinez-Coria, H.; Castello, N.A.; Muller, F.J.; Loring, J.F.; Yamasaki, T.R.; Poon, W.W.; Green, K.N.; LaFerla, F.M. Neural stem cells improve cognition via BDNF in a transgenic model of Alzheimer disease. *Proc. Natl. Acad. Sci. USA* **2009**, *106*, 13594–13599. [CrossRef] [PubMed]
36. Nagahara, A.H.; Merrill, D.A.; Coppola, G.; Tsukada, S.; Schroeder, B.E.; Shaked, G.M.; Wang, L.; Blesch, A.; Kim, A.; Conner, J.M.; et al. Neuroprotective effects of brain-derived neurotrophic factor in rodent and primate models of Alzheimer's disease. *Nat. Med.* **2009**, *15*, 331–337. [CrossRef]
37. Li, Y.; Luikart, B.W.; Birnbaum, S.; Chen, J.; Kwon, C.H.; Kernie, S.G.; Bassel-Duby, R.; Parada, L.F. TrkB regulates hippocampal neurogenesis and governs sensitivity to antidepressive treatment. *Neuron* **2008**, *59*, 399–412. [CrossRef]
38. Bruel-Jungerman, E.; Veyrac, A.; Dufour, F.; Horwood, J.; Laroche, S.; Davis, S. Inhibition of PI3K-Akt signaling blocks exercise-mediated enhancement of adult neurogenesis and synaptic plasticity in the dentate gyrus. *PLoS One* **2009**, *4*, e7901. [CrossRef]
39. Jiang, P.; Zhu, T.; Xia, Z.; Gao, F.; Gu, W.; Chen, X.; Yuan, T.; Yu, H. Inhibition of MAPK/ERK signaling blocks hippocampal neurogenesis and impairs cognitive performance in prenatally infected neonatal rats. *Eur. Arch. Psychiatry Clin. Neurosci.* **2015**, *265*, 497–509. [CrossRef]
40. Tang, G.; Dong, X.; Huang, X.; Huang, X.J.; Liu, H.; Wang, Y.; Ye, W.C.; Shi, L. A natural diarylheptanoid promotes neuronal differentiation via activating ERK and PI3K-Akt dependent pathways. *Neuroscience* **2015**, *303*, 389–401. [CrossRef]

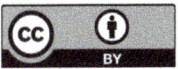

© 2020 by the authors. Licensee MDPI, Basel, Switzerland. This article is an open access article distributed under the terms and conditions of the Creative Commons Attribution (CC BY) license (http://creativecommons.org/licenses/by/4.0/).

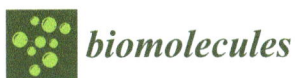

Review

Pro-Resolving Effect of Ginsenosides as an Anti-Inflammatory Mechanism of *Panax ginseng*

Dong-Soon Im [1,2]

1. Laboratory of Pharmacology, College of Pharmacy, Kyung Hee University, 26 Kyungheedae-ro, Dongdaemun-gu, Seoul 02447, Korea; imds@khu.ac.kr; Tel.: +82-2-961-9377; Fax: +82-2-961-9580
2. Department of Life and Nanopharmaceutical Sciences, Graduate School, Kyung Hee University, 26 Kyungheedae-ro, Dongdaemun-gu, Seoul 02447, Korea

Received: 25 February 2020; Accepted: 11 March 2020; Published: 13 March 2020

Abstract: *Panax ginseng*, also known as Korean ginseng, is a famous medicinal plant used for the treatment of many inflammatory diseases. Ginsenosides (ginseng saponins) are the main class of active constituents of ginseng. The anti-inflammatory effects of ginseng extracts were proven with purified ginsenosides, such as ginsenosides Rb1, Rg1, Rg3, and Rh2, as well as compound K. The negative regulation of pro-inflammatory cytokine expressions (TNF-α, IL-1β, and IL-6) and enzyme expressions (iNOS and COX-2) was found as the anti-inflammatory mechanism of ginsenosides in M1-polarized macrophages and microglia. Recently, another action mechanism emerged explaining the anti-inflammatory effect of ginseng. This is a pro-resolution of inflammation derived by M2-polarized macrophages. Direct and indirect evidence supports how several ginsenosides (ginsenoside Rg3, Rb1, and Rg1) induce the M2 polarization of macrophages and microglia, and how these M2-polarized cells contribute to the suppression of inflammation progression and promotion of inflammation resolution. In this review, the new action mechanism of ginseng anti-inflammation is summarized.

Keywords: ginsenoside; anti-inflammation; pro-resolving; ginseng; macrophage; M2 polarization

---

1. Introduction—Ginseng

Ginseng, the root of *Panax ginseng* C.A. Meyer, was used for thousands of years as a tonic herb that provides numerous benefits in Asian countries like Korea and China [1]. As *Panax* means "heals all" in Greek, the effects of ginseng are the longevity and replenishment of vital energy in traditional Chinese medicine [1–3]. In the modern era, ginseng attracts great interest because of its various pharmacological and therapeutic effects on aging, cancer, the cardiovascular system, diabetes, immune-regulatory function, and inflammation [4–8]. There are various components in ginseng, including ginsenosides, gintonin, polysaccharides, polypeptides, glycoconjugate compounds, and other compounds [1]. Over the last decade, extensive studies elucidated ginsenosides (ginseng saponins) as the chief active constituents of ginseng, especially with regard to anti-inflammatory effects [1]. As shown in Figure 1, many papers with two keywords in their abstracts were retrieved, i.e., ginseng plus inflammation (658 papers) or ginsenoside plus inflammation (274 papers), in a public database, PubMed (https://www.ncbi.nlm.nih.gov/pubmed). Since 2010, the number of papers on ginsenosides and inflammation increased.

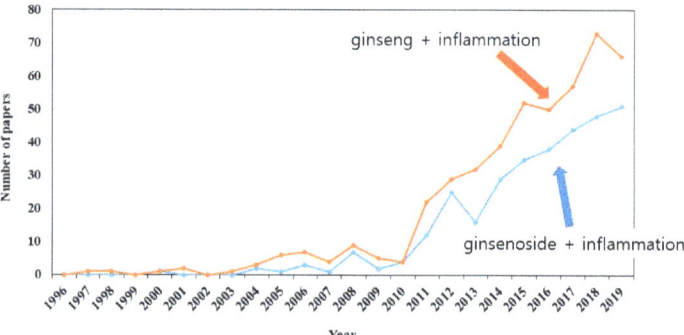

Figure 1. Annual changes in the number of published papers on ginseng, ginsenoside, and inflammation.

2. Ginsenosides in Anti-Inflammation

Inflammation is part of the immunological response in the body to infection or injury, and it is associated with numerous human diseases and conditions [9]. A dynamic balance between pro-inflammatory cytokines (TNF-α and IL-1β) and anti-inflammatory cytokines (IL-2, IL-4, and IL-10) modulates the status of inflammation, while an imbalance or overwhelming production of pro-inflammatory cytokines subsequently results in inflammation-related diseases such as diabetes, cancer, cardiovascular disease, and neurological diseases [10,11]. Inflammation is also essential in the process of repairing tissue and restoring tissue homeostasis [10,11].

Ginsenosides—dammarane-type triterpene glycosides—are the representative active ingredients of ginseng [2]. Almost 100 different types of ginsenosides were isolated from the roots of Korean and American ginseng [12]. Ginsenosides are expressed by Rx, where x is determined by the distance from the origin of thin-layer chromatography [10]. The most polar segment is marked as A and the least polar one is marked as H [10]. Ginsenosides are generally divided into three groups: protopanaxadiols, protopanaxatriols, and oleanane (ginsenoside Ro). Protopanaxadiols have sugar moieties on the C-3 position of dammarane-type triterpene, such as ginsenosides Rb1, Rb2, Rb3, Rc, Rd, Rg3, Rh2, and Rh3. Protopanaxatriols have sugar moieties on the C-6 position of dammarane-type triterpene, such as ginsenosides Re, Rf, Rg1, Rg2, and Rh1 [10,11,13].

The anti-inflammatory effects of ginseng extracts were proven with purified ginsenosides. The negative regulation of pro-inflammatory cytokine expressions (TNF-α, IL-1β, and IL-6) and enzyme expressions (iNOS and COX-2) was found as the anti-inflammatory mechanism of ginsenosides in M1-polarized macrophages and microglia (Figure 2) [10,11]. Among them, the most commonly studied ginsenosides are Rb1, Rg1, Rg3, Re, Rd, and Rh1 [11]. Kim et al. published a review on the role of ginsenosides in inflammatory responses and diseases [10]. The reported pharmacology and signal transduction are well summarized for each ginsenoside, i.e., ginsenosides Rb1, Rb2, Rd, Re, Rg1, Rg3, Rg5, Rh1, Rh2, and Rp1, sulfated Rh2, and compound K [10]. This paper provides an update on the more anti-inflammatory ginsenosides, such as ginsenosides Rc, Rf, Rg5, Rg6, Rh3, Rk1, Ro, and Rz1, as well as ginseng glycopeptides, and it also summarizes a mechanistic viewpoint in anti-inflammatory ginseng pharmacology.

Ginsenoside Rc was found to show the highest inhibitory activity against the expression of TNF-α, IL-1, and IFNs, and it attenuated inflammatory symptoms in type II collagen-induced arthritis, ethanol/HCl-mediated gastritis, and LPS/D-galactosamine-triggered hepatitis [14]. Ginsenoside Rc was also found to exert anti-inflammatory actions by means of suppressing TANK-binding kinase 1/IκB kinase ε/interferon regulatory factor-3 and p38/ATF-2 signaling [15]. Furthermore, ginsenoside Rc significantly enhanced glucose uptake in C2C12 myotubes by inducing ROS generation, which leads to AMPK and p38 MAPK activation, suggesting its potential as an anti-diabetic agent [16]. Later, Kim et al. found that ginsenoside Rc modulates forkhead box O (FoxO1) phosphorylation through the activation of PI3K/Akt and inhibition of AMPK and FoxO1 acetylation, leading to an upregulation of catalase under conditions of oxidative stress in HEK293 cells [17].

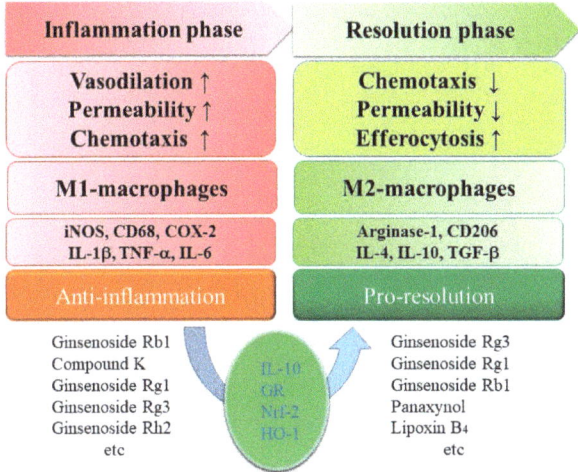

Figure 2. Summarized effects of ginsenosides on M1- and M2-polarized macrophages during inflammatory and resolving phases.

Ginsenoside Rf showed an inhibitory effect on the inflammatory mediators downstream of p38/NF-κB activation, such as the reduction of IL-1β, IL-6, TNF-α, NO, and ROS productions, on TNF-α-stimulated HT-29 intestinal epithelial cells and RAW264.7 mouse macrophage cells [18]. Moreover, its anti-inflammatory activity, along with ginsenoside Rb1 and Rg1, was reported, and anti-oxidation and the inhibition of NO synthesis were proposed as its mechanism [19,20].

Ginsenoside Rf could significantly attenuate Aβ-induced apoptosis in N2A cells, accelerate Aβ clearance, and reduce Aβ level in N2A cells stably transfected with human Swedish mutant APP695 [21]. Daily treatment with ginsenoside Rf improved spatial learning and memory in an Aβ$_{42}$-induced mouse model of Alzheimer's disease [21]. In a surgically induced rat endometriosis model, ginsenoside Rf could decrease the volume of endometriotic implants and the writhing response [22]. Expression levels of VEGF and inflammation-related iNOS, IL-6, IL-1β, and TNF-α were significantly downregulated in the ginsenoside Rf-treated group in a dose-dependent manner [22]. In a rat nerve injury-induced neuropathic pain model, chronic ginsenoside Rf treatment partially reversed the upregulation of pro-inflammatory cytokines in the spinal cord and/or the dorsal root ganglion, but elevated IL-10, an anti-inflammatory factor [23].

Ginsenoside Rg6, a rare ginsenoside from ginseng, was found to have a significant immunosuppressive function on TLR4-induced systemic inflammatory responses, i.e., LPS-induced septic shock, cecal ligation and puncture-induced sepsis [24]. Mechanistically, ginsenoside Rg6 augmented IL-10 expression in bone marrow-derived macrophages, whereas it inhibited NF-κB activation and MAP kinases via induction of miR-146a, an operator microRNA (miRNA) for anti-inflammation [24].

Ginsenosides Rz1, Rk1, and Rg5 were present in heat-treated ginseng in a ratio of 1:2:6 [25]. These converted ginsenosides from primary protopanaxdiol ginsenosides significantly inhibited COX-2 and iNOS gene expression and inhibited TNF-α-induced NF-κB expression [26].

Ginsenoside Rk1 was studied as a mixture form with ginsenoside Rg5 in a 1:1 weight ratio for its effects on atopic dermatitis. In the study, the mixture of ginsenoside Rg5:Rk1 attenuated TNF-α/IFN-γ-induced phosphorylation of p38 MAPK, STAT1, and NF-κB/IKKβ in HaCaT cells and decreased LPS-mediated NO and ROS production in RAW264.7 macrophages [27]. Ginsenoside

Rk1 also inhibited LPS-induced expression of NO, IL-6, IL-1β, TNF-α, and MCP-1 by means of blocking the activation of NF-κB and the Jak2/Stat3 pathway in RAW264.7 cells [28]. Ginsenoside Rk1 was also found to exhibit a strong inhibitory effect on arachidonic acid-induced platelet aggregation [29]. Decreased productions of thromboxane B_2, a key element in platelet aggregation, and 12-hydroxy-5,8,10,14-eicosatetraenoic acid (12-HETE), an arachidonic acid metabolite, were observed in the ginsenoside Rk1-treated platelets via inhibition of COX activity and 12-lipoxygenase translocation resulting from decreased Ca^{2+} levels [29].

Ginsenoside Ro, an oleanane-type saponin, inhibited an increase in vascular permeability in mice, induced by acetic acid, and it reduced acute paw edema in rats induced by compound 48/80 or carrageenan, without suppressing edema in arthritic rats [30]. In experimental models of acute and chronic hepatitis, ginsenoside Ro inhibited the increase of serum AST and ALT levels in D-galactosamine- and CCl_4-induced acute hepatitic rats [31]. Ginsenoside Ro could also suppress IL-1β-induced apoptosis of rat chondrocytes by inhibiting levels of Bax and Bad, decreasing p53 phosphorylation, and promoting the expression of Bcl-xL and PCNA [32]. Ginsenoside Ro also alleviated IL-1β-induced inflammation and matrix degradation by downregulating the expression of MMP 3, MMP 9, and COX-2, and inhibited NF-κB p65 phosphorylation, suggesting its potential for the treatment of osteoarthritis [32]. Recently, ginsenoside Ro was found to decrease inflammatory NO synthase and COX-2 expression induced by LPS and to increase the expression of heme oxygenase-1 (HO-1) in a dose-dependent manner in RAW264.7 macrophages [33].

Ginseng glycopeptides were tested in inflammatory pain models induced by carrageenan and rat pain models induced by Faure Marin [34]. Glycoproteins extracted from ginseng have a molecular weight in the range of 0.4 to 4.4 kDa. Significant differences were found in IL-1β, IL-2, IL-4, TNF-α, and histamine via the treatment of glycoproteins. In the Morris water maze test, the glycopeptides effectively alleviated the memory impairment symptoms of rats induced by $Aβ_{25-35}$, and they showed significant protective activity against the apoptosis of SH-SY5Y neuronal cells induced by $Aβ_{25-35}$ [35].

For the mechanism of ginseng anti-inflammation, several targets were proposed: (1) activation of the glucocorticoid receptor, the target of steroidal anti-inflammatory drugs such as cortisol and dexamethasone (compound K, ginsenosides Rg1 and Re) [36–39]; (2) an anti-oxidation-related mechanism, i.e., inhibition of ROS production and activation of Nrf-2 and HO-1 (compound K, ginsenosides Rg1, Rb1, Ro, and Rg5) [27,33,36,40–42]; (3) blocking of TLR4 interaction with LPS (ginsenosides Re and Rg5) [43,44]; (4) activation of anti-inflammatory PPARγ (ginsenosides Rg3, Re, Rb1, Rg1, and Rf) [40,45–50].

3. Ginsenosides in Pro-Resolution

Macrophages that are widely distributed play an indispensable role in homeostasis and defense as part of the immune system [51,52]. They can be polarized phenotypically by the microenvironment to mount specific functional programs [51,52]. The polarization of mononuclear phagocytes is a useful simplified conceptual framework, describing a continuum of functional states classified according to their phenotypes [51,52]. Classically activated macrophages are called M1-polarized macrophages. Prototypical stimuli are IFN-γ and LPS. Alternatively activated macrophages are called M2-polarized macrophages. Depending on the stimuli, they are subdivided into M2a, M2b, and M2c, induced after exposure to IL-4 or IL-13 (M2a), to immune complexes in combination with IL-1β or LPS (M2b), and to IL-10, TGF-β, or glucocorticoids (M2c), respectively [51,52]. M2-polarized macrophages play a role in the resolution of inflammation through high endocytic clearance capacities and trophic factor synthesis, as well as reduced pro-inflammatory cytokine production (Figure 2) [51,52]. Resolution of inflammation is now considered to be an active process driven by M2-polarized macrophages [53,54]. There are three constituents in ginseng reported to drive M2 polarization, i.e., ginsenosides Rg3, Rb1, and Rg1.

Based on the induction of M2 macrophage polarization, ginsenoside Rg3 was identified as a pro-resolving ginsenoside. Ginsenoside Rg3 not only induced the expression of arginase-1 (a representative M2 marker gene), but also suppressed M1 marker genes, such as inducible NO synthase and NO levels [55]. Previously, anti-inflammatory effects of ginsenoside Rg3 were reported in M1 activated macrophages. Ginsenoside Rg3 suppressed NO, ROS, and prostaglandin E_2 (PGE_2) productions induced by LPS in RAW264.7 macrophages in a concentration-dependent manner [56]. Moreover, ginsenoside Rg3 suppressed matrix MMP 9 activity, COX-2 expression, and pro-inflammatory cytokine production, such as TNF-α, IL-1β, and IL-6 [56]. Similarly, enhanced ginsenoside Rg3 significantly suppressed the expression of IFN-γ and TBX21 in T cells under Th1-skewing conditions [57]. Furthermore, oral administration of enhanced ginsenoside Rg3 suppressed the frequency of Th1 cells in the Peyer's patch and lamina propria cells in vivo [57]. Ginsenoside Rg3-enriched red ginseng extract potently suppressed NO production in murine RAW 264.7 macrophages, without any cytotoxicity across dosages. Additionally, it inhibited the mRNA expression of pro-inflammatory mediators and cytokines such as iNOS, COX-2, IL-1β, IL-6, and TNF-α [58]. Therefore, ginsenoside Rg3 was reported as an anti-inflammatory constituent in M1-polarized macrophages and in vivo conditions. Recently, ginsenoside Rg3 induction of M2 polarization in mouse peritoneal macrophages was initially reported by Kang et al. among 11 tested ginsenosides (Rb1, Rb2, Rc, Rd, Re, Rf, Rg1, Rg2, Rg3, Rh2, and Ro) [55].

In a zymosan-induced peritonitis model, the pro-resolving activity of ginsenoside Rg3 was confirmed in vivo [55]. When ginsenoside Rg3 was administered at peak inflammatory response (12 h after zymosan treatment) into the peritoneal cavity, it accelerated the resolution process, i.e., the rapid disappearance of immune cells. Therefore, ginsenoside Rg3 induces the M2 polarization of macrophages in vitro and accelerates the resolution of inflammation in vivo [55]. Ginsenosides Rg1 and Rh2 were also reported to induce arginase-1 expression in the peritoneal macrophages in a concentration-dependent manner up to 5 μM [55].

In another study, Guo et al. showed a similar observation [59]. Treatment of advanced glycation end products promoted the expression of M1 markers (iNOS and CD86) and pro-inflammatory molecules, whereas ginsenoside Rg3 reversed the M1 polarization to the M2 phenotype expressing arginase 1 and CD206 (i.e., mannose receptor), two M2 markers in vitro [59]. The administration of ginsenoside Rg3 promoted atherosclerotic plaque stability, which was accompanied by increased M2 phenotype macrophages and reduced M1 phenotype macrophages in the plaque [59]. By means of a PPARγ antagonist, GW9662, the important role of PPARγ pathways was suggested in mediating ginsenoside Rg3 effects in macrophage polarization and atherosclerotic plaque stability [59].

Well-known pro-resolving lipids are arachidonic acid-derived lipoxins (lipoxin B_4 and lipoxin A_4) and ω-3 polyunsaturated fatty acid-derived resolvins, protectin, and maresins [53,54]. Previously, ginsenoside Rg3 was reported to increase the level of lipoxin B_4 and to decrease various prostaglandins and HETEs, implying the pro-resolution and anti-inflammatory action of ginsenoside Rg3 [56].

Treatment with ginsenoside Rb1 induced expression of the classic M2 macrophage markers (arginase-1 and CD206), while expression of the M1 macrophage marker, iNOS, was suppressed in primary peritoneal macrophages [60]. Ginsenoside Rb1-induced M2 polarization was found to be achieved partly by the production of IL-4 and/or IL-13 and STAT6 phosphorylation [60]. In an ApoE-deficient atherosclerosis model, the administration of ginsenoside Rb1 increased the M2 macrophage phenotype in atherosclerotic plaque and promoted atherosclerotic lesion stability [60].

Ginsenoside Rg1 significantly improved chemotherapy-induced cognitive impairment-like behavior in the water maze test and suppressed chemotherapy-induced elevation of the pro-inflammatory cytokines TNF-α and IL-6 [61]. In addition, it increased the levels of the anti-inflammatory cytokines IL-4 and IL-10 in multiple sera and brain tissues, and it also inhibited chemotherapy-induced microglial polarization from M2 to M1 phenotypes [61]. Chemotherapy caused an increase in IL-6-labeled M1 microglia, but a decrease in the expression of arginase 1-labeled M2 microglia in both brain tissues and cultured microglial cells [61]. However, ginsenoside Rg1 co-treatment inhibited microglial polarization from M2 to M1 phenotype [61], supporting the observation of peritoneal macrophage M2 polarization by ginsenoside Rg1 [55].

4. Perspective

As mentioned above, three ginsenosides were found to induce M2 polarization of macrophages or microglia, resulting in pro-resolving and anti-inflammatory effects. Based on the available literature, a possibility that more ginsenosides may induce M2 polarization was found. The assumption was based on the following indirect evidence: (1) IL-10 production or glucocorticoid receptor activation could induce M2 polarization, and (2) the anti-oxidative Nrf2–HO-1 pathway could induce M2 polarization.

Because exposure to IL-4, IL-10, or glucocorticoids could induce a type of M2-polarized macrophage [51,52], the previously reported induction of anti-inflammatory cytokine IL-10 by ginsenosides Rg6, Rb1, Rc, Rd, Re, Rf, Rg1, Rh1, Rh2, and Rp1, as well as compound K [14,23,24,41,61–67], or activation of glucocorticoid receptors by compound K, ginsenosides Rg1, and Re [36–39] may imply that those ginsenosides could partly induce the resolution of inflammation through M2 polarization.

Ginsenoside Ro was found not only to inhibit ROS production but also to induce HO-1 expression in RAW264.7 macrophages, with the induction of HO-1 being correlated with decreased pro-inflammatory molecules such as iNOS and COX-2 induced by LPS [33]. Because HO-1 induction could drive the phenotypic shift to M2 macrophages [68], the anti-inflammatory effect of ginsenoside Ro may also be mediated through M2 macrophage polarization.

Nrf2 is a key transcription factor to control the basal and inducible expression of more than 200 genes including antioxidants [69,70]. Nrf2 activation suppressed a set of pro-inflammatory cytokines including iNOS, MCP-1, and MIP-1β while minimally regulating NF-κB activity and the expression of its downstream cytokines, such as IL-6, IL-1β, and TNF-α in macrophages [71]. Recently, Nrf2 activation was linked to M2 polarization in macrophages [72,73]. Panaxynol, one of the major polyacetylenes, was found to be a potent Nrf2 activator, and it activated Nrf2 post-transcriptionally by inhibiting Keap-1-mediated degradation [74]. Therefore, panaxynol suppression of cytokine expression via the activation of Nrf2 may imply that its activation of Nrf2 may induce M2 polarization to exert anti-inflammation [74]. Because HO-1 is one of the target genes of Nrf2, and both Nrf2 and HO-1 could drive M2 polarization, the Nrf2–HO-1 pathway might be considered as a regulatory set for M2 polarization. Furthermore, ginsenoside Rd protected the heart against ischemia/reperfusion injury via enhanced expression of Nrf2 and HO-1 [75]. Additionally, ginsenoside Rd was found to induce CD4$^+$ Foxp3$^+$ CD25$^+$ regulatory T-cell (Treg) differentiation by upregulating Foxp3 expression, and it increased the generation of IL-10, TGF-β1, and IL-35, suggesting that ginsenoside Rd may have the potential to modulate M2 polarization [13]. Ginsenoside Re enhanced the activation of Nrf2 in Aβ-induced SH-SY5Y cells [76]. The activation of the Nrf2–HO-1 pathway for M2 macrophage polarization is also supported by the findings that a red ginseng-derived saponin fraction suppressed inflammatory responses via the Nrf2–HO-1 pathway in an adipocyte–macrophage co-culture system [42], and that saponins from *Panax notoginseng* acted as an extrinsic regulator that activates the Nrf2 antioxidant defense system and inhibits NF-κB inflammatory signaling to attenuate LPS-induced monocyte adhesion on cerebral endothelial cells [77].

As mentioned in Section 1, ginsenosides and ginseng were extensively studied for anti-inflammatory effects in the last decade [1]. Researchers mainly focused on M1-polarized macrophages and microglia to elucidate the negative regulation of pro-inflammatory cytokine expressions (TNF-α, IL-1β, and IL-6) and enzyme expressions (iNOS and COX-2), such as LPS-stimulated RAW264.7 macrophages or BV2 microglia. The resolution of inflammation derived by M2-polarized macrophages is now emerging, with a contribution to the anti-inflammatory mechanism. It will be noteworthy to determine the merged or fused mechanisms of the ginseng anti-inflammatory system in the future.

Funding: This research was supported by the Basic Science Research Program of the Korean National Research Foundation funded by the Korean Ministry of Education, Science, and Technology (NRF-2019R1A2C1005523).

Conflicts of Interest: The author has no conflict of interest to declare. The funder had no role in the writing of the manuscript.

Abbreviations

AMPK 5′—adenosine monophosphate-activated protein kinase, ATF-2—activating transcription factor-2, COX-2—cyclooxygenase 2, FoxO1—forkhead box O1, GR—glucocorticoid receptor, HO-1—heme oxygenase-1, IFN—interferon, IL-1β—interleukin-1β, iNOS—inducible nitric oxide synthase, LPS—lipopolysaccharide, MCP-1—monocyte chemoattractant protein-1, NF-κB—nuclear factor κ-B, Nrf2—nuclear factor erythroid 2-related factor 2, PPARγ—peroxisome proliferator-activating receptor γ, ROS—reactive oxygen species, TGFβ—transforming growth factor β, TLR4—Toll-like receptor 4, TNF-α—tumor necrosis factor-α.

References

1. Im, D.S.; Nah, S.Y. Yin and Yang of ginseng pharmacology: ginsenosides vs. gintonin. *Acta Pharmacol. Sin.* **2013**, *34*, 1367–1373. [CrossRef]
2. Nah, S.Y.; Kim, D.H.; Rhim, H. Ginsenosides: are any of them candidates for drugs acting on the central nervous system? *CNS Drug Rev.* **2007**, *13*, 381–404. [CrossRef]
3. Choi, K.T. Botanical characteristics, pharmacological effects and medicinal components of Korean *Panax ginseng* C A Meyer. *Acta Pharmacol. Sin.* **2008**, *29*, 1109–1118. [CrossRef] [PubMed]
4. Kim, J.H. Pharmacological and medical applications of *Panax ginseng* and ginsenosides: a review for use in cardiovascular diseases. *J. Ginseng Res.* **2018**, *42*, 264–269. [CrossRef] [PubMed]
5. Liu, J.; Nile, S.H.; Xu, G.; Wang, Y.; Kai, G. Systematic exploration of *Astragalus membranaceus* and *Panax ginseng* as immune regulators: Insights from the comparative biological and computational analysis. *Phytomedicine* **2019**, 153077. [CrossRef] [PubMed]
6. Gui, Q.F.; Xu, Z.R.; Xu, K.Y.; Yang, Y.M. The Efficacy of Ginseng-Related Therapies in Type 2 Diabetes Mellitus: An Updated Systematic Review and Meta-analysis. *Medicine (Baltimore)* **2016**, *95*, e2584. [CrossRef]
7. Ong, W.Y.; Farooqui, T.; Koh, H.L.; Farooqui, A.A.; Ling, E.A. Protective effects of ginseng on neurological disorders. *Front. Aging Neurosci.* **2015**, *7*, 129. [CrossRef]
8. Majeed, F.; Malik, F.Z.; Ahmed, Z.; Afreen, A.; Afzal, M.N.; Khalid, N. Ginseng phytochemicals as therapeutics in oncology: Recent perspectives. *Biomed. Pharmacother.* **2018**, *100*, 52–63. [CrossRef]
9. Ferrero-Miliani, L.; Nielsen, O.H.; Andersen, P.S.; Girardin, S.E. Chronic inflammation: importance of NOD2 and NALP3 in interleukin-1b generation. *Clin. Exp. Immunol.* **2007**, *147*, 227–235. [CrossRef]
10. Kim, J.H.; Yi, Y.S.; Kim, M.Y.; Cho, J.Y. Role of ginsenosides, the main active components of *Panax ginseng*, in inflammatory responses and diseases. *J. Ginseng Res.* **2017**, *41*, 435–443. [CrossRef]
11. Lu, J.M.; Yao, Q.; Chen, C. Ginseng compounds: an update on their molecular mechanisms and medical applications. *Curr. Vasc. Pharmacol.* **2009**, *7*, 293–302. [CrossRef] [PubMed]
12. Nag, S.A.; Qin, J.J.; Wang, W.; Wang, M.H.; Wang, H.; Zhang, R. Ginsenosides as Anticancer Agents: *In vitro* and *in vivo* Activities, Structure-Activity Relationships, and Molecular Mechanisms of Action. *Front. Pharmacol.* **2012**, *3*, 25. [CrossRef] [PubMed]
13. Kim, J.; Byeon, H.; Im, K.; Min, H. Effects of ginsenosides on regulatory T cell differentiation. *Food Sci. Biotechnol.* **2018**, *27*, 227–232. [CrossRef] [PubMed]
14. Yu, T.; Rhee, M.H.; Lee, J.; Kim, S.H.; Yang, Y.; Kim, H.G.; Kim, Y.; Kim, C.; Kwak, Y.S.; Kim, J.H.; et al. Ginsenoside Rc from Korean Red Ginseng (*Panax ginseng* C.A. Meyer) Attenuates Inflammatory Symptoms of Gastritis, Hepatitis and Arthritis. *Am. J. Chin. Med.* **2016**, *44*, 595–615. [CrossRef] [PubMed]
15. Yu, T.; Yang, Y.; Kwak, Y.S.; Song, G.G.; Kim, M.Y.; Rhee, M.H.; Cho, J.Y. Ginsenoside Rc from *Panax ginseng* exerts anti-inflammatory activity by targeting TANK-binding kinase 1/interferon regulatory factor-3 and p38/ATF-2. *J. Ginseng Res.* **2017**, *41*, 127–133. [CrossRef]
16. Lee, M.S.; Hwang, J.T.; Kim, S.H.; Yoon, S.; Kim, M.S.; Yang, H.J.; Kwon, D.Y. Ginsenoside Rc, an active component of *Panax ginseng*, stimulates glucose uptake in C2C12 myotubes through an AMPK-dependent mechanism. *J. Ethnopharmacol.* **2010**, *127*, 771–776. [CrossRef]

17. Kim, D.H.; Park, C.H.; Park, D.; Choi, Y.J.; Park, M.H.; Chung, K.W.; Kim, S.R.; Lee, J.S.; Chung, H.Y. Ginsenoside Rc modulates Akt/FoxO1 pathways and suppresses oxidative stress. *Arch. Pharm. Res.* **2014**, *37*, 813–820. [CrossRef]
18. Ahn, S.; Siddiqi, M.H.; Aceituno, V.C.; Simu, S.Y.; Yang, D.C. Suppression of MAPKs/NF-kB Activation Induces Intestinal Anti-Inflammatory Action of Ginsenoside Rf in HT-29 and RAW264.7 Cells. *Immunol. Investig.* **2016**, *45*, 439–449. [CrossRef]
19. Zhou, P.; Lu, S.; Luo, Y.; Wang, S.; Yang, K.; Zhai, Y.; Sun, G.; Sun, X. Attenuation of TNF-a-Induced Inflammatory Injury in Endothelial Cells by Ginsenoside Rb1 via Inhibiting NF-kB, JNK and p38 Signaling Pathways. *Front. Pharmacol.* **2017**, *8*, 464. [CrossRef]
20. Kim, M.K.; Kang, H.; Baek, C.W.; Jung, Y.H.; Woo, Y.C.; Choi, G.J.; Shin, H.Y.; Kim, K.S. Antinociceptive and anti-inflammatory effects of ginsenoside Rf in a rat model of incisional pain. *J. Ginseng Res.* **2018**, *42*, 183–191. [CrossRef]
21. Du, Y.; Fu, M.; Wang, Y.T.; Dong, Z. Neuroprotective Effects of Ginsenoside Rf on Amyloid-b-Induced Neurotoxicity *in vitro* and *in vivo*. *J. Alzheimers Dis.* **2018**, *64*, 309–322. [CrossRef] [PubMed]
22. Qin, X.; Liu, Y.; Feng, Y.; Jiang, J. Ginsenoside Rf alleviates dysmenorrhea and inflammation through the BDNF-TrkB-CREB pathway in a rat model of endometriosis. *Food Funct.* **2019**, *10*, 244–249. [CrossRef] [PubMed]
23. Li, Y.; Chen, C.; Li, S.; Jiang, C. Ginsenoside Rf relieves mechanical hypersensitivity, depression-like behavior, and inflammatory reactions in chronic constriction injury rats. *Phytother. Res.* **2019**, *33*, 1095–1103. [CrossRef] [PubMed]
24. Paik, S.; Choe, J.H.; Choi, G.E.; Kim, J.E.; Kim, J.M.; Song, G.Y.; Jo, E.K. Rg6, a rare ginsenoside, inhibits systemic inflammation through the induction of interleukin-10 and microRNA-146a. *Sci. Rep.* **2019**, *9*, 4342. [CrossRef]
25. Lee, S.M.; Shon, H.J.; Choi, C.S.; Hung, T.M.; Min, B.S.; Bae, K. Ginsenosides from heat processed ginseng. *Chem. Pharm. Bull. (Tokyo)* **2009**, *57*, 92–94. [CrossRef]
26. Lee, S.M. Anti-inflammatory effects of ginsenosides Rg5, Rz1, and Rk1: inhibition of TNF-a-induced NF-kB, COX-2, and iNOS transcriptional expression. *Phytother. Res.* **2014**, *28*, 1893–1896. [CrossRef]
27. Ahn, S.; Siddiqi, M.H.; Aceituno, V.C.; Simu, S.Y.; Zhang, J.; Jimenez Perez, Z.E.; Kim, Y.J.; Yang, D.C. Ginsenoside Rg5:Rk1 attenuates TNF-a/IFN-g-induced production of thymus- and activation-regulated chemokine (TARC/CCL17) and LPS-induced NO production via downregulation of NF-kB/p38 MAPK/STAT1 signaling in human keratinocytes and macrophages. *In Vitro Cell. Dev. Biol. Anim.* **2016**, *52*, 287–295. [CrossRef]
28. Yu, Q.; Zeng, K.W.; Ma, X.L.; Jiang, Y.; Tu, P.F.; Wang, X.M. Ginsenoside Rk1 suppresses pro-inflammatory responses in lipopolysaccharide-stimulated RAW264.7 cells by inhibiting the Jak2/Stat3 pathway. *Chin. J. Nat. Med.* **2017**, *15*, 751–757. [CrossRef]
29. Ju, H.K.; Lee, J.G.; Park, M.K.; Park, S.J.; Lee, C.H.; Park, J.H.; Kwon, S.W. Metabolomic investigation of the anti-platelet aggregation activity of ginsenoside Rk(1) reveals attenuated 12-HETE production. *J. Proteome Res.* **2012**, *11*, 4939–4946. [CrossRef]
30. Matsuda, H.; Samukawa, K.; Kubo, M. Anti-inflammatory activity of ginsenoside Ro. *Planta Med.* **1990**, *56*, 19–23. [CrossRef]
31. Matsuda, H.; Samukawa, K.; Kubo, M. Anti-hepatitic activity of ginesenoside ro1. *Planta Med.* **1991**, *57*, 523–526. [CrossRef] [PubMed]
32. Zhang, X.H.; Xu, X.X.; Xu, T. Ginsenoside Ro suppresses interleukin-1b-induced apoptosis and inflammation in rat chondrocytes by inhibiting NF-kB. *Chin. J. Nat. Med.* **2015**, *13*, 283–289. [PubMed]
33. Kim, S.; Oh, M.H.; Kim, B.S.; Kim, W.I.; Cho, H.S.; Park, B.Y.; Park, C.; Shin, G.W.; Kwon, J. Upregulation of heme oxygenase-1 by ginsenoside Ro attenuates lipopolysaccharide-induced inflammation in macrophage cells. *J. Ginseng Res.* **2015**, *39*, 365–370. [CrossRef] [PubMed]
34. Luo, H.; Zhu, D.; Wang, Y.; Chen, Y.; Jiang, R.; Yu, P.; Qiu, Z. Study on the Structure of Ginseng Glycopeptides with Anti-Inflammatory and Analgesic Activity. *Molecules* **2018**, *23*, 1325. [CrossRef] [PubMed]
35. Luo, H.; Hu, J.; Wang, Y.; Chen, Y.; Zhu, D.; Jiang, R.; Qiu, Z. *In vivo* and *in vitro* neuroprotective effects of *Panax ginseng* glycoproteins. *Int. J. Biol. Macromol.* **2018**, *113*, 607–615. [CrossRef]

36. Cuong, T.T.; Yang, C.S.; Yuk, J.M.; Lee, H.M.; Ko, S.R.; Cho, B.G.; Jo, E.K. Glucocorticoid receptor agonist compound K regulates Dectin-1-dependent inflammatory signaling through inhibition of reactive oxygen species. *Life Sci.* **2009**, *85*, 625–633. [CrossRef]
37. Yang, C.S.; Ko, S.R.; Cho, B.G.; Shin, D.M.; Yuk, J.M.; Li, S.; Kim, J.M.; Evans, R.M.; Jung, J.S.; Song, D.K.; et al. The ginsenoside metabolite compound K, a novel agonist of glucocorticoid receptor, induces tolerance to endotoxin-induced lethal shock. *J. Cell. Mol. Med.* **2008**, *12*, 1739–1753. [CrossRef]
38. Leung, K.W.; Cheng, Y.K.; Mak, N.K.; Chan, K.K.; Fan, T.P.; Wong, R.N. Signaling pathway of ginsenoside-Rg1 leading to nitric oxide production in endothelial cells. *FEBS Lett.* **2006**, *580*, 3211–3216. [CrossRef]
39. Leung, K.W.; Leung, F.P.; Huang, Y.; Mak, N.K.; Wong, R.N. Non-genomic effects of ginsenoside-Re in endothelial cells via glucocorticoid receptor. *FEBS Lett.* **2007**, *581*, 2423–2428. [CrossRef]
40. Yang, Y.; Li, X.; Zhang, L.; Liu, L.; Jing, G.; Cai, H. Ginsenoside Rg1 suppressed inflammation and neuron apoptosis by activating PPARg/HO-1 in hippocampus in rat model of cerebral ischemia-reperfusion injury. *Int. J. Clin. Exp. Pathol.* **2015**, *8*, 2484–2494.
41. Chen, C.; Zhang, H.; Xu, H.; Zheng, Y.; Wu, T.; Lian, Y. Ginsenoside Rb1 ameliorates cisplatin-induced learning and memory impairments. *J. Ginseng Res.* **2019**, *43*, 499–507. [CrossRef] [PubMed]
42. Kim, C.Y.; Kang, B.; Suh, H.J.; Choi, H.S. Red ginseng-derived saponin fraction suppresses the obesity-induced inflammatory responses via Nrf2-HO-1 pathway in adipocyte-macrophage co-culture system. *Biomed. Pharmacother.* **2018**, *108*, 1507–1516. [CrossRef] [PubMed]
43. Lee, I.A.; Hyam, S.R.; Jang, S.E.; Han, M.J.; Kim, D.H. Ginsenoside Re ameliorates inflammation by inhibiting the binding of lipopolysaccharide to TLR4 on macrophages. *J. Agric. Food Chem.* **2012**, *60*, 9595–9602. [CrossRef] [PubMed]
44. Kim, T.W.; Joh, E.H.; Kim, B.; Kim, D.H. Ginsenoside Rg5 ameliorates lung inflammation in mice by inhibiting the binding of LPS to toll-like receptor-4 on macrophages. *Int. Immunopharmacol.* **2012**, *12*, 110–116. [CrossRef] [PubMed]
45. Kwok, H.H.; Guo, G.L.; Lau, J.K.; Cheng, Y.K.; Wang, J.R.; Jiang, Z.H.; Keung, M.H.; Mak, N.K.; Yue, P.Y.; Wong, R.N. Stereoisomers ginsenosides-20(S)-Rg(3) and -20(R)-Rg(3) differentially induce angiogenesis through peroxisome proliferator-activated receptor-g. *Biochem. Pharmacol.* **2012**, *83*, 893–902. [CrossRef]
46. Cao, G.; Su, P.; Zhang, S.; Guo, L.; Zhang, H.; Liang, Y.; Qin, C.; Zhang, W. Ginsenoside Re reduces Ab production by activating PPARg to inhibit BACE1 in N2a/APP695 cells. *Eur. J. Pharmacol.* **2016**, *793*, 101–108. [CrossRef]
47. Mu, Q.; Fang, X.; Li, X.; Zhao, D.; Mo, F.; Jiang, G.; Yu, N.; Zhang, Y.; Guo, Y.; Fu, M.; et al. Ginsenoside Rb1 promotes browning through regulation of PPARg in 3T3-L1 adipocytes. *Biochem. Biophys. Res. Commun.* **2015**, *466*, 530–535. [CrossRef]
48. Shang, W.; Yang, Y.; Jiang, B.; Jin, H.; Zhou, L.; Liu, S.; Chen, M. Ginsenoside Rb1 promotes adipogenesis in 3T3-L1 cells by enhancing PPARg2 and C/EBPa gene expression. *Life Sci.* **2007**, *80*, 618–625. [CrossRef]
49. Zhang, L.; Zhu, M.; Li, M.; Du, Y.; Duan, S.; Huang, Y.; Lu, Y.; Zhang, J.; Wang, T.; Fu, F. Ginsenoside Rg1 attenuates adjuvant-induced arthritis in rats via modulation of PPAR-g/NF-kB signal pathway. *Oncotarget* **2017**, *8*, 55384–55393.
50. Song, H.; Park, J.; Choi, K.; Lee, J.; Chen, J.; Park, H.J.; Yu, B.I.; Iida, M.; Rhyu, M.R.; Lee, Y. Ginsenoside Rf inhibits cyclooxygenase-2 induction via peroxisome proliferator-activated receptor g in A549 cells. *J. Ginseng Res.* **2019**, *43*, 319–325. [CrossRef]
51. Martinez, F.O.; Sica, A.; Mantovani, A.; Locati, M. Macrophage activation and polarization. *Front. Biosci.* **2008**, *13*, 453–461. [CrossRef]
52. Gordon, S.; Martinez, F.O. Alternative activation of macrophages: mechanism and functions. *Immunity* **2010**, *32*, 593–604. [CrossRef] [PubMed]
53. Ariel, A.; Serhan, C.N. New Lives Given by Cell Death: Macrophage Differentiation Following Their Encounter with Apoptotic Leukocytes during the Resolution of Inflammation. *Front. Immunol.* **2012**, *3*, 4. [CrossRef] [PubMed]
54. Serhan, C.N. Discovery of specialized pro-resolving mediators marks the dawn of resolution physiology and pharmacology. *Mol. Aspects Med.* **2017**, *58*, 1–11. [CrossRef] [PubMed]
55. Kang, S.; Park, S.J.; Lee, A.Y.; Huang, J.; Chung, H.Y.; Im, D.S. Ginsenoside Rg3 promotes inflammation resolution through M2 macrophage polarization. *J. Ginseng Res.* **2018**, *42*, 68–74. [CrossRef] [PubMed]

56. Lee, J.W.; Choi, Y.R.; Mok, H.J.; Seong, H.A.; Lee, D.Y.; Kim, G.S.; Yoon, J.H.; Kim, K.P.; Kim, H.D. Characterization of the changes in eicosanoid profiles of activated macrophages treated with 20(S)-ginsenoside Rg3. *J. Chromatogr. B Analyt. Technol. Biomed. Life Sci.* **2017**, *1065–1066*, 14–19. [CrossRef]
57. Cho, M.; Choi, G.; Shim, I.; Chung, Y. Enhanced Rg3 negatively regulates Th1 cell responses. *J. Ginseng Res.* **2019**, *43*, 49–57. [CrossRef]
58. Saba, E.; Jeong, D.; Irfan, M.; Lee, Y.Y.; Park, S.J.; Park, C.K.; Rhee, M.H. Anti-Inflammatory Activity of Rg3-Enriched Korean Red Ginseng Extract in Murine Model of Sepsis. *Evid. Based Complement. Alternat. Med.* **2018**, *2018*, 6874692. [CrossRef]
59. Guo, M.; Xiao, J.; Sheng, X.; Zhang, X.; Tie, Y.; Wang, L.; Zhao, L.; Ji, X. Ginsenoside Rg3 Mitigates Atherosclerosis Progression in Diabetic apoE-/- Mice by Skewing Macrophages to the M2 Phenotype. *Front. Pharmacol.* **2018**, *9*, 464. [CrossRef]
60. Zhang, X.; Liu, M.H.; Qiao, L.; Zhang, X.Y.; Liu, X.L.; Dong, M.; Dai, H.Y.; Ni, M.; Luan, X.R.; Guan, J.; et al. Ginsenoside Rb1 enhances atherosclerotic plaque stability by skewing macrophages to the M2 phenotype. *J. Cell. Mol. Med.* **2018**, *22*, 409–416. [CrossRef]
61. Shi, D.D.; Huang, Y.H.; Lai, C.S.W.; Dong, C.M.; Ho, L.C.; Li, X.Y.; Wu, E.X.; Li, Q.; Wang, X.M.; Chen, Y.J.; et al. Ginsenoside Rg1 Prevents Chemotherapy-Induced Cognitive Impairment: Associations with Microglia-Mediated Cytokines, Neuroinflammation, and Neuroplasticity. *Mol. Neurobiol.* **2019**, *56*, 5626–5642. [CrossRef] [PubMed]
62. Yang, Z.; Chen, A.; Sun, H.; Ye, Y.; Fang, W. Ginsenoside Rd elicits Th1 and Th2 immune responses to ovalbumin in mice. *Vaccine* **2007**, *25*, 161–169. [CrossRef] [PubMed]
63. Su, X.; Pei, Z.; Hu, S. Ginsenoside Re as an adjuvant to enhance the immune response to the inactivated rabies virus vaccine in mice. *Int. Immunopharmacol.* **2014**, *20*, 283–289. [CrossRef] [PubMed]
64. Joh, E.H.; Lee, I.A.; Jung, I.H.; Kim, D.H. Ginsenoside Rb1 and its metabolite compound K inhibit IRAK-1 activation–the key step of inflammation. *Biochem. Pharmacol.* **2011**, *82*, 278–286. [CrossRef]
65. Lee, S.Y.; Jeong, J.J.; Eun, S.H.; Kim, D.H. Anti-inflammatory effects of ginsenoside Rg1 and its metabolites ginsenoside Rh1 and 20(S)-protopanaxatriol in mice with TNBS-induced colitis. *Eur. J. Pharmacol.* **2015**, *762*, 333–343. [CrossRef]
66. Hsieh, Y.H.; Deng, J.S.; Chang, Y.S.; Huang, G.J. Ginsenoside Rh2 Ameliorates Lipopolysaccharide-Induced Acute Lung Injury by Regulating the TLR4/PI3K/Akt/mTOR, Raf-1/MEK/ERK, and Keap1/Nrf2/HO-1 Signaling Pathways in Mice. *Nutrients* **2018**, *10*, 1208.
67. Bae, J.; Koo, J.; Kim, S.; Park, T.Y.; Kim, M.Y. Ginsenoside Rp1 Exerts Anti-inflammatory Effects via Activation of Dendritic Cells and Regulatory T Cells. *J. Ginseng Res.* **2012**, *36*, 375–382. [CrossRef]
68. Naito, Y.; Takagi, T.; Higashimura, Y. Heme oxygenase-1 and anti-inflammatory M2 macrophages. *Arch. Biochem. Biophys.* **2014**, *564*, 83–88. [CrossRef]
69. Kensler, T.W.; Wakabayashi, N.; Biswal, S. Cell survival responses to environmental stresses via the Keap1-Nrf2-ARE pathway. *Annu. Rev. Pharmacol. Toxicol.* **2007**, *47*, 89–116. [CrossRef]
70. Suzuki, T.; Yamamoto, M. Stress-sensing mechanisms and the physiological roles of the Keap1-Nrf2 system during cellular stress. *J. Biol. Chem.* **2017**, *292*, 16817–16824. [CrossRef]
71. Li, B.; Abdalrahman, A.; Lai, Y.; Janicki, J.S.; Ward, K.W.; Meyer, C.J.; Wang, X.L.; Tang, D.; Cui, T. Dihydro-CDDO-trifluoroethyl amide suppresses inflammatory responses in macrophages via activation of Nrf2. *Biochem. Biophys. Res. Commun.* **2014**, *444*, 555–561. [CrossRef] [PubMed]
72. Feng, R.; Morine, Y.; Ikemoto, T.; Imura, S.; Iwahashi, S.; Saito, Y.; Shimada, M. Nrf2 activation drive macrophages polarization and cancer cell epithelial-mesenchymal transition during interaction. *Cell Commun. Signal.* **2018**, *16*, 54. [CrossRef] [PubMed]
73. Wei, J.; Chen, G.; Shi, X.; Zhou, H.; Liu, M.; Chen, Y.; Feng, D.; Zhang, P.; Wu, L.; Lv, X. Nrf2 activation protects against intratracheal LPS induced mouse/murine acute respiratory distress syndrome by regulating macrophage polarization. *Biochem. Biophys. Res. Commun.* **2018**, *500*, 790–796. [CrossRef]
74. Qu, C.; Li, B.; Lai, Y.; Li, H.; Windust, A.; Hofseth, L.J.; Nagarkatti, M.; Nagarkatti, P.; Wang, X.L.; Tang, D.; et al. Identifying panaxynol, a natural activator of nuclear factor erythroid-2 related factor 2 (Nrf2) from American ginseng as a suppressor of inflamed macrophage-induced cardiomyocyte hypertrophy. *J. Ethnopharmacol.* **2015**, *168*, 326–336. [CrossRef] [PubMed]

75. Zeng, X.; Li, J.; Li, Z. Ginsenoside Rd mitigates myocardial ischemia-reperfusion injury via Nrf2/HO-1 signaling pathway. *Int. J. Clin. Exp. Med.* **2015**, *8*, 14497–14504. [PubMed]
76. Liu, M.; Bai, X.; Yu, S.; Zhao, W.; Qiao, J.; Liu, Y.; Zhao, D.; Wang, J.; Wang, S. Ginsenoside Re Inhibits ROS/ASK-1 Dependent Mitochondrial Apoptosis Pathway and Activation of Nrf2-Antioxidant Response in b-Amyloid-Challenged SH-SY5Y Cells. *Molecules* **2019**, *24*, 2687. [CrossRef]
77. Hu, S.; Liu, T.; Wu, Y.; Yang, W.; Hu, S.; Sun, Z.; Li, P.; Du, S. *Panax notoginseng* saponins suppress lipopolysaccharide-induced barrier disruption and monocyte adhesion on bEnd.3 cells via the opposite modulation of Nrf2 antioxidant and NF-kB inflammatory pathways. *Phytother. Res.* **2019**, *33*, 3163–3176. [CrossRef]

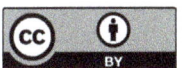

© 2020 by the author. Licensee MDPI, Basel, Switzerland. This article is an open access article distributed under the terms and conditions of the Creative Commons Attribution (CC BY) license (http://creativecommons.org/licenses/by/4.0/).

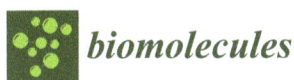

Article

Comparison of Ginsenoside Components of Various Tissues of New Zealand Forest-Grown Asian Ginseng (*Panax Ginseng*) and American Ginseng (*Panax Quinquefolium* L.)

Wei Chen [1,2,3], Prabhu Balan [2,3] and David G Popovich [1,*]

1. School of Food and Advanced Technology, Massey University, Palmerston North 4442, New Zealand; w.chen2@massey.ac.nz
2. Riddet Institute, Massey University, Palmerston North 4442, New Zealand; p.balan@massey.ac.nz
3. Alpha-Massey Natural Nutraceutical Research Centre, Massey University, Palmerston North 4442, New Zealand
* Correspondence: D.G.Popovich@massey.ac.nz; Tel.: +64-6356-9099

Received: 18 February 2020; Accepted: 27 February 2020; Published: 28 February 2020

Abstract: Asian ginseng (*Panax ginseng*) and American ginseng (*Panax quinquefolium* L.) are the two most important ginseng species for their medicinal properties. Ginseng is not only popular to consume, but is also increasingly popular to cultivate. In the North Island of New Zealand, Asian ginseng and American ginseng have been grown in Taupo and Rotorua for more than 15 years. There are no publications comparing the chemical constituents between New Zealand-grown Asian ginseng (NZPG) and New Zealand-grown American ginseng (NZPQ). In this study, fourteen ginsenoside reference standards and LC–MS^2 technology were employed to analyze the ginsenoside components of various parts (fine root, rhizome, main root, stem, and leaf) from NZPG and NZPQ. Fifty and 43 ginsenosides were identified from various parts of NZPG and NZPQ, respectively, and 29 ginsenosides were found in both ginseng species. Ginsenoside concentrations in different parts of ginsengs were varied. Compared to other tissues, the fine roots contained the most abundant ginsenosides, not only in NZPG (142.49 ± 1.14 mg/g) but also in NZPQ (115.69 ± 3.51 mg/g). For the individual ginsenosides of both NZPG and NZPQ, concentration of Rb1 was highest in the underground parts (fine root, rhizome, and main root), and ginsenoside Re was highest in the aboveground parts (stem and leaf).

Keywords: Asian ginseng; American ginseng; *Panax ginseng*; *Panax quinquefolium* L.; ginsenosides

1. Introduction

Ginseng is a perennial herb and belongs to the genus *Panax* (Araliaceae family). There are more than twelve species of ginseng characterized in the genus *Panax*. Among them, Asian ginseng and American ginseng are the two most well-known species and are commonly used for their medicinal properties [1]. Asian ginseng (*Panax ginseng*) root has been used widely as a significant source of natural medicine for thousands of years in East Asia, particularly in China, Korea, and Japan. American ginseng (*Panax quinquefolium* L.), mainly grown in North America, is also well-known in Asian countries. As important Chinese medicine resources, Asian ginseng and American ginseng are considered to possess different properties in clinical applications. Asian ginseng, especially Korean red ginseng, has a warming effect and reinforces 'qi' to promote 'yang' energy, which benefits the spleen and lungs [2], and it was found to modulate the intestinal ecosystem and enhance the gut function [3]. American ginseng is viewed as having a cooling effect and can tonify 'qi' to nourish 'yin' energy, which means it can remove 'heat' and promote the production of body fluids [4]. These functional varieties may be due to differences in chemical composition, particularly in the bioactive triterpenoid saponins, popularly known as ginsenosides [5].

Ginsenosides, also known as triterpenoid saponins with a four-ring skeleton structure, are unique to ginseng species. So far, nearly 200 ginsenosides have been identified in Asian ginseng, and more than 100 in American ginseng; 49 ginsenosides coexist in both plant species [6]. Most of them are classified as members of the dammarane family, including the protopanaxadiol (PPD) type and protopanaxatriol (PPT) type. In chemical analysis of ginseng, ginsenosides Rb1, Rb2, Rb3, Rc, Rd, Re, Rf, Rg1, and p-F11 are the most important compounds to be quantified due to their abundant content in ginseng plants. Among these compounds, ginsenoside Rf is considered to be only present in Asian ginseng, while ginsenoside p-F11 is considered to be only found in American ginseng [7]. Therefore, ginsenosides Rf and p-F11 are used as marker compounds to differentiate Asian ginseng and American ginseng [5,8]. There are some articles about the component analysis of Asian ginseng and American ginseng; they mainly focus on how to differentiate the two ginseng species [9] or the constituent analysis of ginseng roots [10,11]. To our knowledge, there have been no comprehensive analyses of the ginsenoside components of ginseng tissues (fine root, rhizome, main root, stem, and leaf) between Asian ginseng and American ginseng. Furthermore, the vast majority of ginseng used in ginseng studies has been grown in the Northern Hemisphere; there are few reports about how ginseng grows in the Southern Hemisphere, such as those varieties in New Zealand.

New Zealand has a unique geographical environment, with features such as cold winters, temperate summers, adequate rainfall, unique volcanic pumice soil, and high-intensity UV rays. Summer solar radiation in New Zealand is on average 7% higher compared to an equivalent latitude in the Northern Hemisphere [12]. These factors may affect the accumulation and distribution of ginsenosides in ginseng plants. Our previous study found that the average content of total ginsenosides from New Zealand-grown *Panax ginseng* is significantly higher than that of ginseng grown in China or Korea [13]. In this study, we used LC–MS^2 technology to analyze the ginsenoside components of various parts from New Zealand-grown Asian ginseng (NZPG) and New Zealand-grown American ginseng (NZPQ). To our knowledge, this is the first article focusing on ginsenoside component analysis of ginseng tissues between Asian ginseng and American ginseng, particularly for New Zealand-grown ginseng.

2. Materials and Methods

2.1. Ginseng Samples

Eight-year-old Asian ginseng and American ginseng plants were harvested in November 2017 from a Taupo (New Zealand) pine forest. Five parts including fine root (root hair), rhizome (neck between root and stem), main root (root body), stem, and leaf of Asian ginseng and American ginseng were separated, rinsed with water, and lyophilized at –68 °C. The dried ginseng tissues were then powdered using a CG2B coffee grinder (Breville).

2.2. Chemicals and Reagents

Fourteen reference standards of ginsenosides Rb1, Rb2, Rb3, Rc, Rd, Re, Rf, Rg1, Rg2, Rg3, Rh1, Rh2, F2, and 24(R)-pseudoginsenoside F11 (p-F11) were purchased from Star Ocean Ginseng Ltd. (Suzhou, China). The purities of the fourteen standards were no less than 98.0%. Their structures are shown in Figure 1. LC–MS-grade acetonitrile (MeCN) and water were supplied by Merck (Phillipsburg, NJ, USA). LC-grade methanol (MeOH) and formic acid (HCOOH) were purchased from Fisher Chemical (Pittsburgh, PA, USA). Water (for extraction) was obtained from a Milli-Q Ultra-pure water system (Millipore, Billerica, MA, USA). Other reagents used in this study were of analytical grade.

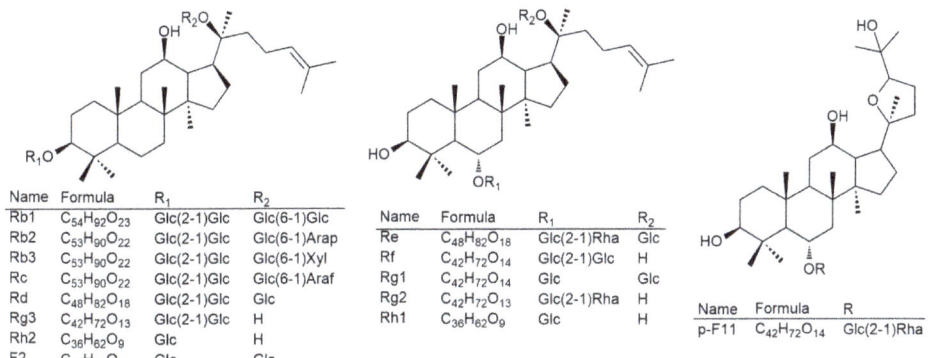

Figure 1. The chemical structures of 14 ginsenoside reference standards.

2.3. Preparation of Samples and Reference Standards

Ginsenosides were ultrasonically extracted three times from each part of the Asian ginseng and American ginseng using a Q700 sonicator (Qsonica, Melville, NY, USA) according to our previous methods [13,14]. Briefly, the fine root, rhizome, main root, stem, and leaf were separately extracted by 70% (v/v) aqueous MeOH at 20 kHz for 10 min at no more than 40 °C. (The extraction was programed for five cycles; each cycle contained ultrasonic extraction at 15% amplitude for 2 min and a cooling period of 1 min between extractions.) The supernatant was collected after centrifugation at 4000 rpm (Thermo Scientific Multifuge 1S-R Centrifuge, Marshall Scientific, Hampton, NH, USA) for 10 min and the sediment was extracted twice more. The three extracts were mixed together and filtered through a 0.22-micron syringe filter before the LC/MS analysis. Fourteen reference standards of ginsenosides Rb1 (0.769 mg/mL), Rb2 (0.846 mg/mL), Rb3 (0.629 mg/mL), Rc (1.077 mg/mL), Rd (0.692 mg/mL), Re (0.923 mg/mL), Rf (1.462 mg/mL), F2 (0.692 mg/mL), p-F11 (0.923 mg/mL), Rg1 (1.154 mg/mL), Rg2 (0.615 mg/mL), Rg3 (1.154 mg/mL), Rh1 (1.000 mg/mL), and Rh2 (1.077 mg/mL) were dissolved and diluted with 70% MeOH to obtain a series of standard solutions of different concentrations. The solutions were filtered through a 0.22-micron syringe filter before the LC–MS^2 analysis.

2.4. High-Performance Liquid Chromatography Coupled with Quadrupole Time-of-Flight Tandem Mass Spectrometry (HPLC-QTOF-MS)

An Agilent 1290 liquid chromatograph (Agilent, Lexington, MA, USA) equipped with an online degasser, a quaternary pump, an auto-sampler, a heated column compartment, a UV detector, and an Agilent 6530 Quadrupole Time-of-Flight Mass Spectrometer (Agilent, Lexington, MA, USA) equipped with an electrospray ionization source were used for LC–MS^2 analysis. The instrument setting was consistent with our previous reports [13,14]. A double end-capped Zorbax Extend-C18 (2.1 × 100 mm, 3.5 μm) column (Agilent, Lexington, MA, USA) was used to separate compounds from the ginseng extract. The column temperature was controlled at 33 °C. The binary gradient eluent consisted of mobile phase A (0.1% formic acid in water) and mobile phase B (0.1% formic acid in acetonitrile). The gradient elution program was as follows: 20% B at 0–4 min, 20–30% B at 6–10 min, 30–32.5% B at 10–25 min, 32.5–60% B at 25–27 min, 60–95% B at 27–39 min, 95% B at 39–40 min. The flow rate was changed with the gradient: 0–27 min, 0.2 mL/min; 27–40 min, 0.25 mL/min. The wavelength was set at 203 nm, and the injected volume was 1 μL. The mass spectrometer data were collected from m/z 100–2200 in negative ion mode, and nitrogen (>99.998%) was used for the nebulizer gas and curtain gas. The gas temperature and flow rate were 350 °C and 10.0 L/min, respectively. The pressure of the nebulizer was 37 psi. The voltages of capillary, fragmentor, and skimmer were 3500 V, 220 V, and 65 V, respectively. The reference masses in negative ion mode were at m/z 121.0509 and 922.0098. The acquisition rates were 4 spectra/s for MS and 1 spectrum/s for MS^2. Mass data were analyzed with

3. Results and Discussion

3.1. Identification of the Detected Ginsenosides in Various Parts of NZPG and NZPQ

To compare the ginsenoside components from various parts of the ginseng plants, Zorbax Extend-C18 column and LC-QTOF-MS/MS were used to separate and determine the ginsenosides extracted from the fine root, rhizome, main root, stem, and leaf of NZPG and NZPQ. Fourteen ginsenosides reference standards (for structures see Figure 1) were used to establish the chromatographic method. The base peak chromatograph (BPC) of the ginsenoside standards is shown in Figure 2. Although ginsenosides Rf and p-F11 are isomeric compounds and have the same retention time, we can differentiate them using mass spectrometry (MS). As shown in Figure 3A,C, ginsenosides Rf and p-F11 had similar [M - H]$^-$ ion at m/z 799.48 and [M + HCOO]$^-$ ion at m/z 845.49 in the negative ESI full scan MS. The abundance of m/z 799.48 [M - H]$^-$ and m/z 845.49 [M + HCOO]$^-$ are almost equal in ginsenoside Rf, while in ginsenoside p-F11, the abundance of m/z 845.59 [M + HCOO]$^-$ is about seven times that of m/z 799.48 [M - H]$^-$. In the MS^2, ginsenosides Rf and p-F11 have the same [M - H]$^-$ ion at m/z 799.48 and distinct product ions at m/z (637.42, 475.38) and (654.42, 491.37), respectively, which were obtained by the successive losses of the two sugar moieties (shown in Figure 3B,D). These distinct ions could be used as the characteristic ions to differentiate and quantify the two ginsenoside isomers.

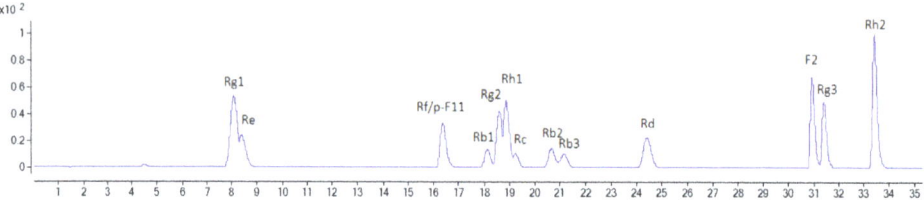

Figure 2. The base peak chromatogram (BPC) of 14 ginsenoside reference standards.

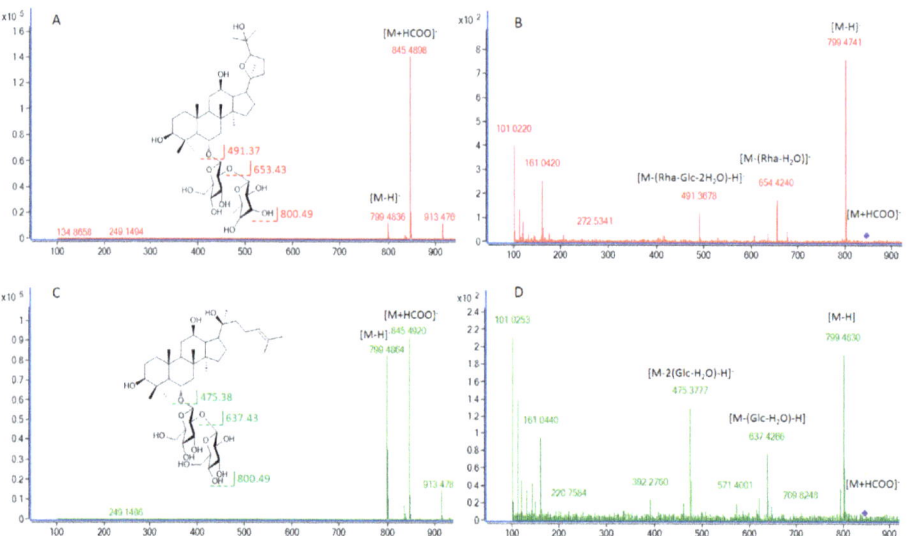

Figure 3. The MS (**A**, **C**) and MS^2 (**B**, **D**) of ginsenosides p-F11 (**A**, **B**) and Rf (**C**, **D**).

The BPC profiles of the various parts of NZPG and NZPQ are shown in Figure 4. A total of 72 potential ginsenosides were detected from the fine root, rhizome, main root, leaf, and stem of NZPG and NZPQ. The potential ginsenosides were identified using the same procedure as our previous report [14]. Briefly, the PPD-type, PPT-type, and oleanolic acid-type ginsenosides could produce [(20S)-protopanaxadiol - H]$^-$ at m/z 459 ($C_{30}H_{51}O_3$), [(20S)-protopanaxatriol - H]$^-$ at m/z 475 ($C_{30}H_{51}O_4$), and [oleanolic acid - H]$^-$ at m/z 455 ($C_{30}H_{47}O_3$) in the negative MS^2 spectra, respectively. Thus, a different type of ginsenoside could be easily differentiated and characterized by finding its [aglycone - H]$^-$. Sugar residues could be identified by calculating the neutral loss molecular mass, for instance, the glucosyl (Glc), rhamnosyl (Rha), and pentosyl [arabinopyranosyl (Arap) or arabinofuranosyl (Araf) or xylosyl (Xyl)] groups correspond to the mass differences of 162, 146, and 132 amu in the MS^2 spectra, respectively. There are some small mass differences, such as 43 and 87 amu, which are mostly acetyl and malonyl groups. These groups are prone to attach with glucose.

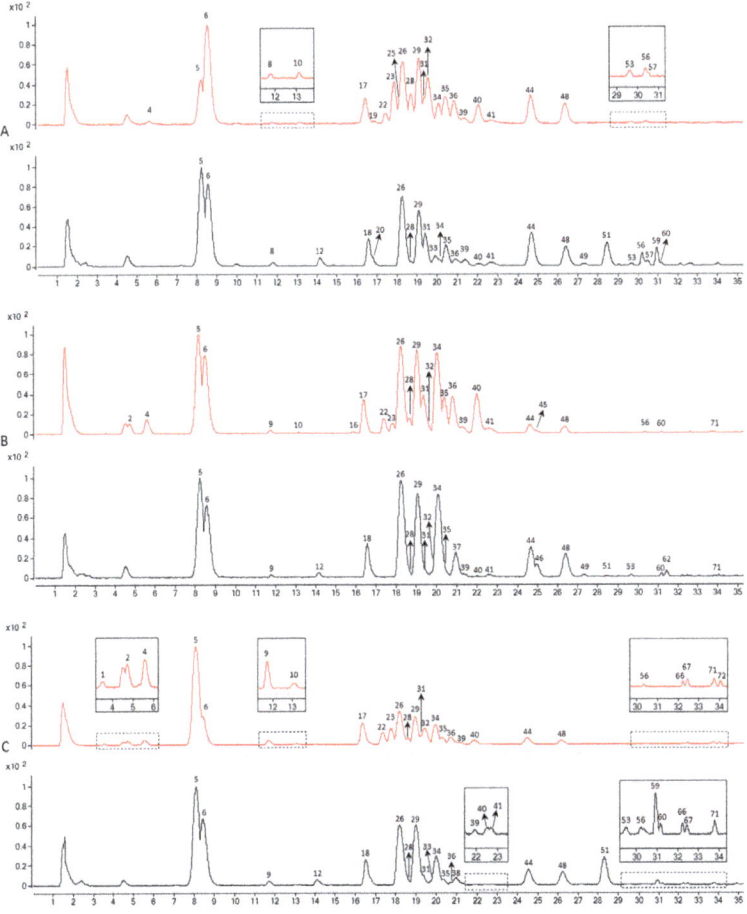

Figure 4. *Cont.*

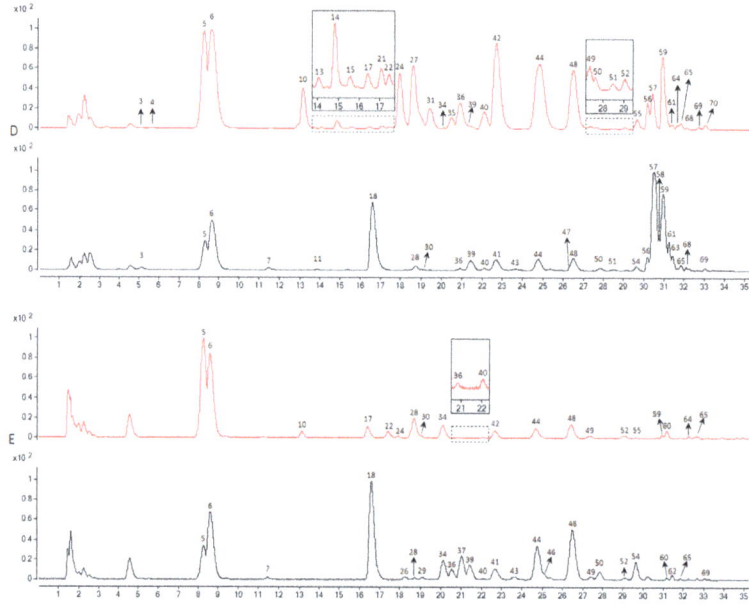

Figure 4. The base peak chromatogram (BPC) profiles of different parts of New Zealand-grown Asian ginseng (NZPG, red line) and New Zealand-grown American ginseng (NZPQ, black line). (**A**) Ginseng fine root, (**B**) ginseng rhizome, (**C**) ginseng main root, (**D**) ginseng leaf, (**E**) ginseng stem.

Fourteen ginsenosides (peaks 5, 6, 17, 18, 26, 28, 30, 31, 36, 39, 44, 59, 61, 70) were unambiguously identified by comparison with their reference standards. The other peaks were allocated by comparing the relative retention time, empirical molecular formulas, and fragmentation information with those in the literature.

The information on 72 detected compounds is summarized in Table 1. Apart from eight unknown compounds, 64 ginsenosides were identified from NZPG and NZPQ. In the ginseng fine root, NZPG and NZPQ contain the same number (26) of ginsenosides, and 18 of them are in both ginsengs (Figure 4A). In the ginseng rhizome, there were 16 ginsenosides found in both ginseng species, and there were 10 and eight ginsenosides found only in NZPG and NZPQ respectively (Figure 4B). As the main source of medicinal material, the chemical constituents of the main root are essential for the pharmacological activity of ginseng. From Figure 4C, we can see that in addition to the common main compounds 5 (Rg1), 6 (Re), 26 (Rb1), 29 (mRb1), 34 (Ro), 44 (Rd), and 48 (mRd) in both ginseng species, NZPG and NZPQ also contain some unique secondary metabolites, such as compounds 17 (Rf), 22 (NG-R2/G-F3/G-F5), and 23 (Ra1/Ra2) in NZPG, and compounds 18 (p-F11), and 51 (Rd isomer) in NZPQ. This may be the reason why Asian ginseng and American ginseng not only have similar bioactive effects, including enhanced physical and sexual functions, general vitality, anti-stress, and anti-aging [4], but also have different medicinal applications. Compared to the underground parts (fine root, rhizome, and main root), ginseng leaf contained more abundant ginsenosides, especially in the less polar areas (Figure 4D). Specifically, 33 and 25 ginsenosides were identified from the leaves of NZPG and NZPQ, respectively; 15 of these ginsenosides were found in both species. In the aboveground parts, there were fewer ginsenosides in stems than in the leaves. Interestingly, NZPQ had more peaks than NZPG had in ginseng stems (Figure 4E), whereas in leaves, NZPG had more peaks than NZPQ. In general, 50 and 43 ginsenosides were identified from various parts of NZPG and NZPQ, respectively, and 29 ginsenosides were found in both ginseng plants. Details about the distribution of ginsenosides are shown in Figure 5.

Table 1. The ginsenosides identified from various parts of New Zealand-grown *Panax ginseng* (PG) and *Panax quinquefolium* L. (PQ).

No.	R.t	Measured Value [ion form]	Formula	Source	Identification	Ref.
1	3.50	815.4775 [M − H]; 861.4822 [M + HCOO]	$C_{42}H_{72}O_{15}$	PG (m)	Ginsenjilinol	[15]
2	4.71	961.5291 [M − H]; 1007.5387 [M + HCOO]	$C_{48}H_{82}O_{19}$	PG (m, r)	20glc-Rf	[11]
3	5.09	931.5215 [M − H]; 977.5257 [M + HCOO]	$C_{47}H_{80}O_{18}$	PG (l); PQ (l)	NG-R1	[11]
4	5.62	931.5162 [M − H]; 977.5212 [M + HCOO]	$C_{47}H_{80}O_{18}$	PG (f, r, m, l)	Re4	[16]
5	8.19	799.4857 [M − H]; 845.4898 [M + HCOO]	$C_{42}H_{72}O_{14}$	PG (f, r, m, s, l); PQ (f, r, m, s, l)	Rg1	std
6	8.55	945.5370 [M − H]; 991.5439 [M + HCOO]	$C_{48}H_{82}O_{18}$	PG (f, r, m, s, l); PQ (f, r, m, s, l)	Re	std
7	11.49	799.4835 [M − H]; 845.4920 [M + HCOO]	$C_{42}H_{72}O_{14}$	PQ (s, l)	Rg1 isomer	[16]
8	11.53	841.4871 [M − H]	$C_{44}H_{74}O_{15}$	PG (f); PQ (f)	Ac-Rg1	[16]
9	11.70	885.4780 [M − H]	$C_{45}H_{74}O_{17}$	PG (m, r); PQ (m, r)	m-Rg1	[11]
10	13.17	1031.5386 [M − H]	$C_{51}H_{84}O_{21}$	PQ (f, r, m, s, l)	m-Re	[11]
11	13.83	799.4821 [M − H]; 845.4770 [M + HCOO]	$C_{42}H_{72}O_{14}$	PQ (l)	Rg1 isomer	[16]
12	14.14	887.4954 [M + HCOO]	$C_{44}H_{74}O_{15}$	PQ (f, m, r)	Yesanchinoside D	[16]
13	14.12	815.4697 [M − H]	$C_{42}H_{72}O_{15}$	PG (l)	Re5	[15]
14	14.81	961.5322 [M − H]; 1007.5338 [M + HCOO]	$C_{48}H_{82}O_{19}$	PG (l)	VG-R4	[17]
15	15.55	829.4839 [M + HCOO]	$C_{42}H_{72}O_{13}$	PG (l)	G-La	[18]
16	15.88	1117.5382 [M − H]	$C_{54}H_{86}O_{24}$	PG (r)	mf-Rd6/isomer	[6]
17	16.40	799.4807 [M − H]; 845.4855 [M + HCOO]	$C_{42}H_{72}O_{14}$	PG (f, r, m, s, l)	Rf	std
18	16.55	799.4772 [M − H]; 845.4862 [M + HCOO]	$C_{42}H_{72}O_{14}$	PQ (f, r, m, s, l)	p-F11	[6]
19	16.84	1325.6255 [M − H]	$C_{62}H_{102}O_{30}$	PG (f)	m-Ra3/m-NG-R4	[6]
20	16.84	653.3698 [M − H]; 699.4271 [M + HCOO]	$C_{36}H_{62}O_{10}$	PQ (f)	G-Kj/G-Km/G-ST2	[16]
21	17.09	799.4497 [M − H]; 845.4817 [M + HCOO]	$C_{42}H_{72}O_{14}$	PG (l)	Rf isomer	[11]
22	17.40	769.4681 [M − H]; 815.4726 [M + HCOO]	$C_{41}H_{70}O_{13}$	PG (f, r, m, s, l)	NG-R2	[16]
23	17.82	1209.6224 [M − H]	$C_{58}H_{98}O_{26}$	PG (f, r, m)	Ra1	[11]
24	17.90	769.4739 [M − H]; 815.4754 [M + HCOO]	$C_{41}H_{70}O_{13}$	PG (s, l)	G-F5	[17]
25	18.02	1239.6273 [M − H]	$C_{59}H_{100}O_{27}$	PG (f)	Ra3/NG-R4	[17]
26	18.22	1107.5929 [M − H]	$C_{54}H_{92}O_{23}$	PG (f, r, m); PQ (f, r, m, s)	Rb1	std
27	18.61	769.4658 [M − H]; 815.4750 [M + HCOO]	$C_{41}H_{70}O_{13}$	PG (l)	G-F3	[17]
28	18.66	783.4858 [M − H]; 829.4930 [M + HCOO]	$C_{42}H_{72}O_{13}$	PG (f, r, m, s); PQ (f, m, s, l)	Rg2	std
29	19.04	1193.5932 [M − H]	$C_{57}H_{94}O_{26}$	PG (f, r, m); PQ (f, r, m, s)	m-Rb1	[11]
30	19.05	683.4329 [M + HCOO]	$C_{36}H_{62}O_{9}$	PG (s); PQ (l)	Rh1	std
31	19.31	1077.5818 [M − H]	$C_{53}H_{90}O_{22}$	PG (f, r, m, l); PQ (f, r, m)	Rc	std
32	19.49	1209.6254 [M − H]	$C_{58}H_{98}O_{26}$	PG (f, r, m)	Ra2	[11]
33	19.75	1193.5849 [M − H]	$C_{57}H_{94}O_{26}$	PQ (f, m)	m-Rb1 isomer	[16]
34	20.01	955.4865 [M − H]	$C_{48}H_{76}O_{19}$	PG (f, r, m, s, l); PQ (f, r, m, s)	Ro	[11]
35	20.38	1163.5798 [M − H]	$C_{56}H_{92}O_{25}$	PG (f, r, m, l); PQ (f, r, m)	m-Rc	[16]
36	20.80	1077.5813 [M − H]	$C_{53}H_{90}O_{22}$	PG (f, r, m, s, l); PQ (f, m, s, l)	Rb2	std
37	20.98	955.4853 [M − H]	$C_{48}H_{76}O_{19}$	PQ (r, s)	Ro isomer	[16]

143

Table 1. *Cont.*

No.	R.t	Measured Value [ion form]	Formula	Source	Identification	Ref.
38	20.95	1193.5892 [M - H]	$C_{57}H_{94}O_{26}$	PQ (m)	m-Rb1 isomer	[16]
39	21.35	1077.5782 [M - H]	$C_{53}H_{90}O_{22}$	PG (f, r, m, l); PQ (f, r, m, s, l)	Rb3	std
40	21.95	1163.5767 [M - H]	$C_{56}H_{92}O_{25}$	PG (f, r, m, s, l); PQ (f, r, m, s, l)	m-Rb2	[11]
41	22.59	1163.5782 [M - H]	$C_{56}H_{92}O_{25}$	PG (f, r, m); PQ (f, r, m, s, l)	m-Rb3	[11]
42	22.69	637.4292 [M - H]; 683.4310 [M + HCOO]	$C_{36}H_{62}O_9$	PQ (s, l)	F1	[17]
43	23.56	1163.5822 [M - H]	$C_{56}H_{92}O_{25}$	PQ (s, l)	m-Rb3 isomer	[16]
44	24.65	945.5364 [M - H]; 991.5469 [M + HCOO]	$C_{48}H_{82}O_{18}$	PG (f, r, m, s, l); PQ (f, r, m, s, l)	Rd	std
45	24.59	1119.5871 [M - H]	$C_{55}H_{92}O_{23}$	PG (r)	Rs1	[19]
46	24.99	793.4306 [M - H]	$C_{42}H_{66}O_{14}$	PQ (r, s)	Zingibroside R1	[11]
47	25.84	1119.5844 [M - H]	$C_{55}H_{92}O_{23}$	PQ (l)	Rs2	[19]
48	26.35	1031.5348 [M - H]	$C_{51}H_{84}O_{21}$	PG (f, r, m, s, l); PQ (f, r, m, s, l)	m-Rd	[11]
49	27.36	987.5413 [M - H]	$C_{50}H_{84}O_{19}$	PG (s, l); PQ (f, r, s)	Ac-Rd	[18]
50	27.76	1031.5348 [M - H]	$C_{51}H_{84}O_{21}$	PG (l); PQ (s, l)	m-Rd isomer	[16]
51	28.41	945.5354 [M - H]; 991.5435 [M + HCOO]	$C_{48}H_{82}O_{18}$	PG (l); PQ (f, r, m, l)	GyXVII	[17]
52	29.12	1117.5369 [M - H]	$C_{54}H_{86}O_{24}$	PG (s, l); PQ (s)	mf-Rd6 isomer	[6]
53	29.56	987.5449 [M - H]	$C_{50}H_{84}O_{19}$	PG (f); PQ (f, r, m)	Ac-Rd isomer	[16]
54	29.63	1117.5314 [M - H]	$C_{54}H_{86}O_{24}$	PQ (s, l)	mf-Rd6 isomer	[6]
55	29.67	987.5436 [M - H]	$C_{50}H_{84}O_{19}$	PG (s, l)	Ac-Rd isomer	[16]
56	30.10	915.5285 [M - H]; 961.5338 [M + HCOO]	$C_{47}H_{80}O_{17}$	PG (f, r, m, l); PQ (f, m, l)	NG-Fe	[17]
57	30.42	915.5226 [M - H]; 961.5279 [M + HCOO]	$C_{47}H_{80}O_{17}$	PG (f, l); PQ (f, l)	VG-R16	[16]
58	30.75	1001.5258 [M + HCOO]	$C_{48}H_{76}O_{19}$	PQ (l)	Ro isomer	[16]
59	30.91	829.4906 [M + HCOO]	$C_{42}H_{72}O_{13}$	PG (s, l); PQ (f, m, l)	F2	std
60	31.15	793.4334 [M - H]	$C_{42}H_{66}O_{14}$	PG (r, s); PQ (f, m, r, s)	Chikusetsusaponin IVa	[11]
61	31.4	783.4806 [M - H]; 829.4874 [M + HCOO]	$C_{42}H_{72}O_{13}$	PG (l); PQ (l)	Rg3	std
62	31.43	793.4301 [M - H]	$C_{42}H_{66}O_{14}$	PQ (r, s)	Chikusetsusaponin IVa isomer	[16]
63	31.43	825.4879 [M - H]; 871.4974 [M + HCOO]	$C_{52}H_{72}O_{11}$	PQ (l)	Unknown	-
64	31.65	675.3529 [M - H]; 721.3579 [M + HCOO]	$C_{40}H_{54}O_9$	PG (s, l)	Unknown	-
65	31.83	675.3505 [M - H]; 721.3589 [M + HCOO]	$C_{40}H_{54}O_9$	PG (s, l); PQ (s, l)	Unknown	-
66	32.23	677.3731 [M - H]; 723.3730 [M + HCOO]	$C_{40}H_{54}O_9$	PG (m); PQ (m)	Unknown	-
67	32.46	677.3743 [M - H]; 723.3746 [M + HCOO]	$C_{40}H_{54}O_9$	PG (m); PQ (m)	Unknown	-
68	32.69	653.3673 [M - H]; 699.3744 [M + HCOO]	$C_{36}H_{62}O_{10}$	PG (l); PQ (l)	G-Kj/G-Km/G-ST2	[6]
69	33.05	513.2942 [M - H]; 559.3044 [M + HCOO]	$C_{27}H_{46}O_9$	PG (l); PQ (s, l)	Unknown	-
70	33.42	667.4373 [M + HCOO]	$C_{36}H_{62}O_8$	PG (l)	Rh2	std
71	33.81	595.2873 [M + HCOO]	$C_{33}H_{42}O_7$	PG (r, m, s); PQ (r, m)	Unknown	-
72	34.05	515.9695 [M - H]; 561.3247 [M + HCOO]	$C_{27}H_{48}O_9$	PG (m)	Unknown	-

Note: f, r, m, s, and l refer to fine root, rhizome, main root, stem, and leaf of ginseng, respectively.

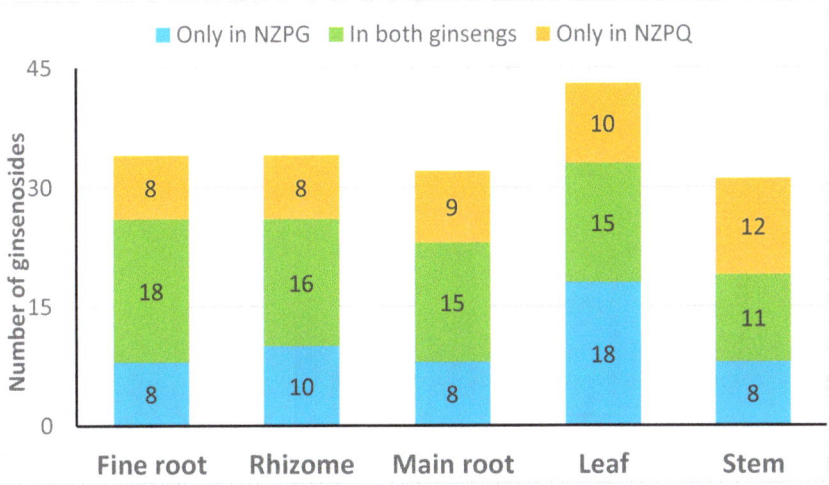

Figure 5. Distribution of ginsenosides in different parts of NZPG and NZPQ.

3.2. Quantification of the Main Ginsenosides in Various Parts of NZPG and NZPQ

To compare the differences in the content of ginsenosides between NZPG and NZPQ, the main ginsenosides in various parts of both ginseng plants were quantified according to our previous methods [14]. Briefly, 14 ginsenosides (Rb1, Rb2, Rb3, Rc, Rd, Re, Rf, p-F11, F2, Rg1, Rg2, Rg3, Rh1, and Rh2) were accurately quantified by their own linear regression equations of standard curves (the regression equations of calibration curves, correlation coefficient, and linear ranges for the ginsenoside standards are shown in supplementary material); some ginsenosides without reference standards, such as ginsenosides mRb1 (m = malonyl), mRb2, mRb3, mRc, mRd, mRe, and mRg1, were relatively quantified by the regression equations of their corresponding neutral ginsenosides.

As shown in Figure 6, ginsenoside concentrations are varied in different ginseng tissues and different ginseng species. The four highest concentration saponins in the underground parts (fine root, rhizome, and main root) are ginsenosides Rb1, mRb1, Re, and Rg1. The ginsenoside contents differ between the two ginseng species. In the fine root (Figure 6A), ginsenoside Rb1 has the highest concentration of saponins in both NZPQ (24.95 ± 2.14 mg/g) and NZPG (27.49 ± 1.57 mg/g). The contents of ginsenosides mRb1, Re, Rg2, Rb2, and mRb2 in NZPG are significantly higher than in NZPQ. The ginsenoside Rg1 content in NZPG is significantly lower than that in NZPQ. In the rhizome (Figure 6B), ginsenosides Rb1, mRb1, Re, and Rg1 have the four highest concentration saponins, and there are no significant differences in their concentrations between NZPQ and NZPG. However, the contents of PPD-type ginsenosides Rc, Rb2, Rb3, and their corresponding malonyl ginsenosides (mRc, mRb2, and mRb3) in NZPG are significantly higher than those in NZPQ. The contents of ginsenosides Rb1, mRb1, Re, and Rd in NZPG are significantly lower than those in NZPQ in the main root (Figure 6C), and the concentrations of ginsenosides Rg1, Rb2, and mRb2 in NZPG are more than those in NZPQ. Compared to the underground parts, the distribution of ginsenosides in the aboveground parts (stem and leaf) is much different. Ginsenoside Re has the highest level of compound in the leaf and stem of both NZPG and NZPQ. Ginsenosides Rd and m-Rd became the second and third highest ingredients in NZPG leaves, while in NZPQ leaves, compound p-F11 became the major constituent, with the concentration ranking just after Re. Interestingly, ginsenosides Rb1 and mRb1, which are the main components in the underground parts, are very low and could not be quantified in some aboveground parts due to the low concentration (Figure 6D,E). As for the total ginsenoside content, the fine roots contain the most abundant ginsenosides not only in NZPG (142.49 ± 1.14 mg/g), but also in NZPQ (115.69 ± 3.51 mg/g); stems have the fewest ginsenosides. From the point of the total amount of ginsenoside, the main roots have similar concentrations between NZPG and NZPQ, while there is greater difference in the aboveground parts, especially in the ginseng leaves of both species (37.40 ± 3.35 mg/g in NZPQ vs. 91.51 ± 7.20 mg/g in NZPG).

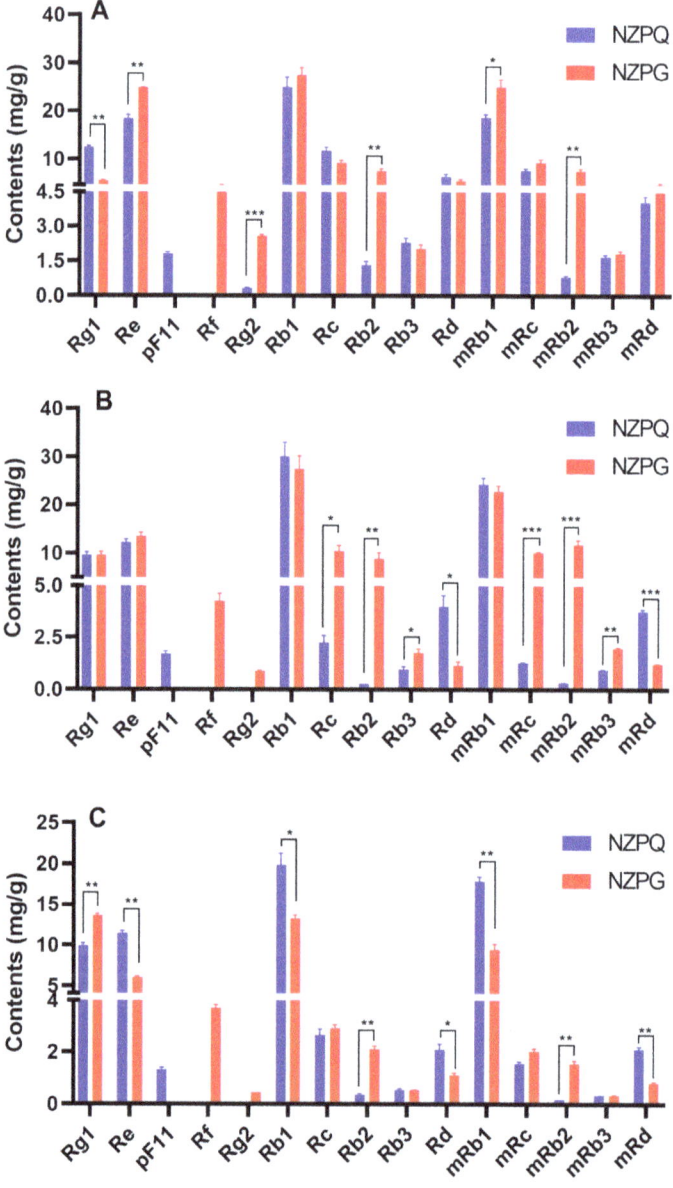

Figure 6. *Cont.*

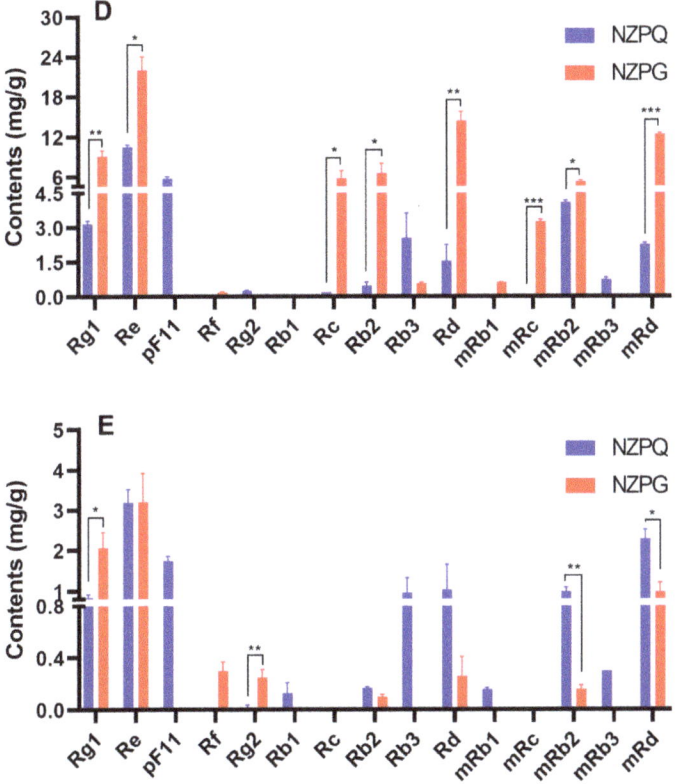

Figure 6. The ginsenoside contents from different parts of NZPQ and NZPG. (**A**) Fine root; (**B**) rhizome; (**C**) main root; (**D**) leaf; (**E**) stem. Data were expressed as mean ± SD and analyzed by t-test using Graph pad 8 software. * $p < 0.05$, ** $p < 0.01$, *** $p < 0.001$. Differences were considered significant if $p < 0.05$.

Apart from the individual ginsenoside content and the total ginsenoside amount, the ratio of PPD-type to PPT-type (PPD/PPT), the ratio of neutral ginsenoside to malonyl ginsenoside (G/m-G), and the ratios of Rb1/Rg1, Rg1/Re, and Rb2/Rc are also described in this study. These ratios in the five ginseng parts vary in both ginseng species. The Rb1/Rg1 of NZPG (4.94 ± 0.31) is much higher ($p < 0.05$) than that of NZPQ (2.01 ± 0.07) in the fine roots (Figure 7A). There are similar ratios of ginsenosides in the rhizome of both ginseng species (Figure 7B). In the main root, the Rb1/Rg1 in NZPG (0.97 ± 0.03) is significantly lower than in NZPQ (2.00 ± 0.11); the ratios of Rg1/Re and Rb2/Rc in NZPG are significantly higher than in NZPQ (Figure 7C). In the aboveground parts, NZPQ (2.67 ± 0.13) has a significantly higher ratio of Rb2/Rc compared to NZPG (1.13 ± 0.09) in the ginseng leaves (Figure 7D), and the ratio of PPD/PPT in NZPQ stems is remarkably higher than that in NZPG stems (Figure 7E).

Consistent with other reports [7], we found ginsenoside Rf only in NZPG, and p-F11 only in NZPQ. They can be used as a reference marker to differentiate between Asian ginseng and American ginseng. We need to note that the two ginsenosides have very similar retention times in HPLC, and often co-elute. Thus, they are easily confused if identifications are made only according to the retention time of compounds. However, ginsenosides Rf and p-F11 can produce unique ions at m/z (637, 475) and (653, 491) in negative MS^2 spectrum, respectively, due to fragmentation differences in their sugar moieties. Therefore, LC–MS^2 can be an effective and sensitive method to identify ginsenoside Rf and p-F11 and further distinguish Asian ginseng and American ginseng, even without reference standards.

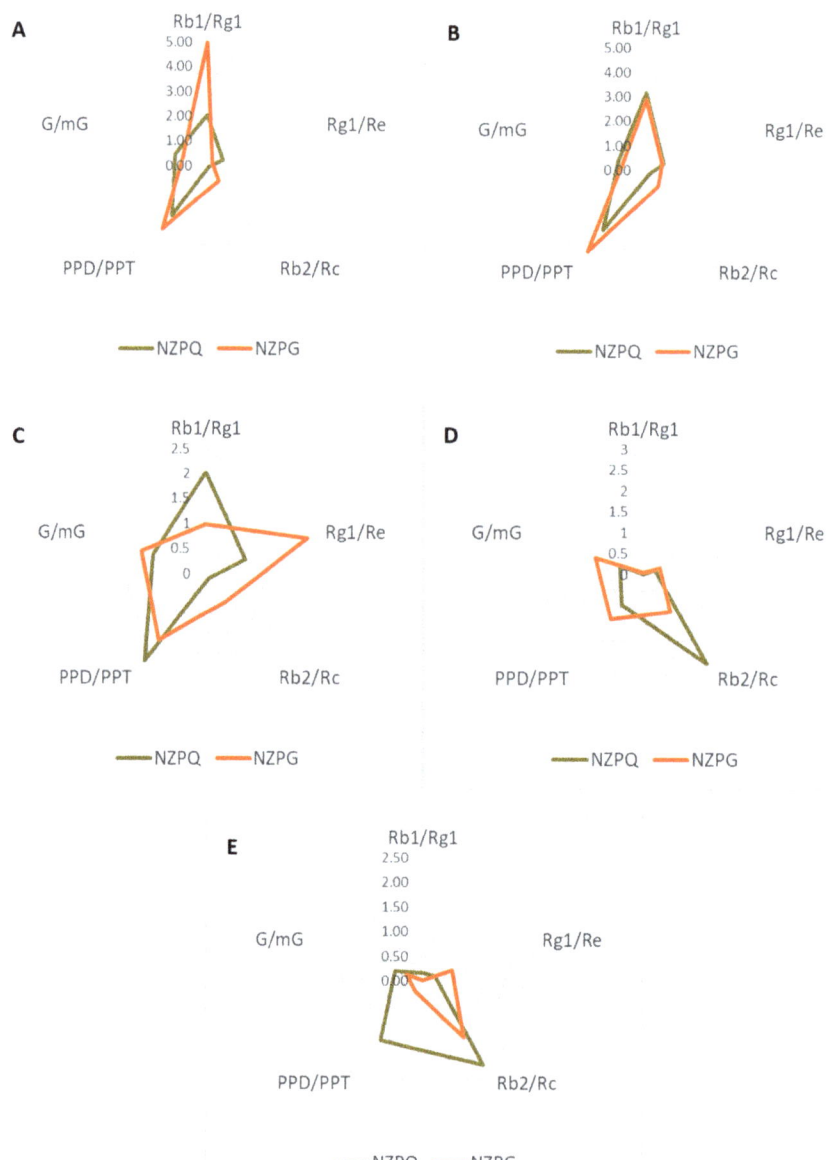

Figure 7. The ratios of Rb1/Rg1, Rg1/Re, Rb2/Rc, protopanaxadiol/protopanaxatriol (PPD/PPT), and G/mG in NZPQ and NZPG. (**A**) Fine root; (**B**) rhizome; (**C**) main root; (**D**) leaf; (**E**) stem. The PPD-type amount and PPT-type amounts are the sum of all the quantified PPD-type ginsenosides and PPT-type ginsenosides, respectively. G/mG is the ratio of neutral ginsenoside amount to malonyl ginsenoside amount; the malonyl ginsenoside amount is the sum of five quantified malonyl ginsenosides (mRb1, mRb2, mRb3, mRc, and mRd), and the neutral ginsenoside amount is the sum of corresponding neutral ginsenosides (Rb1, Rb2, Rb3, Rc, and Rd).

The literature reports that the contents of ginsenosides Rg1, Rb2, and Rc in Asian ginseng are higher than they are in American ginseng, and in Asian ginseng, the contents of Rb1, Re, and Rd are lower than they are in American ginseng [4]. In this study, we found that the contents of Rg1, Rb2, and Rc in NZPG are higher than they are in NZPQ only in the main root, and the contents of Rb1, Re, and Rd in NZPG are lower compared to the contents in NZPQ. However, in other parts, this rule has not been maintained. A few ginsenosides in the fine root (Rb2, Rd) and rhizome (Rg1, Re) do not comply with this rule, while, particularly in the leaf, the contents of these ginsenosides in NZPG are higher than that in NZPQ. A recent publication found the ratios of Rg1/Re < 0.15, Rb1/Rg1 > 2.15, and Rb2/Rc < 0.26 as the ginsenoside markers of American ginseng (as opposed to Asian ginseng) [9]. In the main root of New Zealand-grown ginseng, we found that Rb1/Rg1 > 2.15 and Rb2/Rc < 0.26 are in American ginseng and Rb1/Rg1 < 2.15, Rb2/Rc > 0.26, and Rg1/Re > 0.15 are in Asian ginseng, which is in line with the published report. In the rhizome, the ratios of these ginsenosides are similar between the two ginseng species. However, in other tissues, these ratios are waved and do not exhibit an obvious rule. This may be due to the uninterrupted interaction between the fine roots (root hair) and soil (microorganism), and the leaves and atmosphere (solar energy) leading to variation in ginsenosides in these parts. The transport of ginsenosides from various tissue parts needs to be explored in future experiments. Moreover, ginseng is typically grown in a farm setting under artificial shade conditions often involving pesticides and fertilizers [20,21], and managed by unified practice. Whereas this ginseng is certified organic grown under the shade of a pine forest, accumulation of ginsenosides can be affected by some uncontrolled factors, including soil, moisture, and light [22].

4. Conclusions

This study systematically investigated the composition of ginsenosides in various tissues of NZPG and NZPQ through qualitative and quantitative analysis. The number of ginsenosides and the total contents of ginsenosides in different parts between two ginseng variations is summarized in Figure 8. The ginsenoside composition and content of the two kinds of ginseng are very different in the aboveground parts (leaf and stem), and in the underground parts (main root, fine root, and rhizome); Asian ginseng and American ginseng have relatively similar ginsenoside constituent in the number of ginsenosides as well as the total ginsenoside amounts.

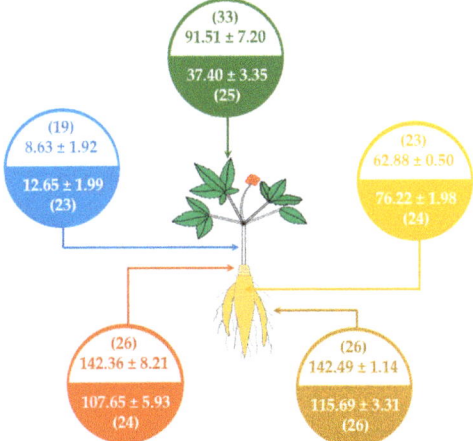

Figure 8. Comparison of ginsenoside components between New Zealand-grown Asian ginseng (colorless background) and New Zealand-grown American ginseng (colored background) in leaf (green), stem (blue), rhizome (red), fine root (brown), and main root (yellow). The numbers in parentheses refer to the number of ginsenosides identified by qualitative analysis, and the other numbers refer to the total content of ginsenosides (mg/g) quantified by quantitative analysis.

Supplementary Materials: The following are available online at http://www.mdpi.com/2218-273X/10/3/372/s1: Table S1: The regression equations, linear ranges, limits of detection and limits of quantification of 14 ginsenosides.

Author Contributions: W.C. and D.G.P. conceived and designed the experiments; W.C. performed the experiments, analyzed the data, and wrote the original manuscript; P.B. and D.G.P. reviewed and edited the manuscript. All authors have read and agreed to the published version of the manuscript.

Funding: This research was funded by the Alpha–Massey Natural Nutraceutical Research Centre: RM18873.

Acknowledgments: The authors thank the Kiwiseng Co. Ltd. for providing the NZ-grown ginseng. We would like to acknowledge Maggie Zou for her help to acquire the LC–MS/MS data.

Conflicts of Interest: The authors declare no conflicts of interest.

References

1. Qi, L.W.; Wang, C.Z.; Yuan, C.S. Ginsenosides from American ginseng: Chemical and pharmacological diversity. *Phytochemistry* **2011**, *72*, 689–699. [CrossRef]
2. Angelova, N.; Kong, H.W.; van der Heijden, R.; Yang, S.Y.; Choi, Y.H.; Kim, H.K.; Wang, M.; Hankemeier, T.; van der Greef, J.; Xu, G.; et al. Recent methodology in the phytochemical analysis of ginseng. *Phytochem. Anal.* **2008**, *19*, 2–16. [CrossRef]
3. Han, K.S.; Balan, P.; Hong, H.D.; Choi, W.I.; Cho, C.W.; Lee, Y.C.; Moughan, P.J.; Singh, H. Korean ginseng modulates the ileal microbiota and mucin gene expression in the growing rat. *Food Funct.* **2014**, *5*, 1506–1512. [CrossRef]
4. Chen, C.F.; Chiou, W.F.; Zhang, J.T. Comparison of the pharmacological effects of *Panax ginseng* and *Panax quinquefolium*. *Acta Pharmacol. Sin.* **2008**, *29*, 1103–1108. [CrossRef] [PubMed]
5. Yang, W.; Qiao, X.; Li, K.; Fan, J.; Bo, T.; Guo, D.A.; Ye, M. Identification and differentiation of *Panax ginseng*, *Panax quinquefolium*, and *Panax notoginseng* by monitoring multiple diagnostic chemical markers. *ActaPharmaceutica Sinica. B* **2016**, *6*, 568–575. [CrossRef] [PubMed]
6. Chen, W.; Balan, P.; Popovich, D.G. Chapter 6—Comparison of the ginsenoside composition of Asian ginseng (*Panax ginseng*) and American ginseng (*Panax quinquefolius* L.) and their transformation pathways. In *Studies in Natural Products Chemistry*; Atta ur, R., Ed.; Elsevier: Amsterdam, The Netherlands, 2019; Volume 63, pp. 161–195.
7. Leung, K.S.-Y.; Chan, K.; Bensoussan, A.; Munroe, M.J. Application of atmospheric pressure chemical ionisation mass spectrometry in the identification and differentiation ofPanax Species. *Phytochem. Anal.* **2007**, *18*, 146–150. [CrossRef]
8. Li, L.; Luo, G.A.; Liang, Q.L.; Hu, P.; Wang, Y.M. Rapid qualitative and quantitative analyses of Asian ginseng in adulterated American ginseng preparations by UPLC/Q-TOF-MS. *J. Pharm. Biomed. Anal.* **2010**, *52*, 66–72. [CrossRef]
9. Wu, R.; Chen, X.; Wu, W.J.; Wang, Z.; Wong, Y.E.; Hung, Y.W.; Wong, H.T.; Yang, M.; Zhang, F.; Chan, T.D. Rapid Differentiation of Asian and American Ginseng by Differential Ion Mobility Spectrometry-Tandem Mass Spectrometry Using Stepwise Modulation of Gas Modifier Concentration. *J. Am. Soc. Mass. Spectrom.* **2019**, *31*, 2212–2221. [CrossRef]
10. Cui, S.; Wu, J.; Wang, J.; Wang, X. Discrimination of American ginseng and Asian ginseng using electronic nose and gas chromatography-mass spectrometry coupled with chemometrics. *J. Ginseng Res.* **2017**, *41*, 85–95. [CrossRef]
11. Chen, Y.; Zhao, Z.; Chen, H.; Yi, T.; Qin, M.; Liang, Z. Chemical differentiation and quality evaluation of commercial Asian and American ginsengs based on a UHPLC-QTOF/MS/MS metabolomics approach. *Phytochem. Anal.* **2015**, *26*, 145–160. [CrossRef]
12. Smallfield, B.M.; Follett, J.M.; Douglas, M.H.; Douglas, J.A.; Parmenter, G.A. Production of *Panax* SPP. in New Zealand. *Acta Hortic.* **1995**, *390*, 83–91. [CrossRef]
13. Chen, W.; Balan, P.; Popovich, D.G. Analysis of Ginsenoside Content (*Panax ginseng*) from Different Regions. *Molecules* **2019**, *24*, 3491. [CrossRef]
14. Chen, W.; Balan, P.; Popovich, D.G. Ginsenosides analysis of New Zealand–grown forest *Panax ginseng* by LC-QTOF-MS/MS. *J. Ginseng Res.* **2019**, in press. [CrossRef]

15. Wang, H.P.; Yang, X.B.; Yang, X.W.; Liu, J.X.; Xu, W.; Zhang, Y.B.; Zhang, L.X.; Wang, Y.P. Ginsenjilinol, a new protopanaxatriol-type saponin with inhibitory activity on LPS-activated NO production in macrophage RAW 264.7 cells from the roots and rhizomes of *Panax ginseng*. *J. Asian Nat. Prod. Res.* **2013**, *15*, 579–587. [CrossRef]
16. Wang, H.P.; Zhang, Y.B.; Yang, X.W.; Zhao, D.Q.; Wang, Y.P. Rapid characterization of ginsenosides in the roots and rhizomes of *Panax ginseng* by UPLC-DAD-QTOF-MS/MS and simultaneous determination of 19 ginsenosides by HPLC-ESI-MS. *J. Ginseng Res.* **2016**, *40*, 382–394. [CrossRef] [PubMed]
17. Lee, J.W.; Choi, B.R.; Kim, Y.C.; Choi, D.J.; Lee, Y.S.; Kim, G.S.; Baek, N.I.; Kim, S.Y.; Lee, D.Y. Comprehensive Profiling and Quantification of Ginsenosides in the Root, Stem, Leaf, and Berry of *Panax ginseng* by UPLC-QTOF/MS. *Molecules* **2017**, *22*, 2147. [CrossRef]
18. Li, X.; Yao, F.; Fan, H.; Li, K.; Sun, L.; Liu, Y. Intraconversion of Polar Ginsenosides, Their Transformation into Less-Polar Ginsenosides, and Ginsenoside Acetylation in Ginseng Flowers upon Baking and Steaming. *Molecules* **2018**, *23*, 759. [CrossRef]
19. Zhang, Y.; Pi, Z.; Liu, C.; Song, F.; Liu, Z.; Liu, S. Analysis of Low-polar Ginsenosides in Steamed *Panax Ginseng* at High-temperature by HPLC-ESI-MS/MS. *Chem. Res. Chin. Univ.* **2012**, *28*, 31–36.
20. Cho, E.J.; Lee, D.J.; Wee, C.D.; Kim, H.L.; Cheong, Y.H.; Cho, J.S.; Sohn, B.K. Effects of AMF inoculation on growth of *Panax ginseng* C.A. Meyer seedlings and on soil structures in mycorrhizosphere. *Sci. Hortic.* **2009**, *122*, 633–637. [CrossRef]
21. Khan Chowdhury, E.; Jeon, J.; Ok Rim, S.; Park, Y.H.; Kyu Lee, S.; Bae, H. Composition, diversity and bioactivity of culturable bacterial endophytes in mountain-cultivated ginseng in Korea. *Sci. Rep.* **2017**, *7*, 10098. [CrossRef]
22. Szakiel, A.; Pączkowski, C.; Henry, M. Influence of environmental abiotic factors on the content of saponins in plants. *Phytochem. Rev.* **2011**, *10*, 471–491. [CrossRef]

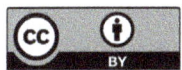

© 2020 by the authors. Licensee MDPI, Basel, Switzerland. This article is an open access article distributed under the terms and conditions of the Creative Commons Attribution (CC BY) license (http://creativecommons.org/licenses/by/4.0/).

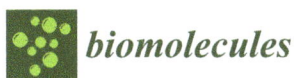

Article

Exploration and Characterization of Novel Glycoside Hydrolases from the Whole Genome of *Lactobacillus ginsenosidimutans* and Enriched Production of Minor Ginsenoside Rg3(*S*) by a Recombinant Enzymatic Process

Muhammad Zubair Siddiqi [1,2], Sathiyaraj Srinivasan [3], Hye Yoon Park [4] and Wan-Taek Im [1,2,*]

[1] Department of Biotechnology, Hankyong National University, 327 Jungang-ro Anseong-si, Gyeonggi-do 17579, Korea; mzsiddiqi1988@gmail.com
[2] AceEMzyme Co., Ltd., Academic Industry Cooperation, 327 Jungang-ro Anseong-si, Gyeonggi-do Anseong-si, Gyeonggi-do 17579, Korea
[3] Department of Bio & Environmental Technology, Division of Environmental & Life Science, College of Natural Science, Seoul Women's University, 623 Hwarangno, Nowon-gu, Seoul 139-774, Korea; sathiya.micro@gmail.com
[4] National Institute of Biological Resources, Incheon 22689, Korea; rejoice077@korea.kr
* Correspondence: wandra@hknu.ac.kr; Tel.: +82-31-6705335; Fax: +82-31-6705339

Received: 21 December 2019; Accepted: 7 February 2020; Published: 12 February 2020

Abstract: Background: Several studies have reported that ginsenoside Rg3(*S*) is effective in treating metastatic diseases, obesity, and various cancers, however, its presence in white ginseng cannot be estimated, and only a limited amount is present in red ginseng. Therefore, the use of recombinant glycosidases from a Generally Recognized As Safe (GRAS) host strain is a promising approach to enhance production of Rg3(*S*), which may improve nutritional activity, human health, and quality of life. Method: *Lactobacillus ginsenosidimutans* EMML 3041^T, which was isolated from Korean fermented pickle (kimchi), presents ginsenoside-converting abilities. The strain was used to enrich the production of Rg3(*S*) by fermenting protopanaxadiol (PPD)-mix-type major ginsenosides (Rb1, Rb2, Rc, and Rd) in four different types of food-grade media (1, MRS; 2, Basel Food-Grade medium; 3, Basel Food-Grade medium-I, and 4, Basel Food-Grade medium-II). Due to its tendency to produce Rg3(*S*), the presence of glycoside hydrolase in *Lactobacillus ginsenosidimutans* was proposed, the whole genome was sequenced, and the probable glycoside hydrolase gene for ginsenoside conversion was cloned. Results: The *L. ginsenosidimutans* EMML 3041^T strain was whole genome sequenced to identify the target genes. After genome sequencing, 12 sets of glycoside hydrolases were identified, of which seven sets (α,β-glucosidase and α,β-galactosidase) were cloned in *Escherichia coli* BL21 (DE3) using the pGEX4T-1 vector system. Among the sets of clones, only one clone (BglL.gin-952) showed ginsenoside-transforming abilities. The recombinant BglL.gin-952 comprised 952 amino acid residues and belonged to glycoside hydrolase family 3. The enzyme exhibited optimal activity at 55 °C and a pH of 7.5 and showed a promising conversion ability of major ginsenoside Rb1→Rd→Rg3(*S*). The recombinant enzyme (GST-BglL.gin-952) was used to mass produce Rg3(*S*) from major ginsenoside Rb1. Scale-up of production using 50 g of Rb1 resulted in 30 g of Rg3(*S*) with 74.3% chromatography purity. Conclusion: Our preliminary data demonstrated that this enzyme would be beneficial in the preparation of pharmacologically active minor ginsenoside Rg3(*S*) in the functional food and pharmaceutical industries.

Keywords: *Lactobacillus ginsenosidimutans*; complete genome sequence; novel glycoside hydrolases; bioconversion; recombinant enzyme; ginsenoside Rg3(*S*); gram unit production

1. Introduction

Natural products (especially secondary metabolites of herbal medicinal plants) play therapeutic roles in treating numerous human diseases. Among these natural products, the biologically active compounds of Panax ginseng are famous around the world because of their strong pharmacological effects against numerous human diseases [1–6]. Historically, to produce biologically active minor ginsenosides, the ginseng plant was treated with heat or steam and was commonly known as red or black ginseng. However, in recent years, due to new technology, these two traditional methods (steaming and heating) were replaced by more conventional ginsenoside transformation methods such as bacterial transformation, fungal enzyme transformation, and recombinant enzyme biotransformation [5,7,8]. Due to the presence of several biologically active compounds in ginseng extract, the popularity of ginseng products became not only limited to Asian countries (e.g., South Korea, Japan, China, Vietnam, India, and Pakistan), but recently also gained immense attention in Western countries. More than 80% of ginseng extract is composed of the major ginsenosides Rb1, Rc Rd, Re, and Rg1, which are categorized as protopanaxadiol (PPD)- and protopanaxatriol (PPT)-type ginsenosides based on the structure of the aglycon [9,10]. However, these major ginsenosides can be transformed into pharmacologically active minor ginsenosides, such as Rg3(S), F2, C-K, CM-c1, and Rh2, by microorganisms or recombinant enzymes [4,6–8]. Minor ginsenosides exhibit various antitumor, antistress, anti-inflammatory, anticancer, immunomodulatory, anti-atherosclerotic, anti-allergic, anti-osteoporosis, antiproliferation, antidiabetic, antigenotoxic, and antihypertensive properties [1–6].

Among the minor ginsenosides (e.g., C-Mc1, C-Mx1, Rh2, Rh1, F2, C-K, Rk1, Rg5, Rh3, Rg6, and Rg4), Rg3(S) is widely used due to its strong pharmacological effects against several cancers and lung metastasis [11]. Additionally, Rg3(S) is known to exert antitumor [12] and anti-obesity effects involving the AMPK signaling pathway and PPAR-c inhibition [13], decrease intracellular calcium levels [14], reduce cytotoxicity in colon cancer, which depends on several mechanisms including apoptosis [15], inhibit prostate cancer cell proliferation [16], and significantly inhibit the growth and angiogenesis of ovarian cancer cells when used alone or in combination with cyclophosphamide [17]. It has been reported that ginsenoside Rg3 prevents the opening of MPTP through free radical-scavenging action in the brain and may contribute to its neuroprotective effect [18]. The protective effects of ginsenoside Rg3 are mainly related to the induction of apoptosis and the inhibition of proliferation, metastasis, and angiogenesis, as presented in Table S1.

Rg3(S) is present in very small amounts in total ginseng extract, therefore, two conventional methods (the steaming method and heat acid treatment) were developed to increase production [19]. However, these two practices generate byproducts, such as Rg3(R), Rg2, Rh1, Rk1, Rg5, Rg4, and Rg6, thereby decreasing the concentration of Rg3(S). As a result, researchers recently introduced microorganism- and recombinant enzyme-based methods, which are considered to be more suitable processes compared to the steaming method and heat acid treatment for the production of target minor ginsenosides.

Accordingly, the present study aimed to explore the efficient novel glycoside hydrolases from a Generally Recognized As Safe (GRAS) host, *Lactobacillus ginsenosidimutans* EMML 3041^T, through whole genome sequencing to enrich and produce ginsenoside Rg3(S) up to the gram scale from the PPD-mix-type ginsenosides Rb1 and Rd.

2. Materials and Methods

2.1. Materials

The ginsenoside standards, Rb1, Rb2, Rc, Rd, and Rg3(S), as well as the PPD mixtures (mainly composed of Rb1, Rb2, Rc, and Rd) were purchased from AceEMzyme Co., Ltd., Republic of Korea. Fifteen different kinds of glucose substrates (with para- (*p*-) and ortho- (*o*-) nitrophenol configurations) as well as the other chemicals used in this study were purchased from Sigma (St. Louis, MO, USA).

2.2. Strain Isolation and Fermentation of PPD-Mix-Type Major Ginsenosides

The strain *L. ginsenosidimutans* EMML 3041^T, which belongs to the family Lactobacillaceae, was isolated from Korean fermented pickle (kimchi) [20]. The strain was positive for its β-glucosidase activity and was responsible for the hydrolysis of PPD-type major ginsenosides (PPD-mix ginsenosides (Rb1 and Rd)) into minor ginsenosides Rg3(S). The PPD-mix-type major ginsenosides, which were extracted from Korean red ginseng, were dissolved in MRS and three different food-grade media (i.e., Basel Food-Grade (BFG), Food-Grade medium I (FG-I) and Food-Grade medium II (FG-II)) [21], with certain modifications, as presented in Table S2. The PPD-mix solutions were sterilized using 0.20 μm ADVANTEC filter paper and *L. ginsenosidimutans* was inoculated in the PPD-mix solutions (PPD-mix in MRS and three food-grade media). Next, the samples were incubated for 1–3 days at 30 °C.

2.3. Exploration of Glycoside Hydrolase Gene Through Complete Genome Sequencing

2.3.1. Identification of Target Functional Genes

In the taxonomic characterization of novel bacterial strains and target gene identification, complete genome sequence (CGS) plays a pivotal role in determining a target functional gene at a single time. Therefore, for target functional gene identification, the whole genome of *L. ginsenosidimutans* EMML 3041^T was sequenced by Macrogen Korea, and the whole genome sequence was processed as described previously for genome annotation [22]. Moreover, the complete genome sequence was submitted to NCBI GenBank; the project information of *L. ginsenosidimutans* EMML 3041^T is available at the Genomes OnLine Database (GOLD).

2.3.2. NCBI Accession Number

After CGS analysis, the CGS of *L. ginsenosidimutans* EMML 3041^T was deposited into DDBJ/EMBL/GenBank under the accession number CP012034. The strain *L. ginsenosidimutans* was collected from the Korean Agricultural Culture Collection, South Korea, with the accession number KACC 14527^T and with the host institution.

2.4. Multilocus Sequence Typing for Identification of Species-Specific Genes

Multilocus sequence typing (MLST) is a molecular epidemiology tool which has been used extensively in recent years to differentiate between molecular subtypes of bacteria using whole genome sequencing. MLST is usually based on 6–7 species-specific genes that can be stored in Internet-based databases to easily compare isolates from different geographical areas of the world more conveniently. In the present study, an online web server (Automated Multi-Locus Species Typing) was used to identify species-specific genes of *L. ginsenosidimutans* EMML 3041^T to help other researchers compare the genome of the GRAS host *Lactobacillus* species.

2.5. Target Gene Identification, Cloning, and Expression and Biotransformation of Ginsenosides

The Carbohydrate-Active enZYmes (CAZY) database (http://www.cazy.org/b4765.html) revealed that the glycoside hydrolase genes annotated via NCBI IMG/ER belong to different glycoside hydrolase families (GH1, GH2, GH3, GH13, GH23, GH36, GH65, and GH75). Thus, from the complete genome sequence analysis, a total of 12 glycoside hydrolases (3 β-glucosidase, 1 α-glucosidase, 2 α-galactosidase, 1 β-galactosidase, and 1 each of ribose pyranase, galactopyranose mutase, β-xylanase, glucosidase, and β-D-ribofuranosyl) were identified (Table 1 and Table S3), of which 7 glycoside hydrolases (1 α-glucosidase, 3 β-glucosidase, 2 β-galactosidase, and 1 α-galactosidase) were selected for cloning. A set of forward and reverse (5′–3′) primers (Table 1) were designed by Macrogen Co. Ltd., Korea to target the functional genes. After PCR amplification, the fragments were purified and introduced into the pGEX 4T-1 GST fusion vector using an EzCloning Kit (Enzynomics Co. Ltd., Daejeon, Korea) with BamHI and XhoI restriction sites. After Ezcloning, the resultant recombinants, named AglL.gin-556,

BglL.gin-484, BglL.gin-902, BglL.gin-952, AgalL.gin-556, and BgalL.gin-629, were used to transform *Escherischia coli* BL21 (DE3) competent cells and were grown in an LB-ampicillin medium at 37 °C until the culture achieved an OD_{600} value of 0.4–0.6. At this point, the cultures were cooled with an ice water bath and the optimum enzyme activity was attained by induction with various concentrations of 0.1 mM isopropyl-β-ᴅ-thiogalactopyranoside (IPTG); the cells were the further incubated for 18 h at 25 °C. After 24 h, the cells were collected via centrifugation and were washed twice with 1% Triton solution. After washing, the pellets were dissolved in 100 mM sodium phosphate (pH 7.0) and were ultrasonicated (Branson Digital Sonifier 450, CT, Danbury, Mexico) to obtain intercellular enzymes. To obtain the crude soluble enzymes, undesirable cell debris was removed by centrifugation (8000 rpm for 15 min at 4 °C). The recombinant enzyme activity and expression were confirmed by hydrolysis of 16 different glucose substrates, as listed in Table S4. SDS-PAGE analysis was performed, which revealed that the molecular weights of the well-localized proteins in the gels were the same as those calculated via amino acid sequence analysis.

The initial biotransformations of seven recombinant enzymes (AglL.gin-556, BglL.gin-484, BglL.gin-902, BglL.gin-952, AgalL.gin-556, AgalL.gin-319, and BgalL.gin-629) were carried out using the PPD-mix-type major ginsenosides Rb1, Rc, and Rd. However, this analysis revealed that only one recombinant enzyme (BglL.gin-952) was responsible for the conversion of the PPD-mix-type of major ginsenosides into minor ginsenosides, as illustrated in Figure 1. Furthermore, the recombinant BglL.gin-952 was characterized and used for the gram unit production of ginsenoside Rg3(*S*) from Rb1.

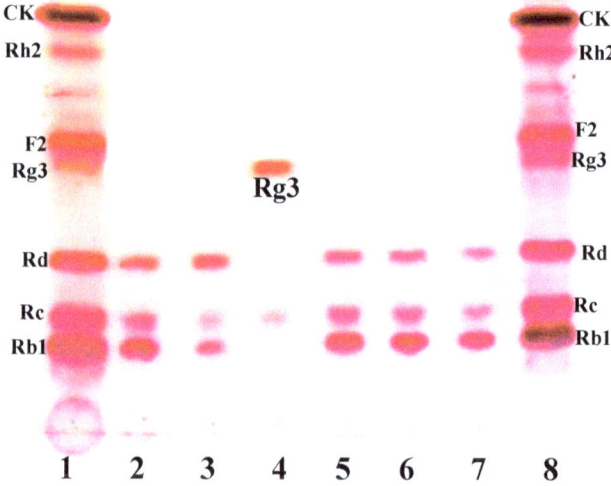

Figure 1. Conversion of protopanaxadiol (PPD)-mix-type ginsenosides by seven different glycoside hydrolases. 1, Ginsenoside standard; 2, AglL.gin-556; 3, BglL.gin-484; 4, BglL.gin-952; 5, BglL.gin-902; 6, AgalL.gin-556; 7, AgalL.gin-319; 8, ginsenoside standard.

Table 1. Set of primers (forward (F) and reverse (R)) used to clone the target functional gene.

Sets of Total Clones	Names of Clone Gene	Total Amino Acids	Common Name	Ginsenoside Conversion Activity	Primers Sequences (F, R)	Vector
1	α-glucosidase-556	556	(AglL.gin-556)	-	GGTTCCGCGTGGATCCACAAAAAATTGGTGGCAAGGTT_F AACCTTGCCACCAATTTTTTGTGGATCCACGCGGAACC_R	pGEX 4T-1
2	β-glucosidase-484	484	(BglL.gin-484)	-	GGTTCCGCGTGGATCCGCAAAAATGAGTATCCTTATT_F AATAAGGATACTCATTTTTGCGGATCCACGCGGAACC_R	
3	β-glucosidase-902	902	(BglL.gin-902)	-	GGTTCCGCGTGGATCCGAAAGCGAAATGTCACAACGAG_F CTCGTTGTGACATTTCGCTTTCGGATCCACGCGGAACC_R	
4	β-glucosidase-952	952	(BglL.gin-952)	+	GGTTCCGCGTGGATCCGATAAAAAACAGAAGAGGATTG_F CAATCCTCTTCTGTTTTTTATCGGATCCACGCGGAACC_R	
5	α-galactosidase-556	556	(AgalL.gin-556)	-	GGTTCCGCGTGGATCCTCTTGTTAATGTTAATCAAAGTA_F TACTTTGATTAACATTAACAGAGGATCCACGCGGAACC_R	
6	α-galactosidase-319	319	(AgalL.gin-319)	-	GGTTCCGCGTGGATCCGATTACACAAATAATAAGTTGC_F GCAACTTATTATTTGTGTAATCGGATCCACGCGGAACC_R	
7	β-galactosidase-629	629	(BgalL.gin-629)	-	GGTTCCGCGTGGATCCAAGCTGATATTAACTGGCTCG_F CGAGCCAGTTAATATCAGCTTGGGATCCACGCGGAACC_R	

Phylogenetic Analysis of BglL.gin-952

To identify the exact position of BglL.gin-952 in the different glycoside hydrolase families (e.g., GH1, GH2, and GH3), a database homology search was performed using the BLAST program provided by NCBI, and the sequences of the characterized glycosyl hydrolases were obtained from the CAZY database (http://www.cazy.org). Multiple alignments were performed using the CLUSTAL_X program [23], gaps were edited in the BioEdit program [24], and evolutionary distances were calculated using the Poisson model. A phylogenetic tree was constructed using the neighbor-joining algorithm [25] obtained from the MEGA6 Program [26], with bootstrap values based on 1000 replicates [27].

2.6. Characterization of Novel Recombinant Bgll.Gin-952 and Purification

Optimum enzyme activity (recombinant BglL.gin-952) was determined by culturing the recombinant *Escherichia coli* in LBA (Luria-Bertani supplemented with 100 mg/mL ampicillin) broth and incubating the flasks at 37 °C. After the OD_{600} reached 0.4, the optimum induction of recombinant BglL.gin-952 was determined with various concentrations (0.1, 0.5, and 1 mM) of IPTG (Isopropyl β-D-1-thiogalactopyranoside) at 28 °C. After IPTG optimum induction, the effects of various temperatures (18 °C, 22 °C, 25 °C, and 28 °C) were also identified for optimum enzyme activity using the optimum induced concentration of IPTG (0.1 mM). After 18 h of incubation at 18 °C, 22 °C, 25 °C, and 28 °C, the cells were harvested and washed twice with 1% Triton solution and the pellets (10 g/100 mL) were dissolved in 50 mM sodium phosphate buffer (pH 7.0). Enzymes were extracted from the cells using the Branson Digital Sonifier (400 W, 70% power, Branson Digital Sonifier 450, CT, Danbury, Mexico) at the following settings: low power (36%) output, 2 s ON/2 s OFF pulses, and ±4 °C ice-water bath. The total sonication time was 5 min. The crude cell extract was retained and the unwanted cell debris was removed by centrifugation (5000 rpm for 10 min at 4 °C). The GST tag was purified using GST·Bind agarose resin (Elpisbiotech Co. Ltd., Korea), and the homogeneity of the protein was assessed using 8% and 10% SDS-PAGE and an EZStain Aqua solution (ATTO Corporation, Tokyo, Japan). The SDS-PAGE analysis revealed the exact molecular weights of the well-localized proteins as presented by the amino acid sequence analysis (131 kDa).

2.6.1. Effect of pH, Temperature, and Metal Ions on Recombinant Enzyme Activity

To identify the specific enzyme activity of BglL.gin-952, the samples were incubated in 50 mM sodium phosphate buffer (pH 7.0), with *p*-nitrophenyl-β-D-glucopyranoside (*p*NPG) as a surrogate substrate for 15 min at 37 °C. After 15 min, the reaction was stopped with 0.5 M (final concentration) Na_2CO_3 and the amount of *p*-nitrophenol released was immediately measured by a microplate reader at 405 nm (Bio-Rad model 680; Bio-Rad, Hercules, CA, USA). The amount of recombinant enzyme required to generate 1 μmol of *p*-nitrophenol in one min is known as one unit of enzyme activity. The specific activity of the enzyme was expressed as units per milligram of enzyme. The protein concentration was determined using the Bio-Rad protein assay (catalog number 500-0006) with bovine serum albumin (Sigma, St. Louis, Missouri, USA) as the standard. All assays were performed in triplicate.

In general, enzymes are quite sensitive to environmental conditions and even small changes in the environment may markedly affect enzyme activity. Thus, in this study, we investigated the effect of pH, temperature, and some commonly known metal ions and chemicals.

The effect of pH on the enzyme activity of BglL.gin-952 was confirmed using various types of buffer solutions. Briefly, 1.0 mM *p*NPG was used a substrate in the following buffers with a final concentration of 100 mM: KCl–HCl and glycine–HCl or citrate were used for pH 2.0 and 3.0, respectively, sodium acetate and sodium phosphate were used for pH 4.0–7.5, and Tris–HCl and glycine–sodium hydroxide or carbonate were used for pH 8.0–10.0. Similarly, pH stability was determined as previously stated by Siddiqi et al. [22]. To investigate the effect of optimum temperature on the enzyme activity of BglL.gin-952, the samples were incubated at optimum pH for 10 min in 100 mM sodium phosphate buffer with 2.0 mM pNPG under various temperatures (5 °C–80 °C, with intervals of 2 °C (e.g., 35 °C, 37 °C) and 5 °C). As BglI.gIN-952 was extremely sensitive to temperature, the thermostability of the enzyme was observed by incubating the samples in 100 mM sodium phosphate buffer for different periods of time (5 min, 10 min, 30 min, and 1 h) at various temperatures (5.0–80 °C). After the preset time intervals, the samples were collected and enzymatic activity was determined using pNPG as the substrate.

Several studies have reported that naturally occurring elements, such as metals and heavy metals at various concentrations, affect enzyme activity. Therefore, high concentrations of heavy metals are toxic to enzyme active sites and may inhibit activity. Thus, the effects of metals and other chelating agents or chemicals on the enzyme activity of BglL.gin-952 were determined. BglL.gin-952 activity was evaluated in the presence of 1 and 10 mM (as the final concentration) of KCl, $CaCl_2$, $CoCl_2$, NaCl, $MgCl_2$, $MnSO_4$, $MgSO_4$, EDTA, and β-mercaptoethanol for 15 min at 55 °C. Next, enzyme activity was determined using pNPG as a substrate, with the results expressed as a percentage of the activity in the absence of metals and other chemicals.

Typically, all enzyme types prefer to hydrolyze specific substrates and do not yield positive results for the hydrolysis of other substrates. Therefore, in this study, the substrate preference of BglL.gin-952 was determined using 2.0 mM (as final concentration) of 15 different sugar substrates (all from Sigma, as presented in Table S5) with o-nitrophenyl (oNP) and p-nitrophenyl (pNP) configurations. Next, the samples were incubated at 37 °C (stable temperature) and 55 °C (optimum temperature) for 5 and 10 min, and enzymatic activity was observed. The amount of enzyme required to release 1 µmol of oNP or pNP in 1 min is known as one unit (U) of enzyme.

2.6.2. Enzymatic Transformation of Major Ginsenosides by Bgll.Gin-952

To assess the effect of the fused GST tag on the recombinant enzyme activity of BglL.gin-952, the initial biotransformation of Rb_1, Rd, and Re was tested. The analysis revealed that the fused GST tag did not affect the activity of the recombinant BglL.gin-952, thus, the GST-fused enzyme (GST-BglL.gin-952) was used to determine the specificity and selectivity of BglL.gin-952 for removing glucose molecules attached to the C3, C6, and C20 positions in four PPD-type (Rb_1, Rb_2, Rc, and Rd) and two PPT-type (Re and Rg_1) major ginsenosides. An equal volume of enzyme solution (concentration of 0.5 mg mL^{-1}) in 100 mM sodium phosphate buffer (pH 7.0) was mixed with Rb_1, Rb_2, Rc, Rd, Re, and Rg_1 at a concentration of 1000 ppm at 37 °C for 24 h. After regular time intervals, the samples were collected and analyzed by thin-layer chromatography (TLC) to evaluate the enzymatic conversion of the PPD- and PPT-type ginsenosides.

2.7. Chromatography

2.7.1. TLC analysis

Thin-layer chromatography (TLC) was performed using 60F254 silica gel plates (Merck, Darmstadt, Germany) with $CHCl_3$–CH_3OH–H_2O (65:35:10, lower phase) as the solvent. The spots on the TLC plates were visualized by spraying H_2SO_4 (10%, v/v) and heating at 110 °C for 5 min. The results were compared with the ginsenoside standards.

2.7.2. HPLC analysis

HPLC analysis of the ginsenosides was carried out using an HPLC system (Young Lin Co. Ltd., Anyang, Korea). Ginsenoside separation and peaks were achieved using a C_{18} column (5 µm, 150 × 4.6 mm i.d.; Phenomenex, Torrance, California, United States) with a guard column (Eclipse XDB C_{18}, 5 µm, 12.5 × 4.6 mm i.d.). The mobile phases were water (A) and acetonitrile (B) with a gradient as follows: 0–11 min, 32%–65% B; 12–18 min, 100% B; and 15–26 min, 32% B. The flow rate was maintained at 1.0 mL/min and the sample injection volume was 25 µL. Detection was performed by monitoring the absorbance at 203 nm.

3. Results

3.1. Bioconversion of PPD Mixtures by L. Ginsenosidimutans EMML 3041^T

The strain *L. ginsenosidimutans*, which was isolated from Korean fermented pickle (kimchi), efficiently converted the major ginsenosides Rb1 and Rd to the minor ginsenoside Rg3(S) in MRS medium. For the edible and economic production of Rg3(S), three different types of food-grade media (BFG, FG-1, and FG-II) were used. Briefly, *L. ginsenosidimutans* was grown in BFG, FG-1, and FG-II broths and the growth of culture of the food-grade media were compared with the strain grown in MRS medium (broth). The results indicated that BFG medium was more suitable for the growth of *L. ginsenosidimutans* compared to FG-I and FG-II media (as presented in Figure S1), therefore, this medium was selected for the bioconversion of major ginsenosides into minor ginsenosides. Interestingly, the strain did not produce Rg3(S) in the BFG medium, but the initial bioconversion of the major ginsenosides (which were extracted from Korean red ginseng, American leaf saponins, and Chinese ginseng) revealed that the *L. ginsenosidimutans* powerfully transformed the PPD-mix ginsenosides to Rd and the target minor ginsenoside Rg3(S) in the BFG and MRS media, respectively (Figure 2A,B). Thus, based on the initial fermentations and quality of the ginseng extracts (Korean, American, and Chinese ginseng extracts), the American leaf saponins were selected for the edible production of the target minor ginsenoside Rg3(S) (Figure 2B). The ginsenoside bioconversion pathways for *L. ginsenosidimutans* in two different media are presented in Figure S2.

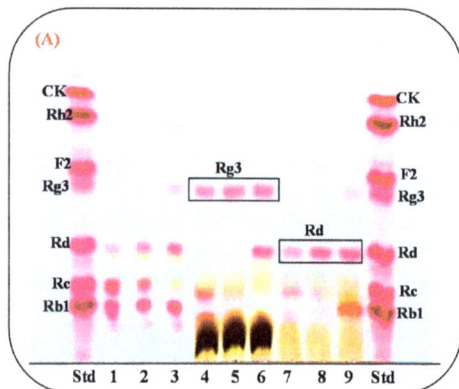
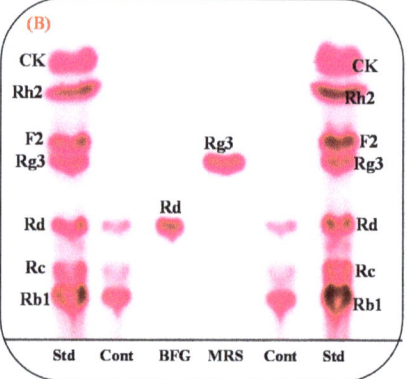

Figure 2. (**A**) Thin-layer chromatography (TLC) analysis showed the conversion of the PPD-mix extracts by *Lactobacillus ginsenosidimutans* EMML 3041^T from Korean ginseng, American leaf saponins, and Chinese ginseng. Std, ginsenosides standards; 1. Korean ginseng extract (KGE) control; 2, American leaf extract (ALE) control; 3, Chinese ginseng extract (CGE) control; 4–6, conversion of KGE, ALE, and CGE in MRS broth; 7–9, conversion of KGE, ALE, and CGE in Basel Food-Grade broth. (**B**) The effect of two different media (MRS and BFG) on the bioconversion of PPD-mix-type ginsenosides. Std, ginsenoside standard; cont, control of PPD-mix ginsenosides (Rb1, Rc, and Rd).

3.2. Genome Properties

The complete genome of *L. ginsenosidimutan* EMML 3041^T was a presumptive circular chromosome of 2,590,556 base pairs (Figure S3) with a G + C content of 36.71%. A total of 2574 genes, 2486 CDS, and 62 RNA genes were assigned a putative function, and the remainder were annotated as hypothetical or conserved hypothetical proteins (Table 2). The total counts of different functional genes and predicted COG and KOG functional genes are depicted in Figure S3 and Table S6. Based on the complete genome annotation, it was evident that the genome comprised numerous glycoside hydrolase metabolism genes clusters, including β-glucosidase, which may be responsible for ginsenoside conversion. Furthermore, from the whole genome analysis, a total of 58 (10.38%) genes were annotated as being involved in carbohydrate transport and metabolism (Table S6).

Table 2. General features of *Lactobacillus ginsenosidimutan* EMML 3041^T.

Features	Chromosome
Length (bp)	2,590,556
DNA coding region (bp)	2,271,180
G + C content (%)	36.71
Genes	2574
Pseudogenes	26
CDS	2486
rRNA gene	9
tRNA genes	53

The auto-MLST revealed 87 characterized, known and uncharacterized, or unknown species-specific genes, which are listed in Table S7. The main advantage of this technique was that it provided unambiguous data that are reproducible among laboratories. For individual species-specific (or housekeeping) genes, the different sequences present within a bacterial species were assigned as distinct alleles; for each isolate, the alleles at each of the loci defined the allelic profile or sequence type (ST).

3.3. Phylogenetic Analysis of Sequence of BglL.Gin-952

The β-glycosidase gene (BglL.gin-952, GenBank accession number: WP_053084464) comprised 2859 bp encoding 952 amino acids with a molecular mass of 131.0 kDa. The hypothetical pI value of of BglL.gin-952 is 4.89 (http://web.expasy.org/compute_pi/). Amino acid sequence analysis of BglL.gin-952 indicated that it possesses less than 82.4% similarity to the glycoside hydrolase of *Lactobacillus* sp. 256–3 (GenBank number WP_125704743) and other uncharacterized glycoside hydrolases, suggesting that BglL.gin-952 has a domain similar to glycoside hydrolase family 3 (GH3). However, GH3 is subdivided into several subfamilies. In order to identify the evolutionary position of BglL.gin-952 within the characterized enzymes in GH3, a phylogenetic analysis was constructed using the maximum-likelihood method from the MEGA-6 Program with bootstrap values of 1000 replications. This analysis revealed that BglL.gin-952 was clustered within subfamily 5 in GH3, forming a separate but well-supported group with the β-glucosidase derived from other *Lactobacillus* species (Figure 3).

3.4. Molecular Cloning

The oligonucleotide primer sequences used for gene cloning were based on the DNA sequences of the aforementioned genes, as listed in Table 2. The primers were designed and synthesized by Macrogen Co. Ltd. (Seoul, Korea) with BamHI and XhoI restriction sites.

After functional gene cloning, a few sets of the clones presented positive and weakly positive activities for *p*NP-β-D-glucopyranoside, pNP-β-D-galactopyranoside, oNP-β-D-glucopyranoside, and oNP-β-D-galactopyranoside. Among these seven sets of clones, only one gene (BglL.gin-952) was responsible for the conversion of the ginsenosides (Table S4).

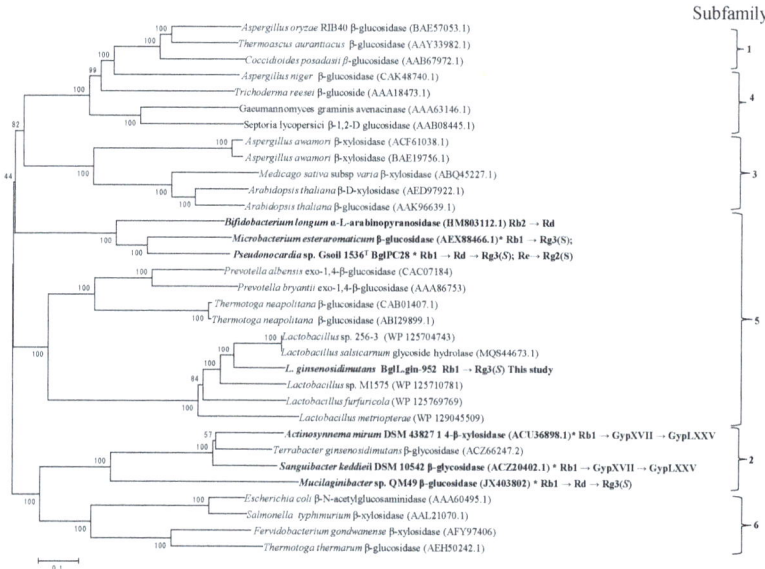

Figure 3. Phylogenetic tree analysis showing the position of the novel BglL.gin-952 in the glycoside hydrolases of family 3 (GH3). The tree was constructed using the maximum-likelihood algorithm alongside a Poisson model and pairwise deletion. Bootstrap values expressed as percentages of 1000 replications greater than 50% are shown at the branch points. The bar represents 10 amino acid residue substitutions per 100 amino acid residues.

3.5. Protein Expression and Biotransformation of Ginsenosides by BglI.Gin-952

The recombinant pGEX- AglL.gin-556, BglL.gin-484, BglL.gin-952, BglL.gin-902, AgalL.gin-556, and AgalL.gin-319 enzymes were used to transform *E. coli* BL21 (DE3). To maximize the yield and expression of the fusion protein, the protein was induced by adding 0.1 mM IPTG. The clone samples of the recombinant *E. coli* BL21 (DE3) grown in LBAmp (1 g mL^{-1}) broth were preserved at different temperatures (18 °C, 22 °C, 25 °C, and 28 °C) with varying induction conditions (0.05, 0.1, and 0.5 mM IPTG (data not shown)). Incubation with 0.1 mM IPTG at 18 °C for 18 h produced the maximum level of soluble, active, fused enzyme, as depicted in Figure 4A,B. The ability of recombinant pGEX-AglL.gin-556, BglL.gin-484, BglL.gin-952, BglL.gin-902, AgalL.gin-556, and AgalL.gin-319 to convert PPD-type ginsenosides (Rb1, Rb2, Rc, and Rd) was assessed by performing TLC analysis of the enzyme hydrolysates at regular intervals. Based on the Rf values, it was evident that BglL.gin-952 converted the PPD-type (Rb1 and Rb2) major ginsenosides into Rg3(*S*) (Figure 1). Thus, the results indicated that only the BglL.gin-952 efficiently hydrolyzed the glucose attached to the C3 and C20 positions of the PPD-type ginsenosides. The proposed pathway for the biotransformation of the PPD-type ginsenosides (2 mg mL^{-1}) by BglL.gin-952 is Rb1 and Rd to Rg3(*S*), where the conversion of PPD-mix type ginsenosides occurs through the stepwise hydrolysis of the inner and outer glucose attached at the C3 and C20 positions of aglycon (Figure 5). Furthermore, the incubation of Rg3(*S*) along with the recombinant enzyme (BglL.gin-952) did not lead to hydrolysis of Rg3(*S*), indicating that the recombinant BglL.gin-952 preferred the outer and inner glucose moiety at the C20 position.

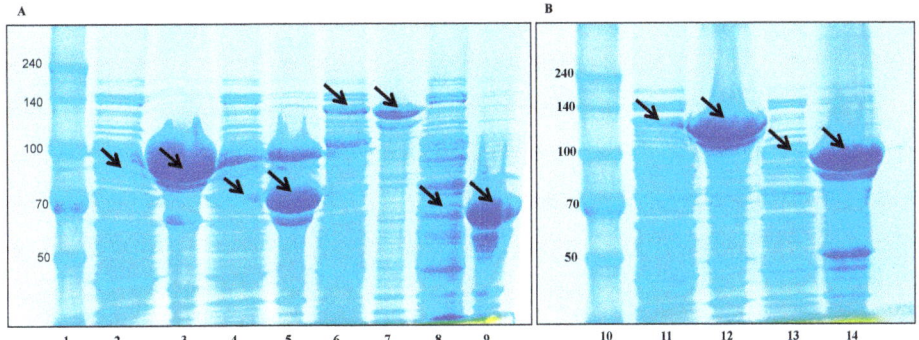

Figure 4. (**A,B**). SDS-PAGE analysis of recombinant glycoside hydrolase genes of *L. ginsenosidimutans*. Lanes 1 and 10, protein marker (50–240 kDa); Lanes 2 and 3, soluble and precipitate enzyme of AglL.gin-556 (87 kDa), respectively; Lanes 4 and 5, soluble and precipitated enzymes of BglL.gin-484 (79 kDa), respectively; Lanes 6 and 7, soluble and precipitated enzymes of BglL.gin-952; Lanes 8 and 9, soluble and precipitated enzymes of AgalL.gin-319, respectively.

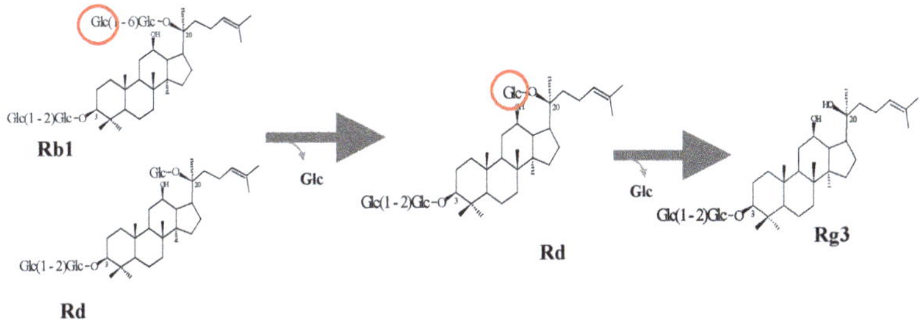

Figure 5. Conversion pathway of ginsenosides Rb1 and Rd to Rg3(S) by recombinant BglL.gin-952.

Characterization of BglL.Gin952

The cell lysate of the recombinant BglL.gin-952 was purified via the GST·bind agarose resin, and the purified protein was subjected to 8% and 10% SDS-PAGE analysis, which confirmed that the exact molecular weight was presented by the full-length sequence (131 kDa), as depicted in Figure S4. The molecular weight (131.0 kDa) of the recombinant protein BglL.gin-952, which was calculated from amino acid-sequence analysis, was similar to that calculated after protein purification.

The optimum temperature and pH values for the bioconversion of the PPD-mix-type major ginsenosides were determined using a crude recombinant BglL.gin-952 enzyme, which exhibited optimal activity at pH 7.5 in sodium phosphate buffer and stability at pH 6.0–8.0 (Figure 6A). When the pH was less than 6.0 or more than 8.0, the enzyme stability decreased markedly, and at pH 4.0 and 10.0, the enzyme activity decreased rapidly to 0% of the optimum activity (Figure 6A). The optimal temperature was found to be 55 °C, whereas the thermostability decreased significantly below 37 °C and the enzyme activity reached 0% when it was further incubated at 55–75 °C for 2 h (Figure 6B). BglL.gin-952 was stable below 37 °C, and about 60% of the activity was lost after incubation at 45 °C for 1 h. Thus, the optimal temperature for the activity of BglL.gin-952 was higher than that of β-glucosidase (45 °C), which was isolated from *Arachidicoccus ginsenosidimutans* and *Terrabacter ginsenosidimutans*, but similar to that of β-glucosidase from *Pyrococcus furiosus* (55 °C), indicating that BglL.gin-952 is mesophilic and stable at a neutral pH range. In addition, the near-neutral optimal pH and the mild optimal temperature of BglL.gin-952 were similar to those of ginsenoside-hydrolyzing GH3 from other bacteria [28–30]. Even though the optimum temperature of BglL.gin-952 against pNPGlc was 55 °C, during prolonged and stable transformation, the ginsenoside bioconversion reaction occurred at 37 °C, with an optimum pH of 7.0–7.5.

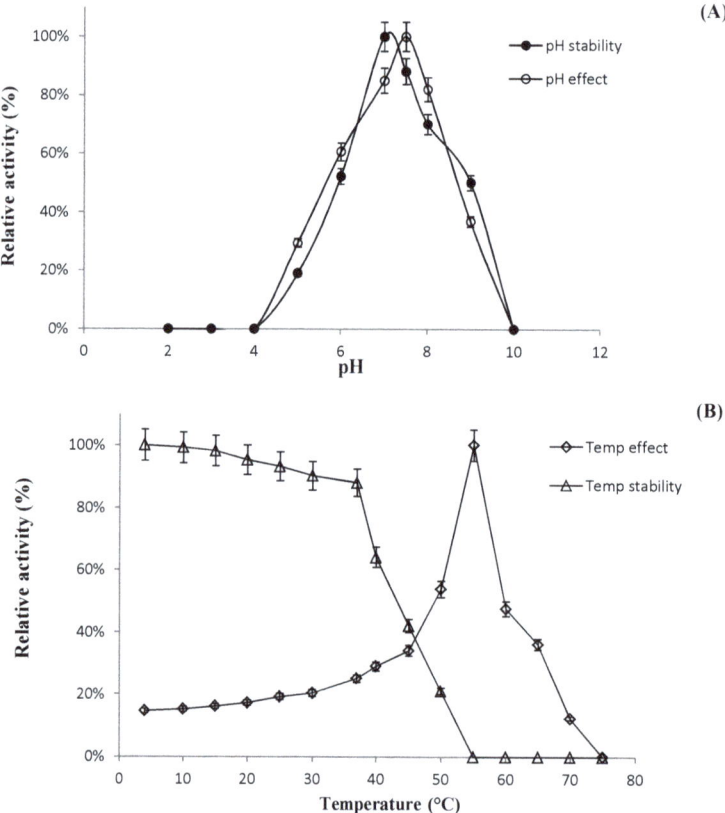

Figure 6. (**A**). Effect of pH on enzyme activity. Enzyme activity was measured under standard assay conditions. Enzyme solutions containing 2.0 mM pNPGlc were incubated with various buffers at pH 2.0–10.0 for 12 h at 4 °C. To assess the stability of BglAg-762, the enzymes were incubated for 30 min at 50 °C in various buffers at pH 2.0–10.0, and the residual activities were measured. (**B**) The effect of temperature on the stability and activity of recombinant BglAg-762 was measured under standard assay conditions. The thermodependence of BglAg-762 was assayed using 50 mM potassium phosphate buffer (pH 7.5) at varying temperatures ranging from 4–60 °C. Thermostability was tested by incubating aliquots of the enzyme in 50 mM potassium phosphate buffer (pH 7.5) for different periods of time at various temperatures. After cooling the sample, the residual activity was determined.

As mentioned previously, heavy metals are atoms with high molecular weights, and changes in metal concentrations may affect enzyme activity. Therefore, the effects of various metal ions and some chemicals (EDTA and β-mercaptoethanol) on the activity of BglL.gin-952 were investigated. The results were expressed as percentages of activity in the absence of the test compound (Table 3). The activity of BglL.gin-952 was not affected by 1 and 10 mM of metal ions (Na^+, K^+, Mg^{2+}, Mn^+, Co^{2+}, Mn^{2+}, and Mg^{2+}) or chemicals (EDTA and β-mercaptoethanol); however, enzyme activity was enhanced by the addition of 10 mM Ca^{2+}, Co^{2+}, and Mn^{2+} ions. Thus, the BglL.gin-952 recombinant enzyme was found to be less affected by metal ions and chelating agents compared to our previously described recombinant enzyme [30].

Table 3. Substrate hydrolysis activity of BglL.gin-952.

Substrates	Relative Activity ± SD (%)
pNP-β-D-glucopyranoside	100.0 ± 3.3
pNP-β-D-galactopyranoside	17.0 ± 1.0
pNP-β-D-fucopyranoside	5.3 ±0.3
pNP-β-N-glucosaminide	ND
pNP-β-L-arabinopyranoside	ND
pNP-β-D-mannopyranoside	ND
pNP-β-D-xylopyranoside	ND
pNP-α-D-glucopyranoside	ND
pNP-α-D-arabinofuranoside	ND
pNP-α-D-arabinopyranoside	14.5 ± 0.67
pNP-α-D-mannopyranoside	ND
pNP-α-D-mannopyranoside	ND
oNP-β-D-glucopyranoside	ND
oNP-β-D-fucopyranoside	ND
oNP-α-D-galactopyranoside	ND

The substrate specificity of BglL.gin-952 was investigated with α- and β-configurations of 1.0 mM pNP- and oNP-glycosides. The analysis revealed that BglL.gin-952 exhibited the highest activity against pNP-β-D-glucopyranoside (100.0%), weak activity against pNP-β-D-galactopyranoside and pNP-α-L-arabinopyranoside, and no effect on any of the other pNP- and oNP-glycosides (Table 4).

Table 4. Effects of 1 and 10 mM β-mercaptoethanol, EDTA, and some metal ions.

Metal Ions or Reagents	Relative Activity ± SD (%) at:	
	1 mM	10 mM
NaCl	80.0 ± 6.7	85.6 ± 1.3
KCl	87.0 ± 0.7	85.3 ± 3.7
CaCl$_2$	81.3 ± 6.1	122.1 ± 0.9
MgCl$_2$	82.9 ± 0.2	71.6 ± 3.3
CoCl$_2$	84.2 ± 0.4	132.0 ± 3.9
MnSO$_4$	88.3 ± 4.0	155.5 ± 5.8
MgSO$_4$	91.6 ± 2.4	79.8 ± 0.3
β-Mercaptoethanol	88.6 ± 3.0	93.9 ± 0.3
EDTA	84.4 ± 3.8	78.7± 3.7
Control	100.0 ± 2.1	100.0 ± 5.1

3.6. Scaled-Up Biotransformation of Rg3(S)

3.6.1. Preparation of High-Cell Density Culture of Recombinant Bgll.Gin-952

A high-cell density culture of the recombinant *E. coli* BL21 (DE3) harboring the pGEX-4T-BglL.gin-952 gene was obtained by inoculating the strain in 5 L of LBA broth (LB broth containing 100 mg ampicillin/mL as the final concentration) at 37 °C and 500 rpm in a 10 L stirred-tank reactor (Biotron GX, Hanil Science Co., Incheon, Korea). The pH of the medium was adjusted to 7.0 using 0.1 M sodium phosphate buffer. When the OD$_{600nm}$ reached 3.0, the culture was allowed to cool, and the protein was induced by 0.1 mM IPTG (final concentration). The culture was further incubated at 18 °C along with glucose (with a final concentration of 10 g/L) until the cell density reached to an OD of 20~25 at 600 nm. The cells were then harvested via centrifugation at 8000 rpm for 10 min and the enzyme was extracted using a Branson Digital Sonifier (Danbury, Mexico). Unwanted cell debris was removed by centrifugation at 4 °C, and the crude soluble enzyme fraction was used for the conversion of ginsenoside Rb1 to Rg3(S).

3.6.2. Gram Unit Production of Rg3(*S*)

To enhance the production of ginsenoside Rg3(*S*), the reaction (Rb1 + BglL.gin-952) was performed in a 10 L stirred-tank reactor with 5 L of working volume. The reaction mixture was prepared with equal volumes (1:1 v/v) of recombinant enzyme solution (30 mg/mL of crude recombinant BglL.gin-952 in 0.1 M of sodium phosphate buffer (pH 7.0 ± 0.2)) and 10 mg/mL (final concentration) of ginsenosides Rb1 (total 50 g). The reaction was completed under optimal conditions at 37 °C and pH 7.0 ± 0.5 at 350 rpm for 24 h. Samples were collected at regular intervals and analyzed using TLC and HPLC to determine the time-course of the biotransformation of ginsenoside Rb1 to Rg3(*S*). After 24 h, Rb1 was completely converted to ginsenoside Rg3(*S*) (Figure 7). The unwanted substances from the reaction mixture were removed by centrifugation at 8000 rpm for 10 min, and Rg3(*S*) was precipitated to a solid form. The precipitated Rg3(*S*) was then dissolved twice in 3 L of a 95% ethanol solution and the Rg3(*S*) supernatant was evaporated in a vacuum to obtain 30 g of powdered Rg3(*S*) (Figure 8, Figure S5).

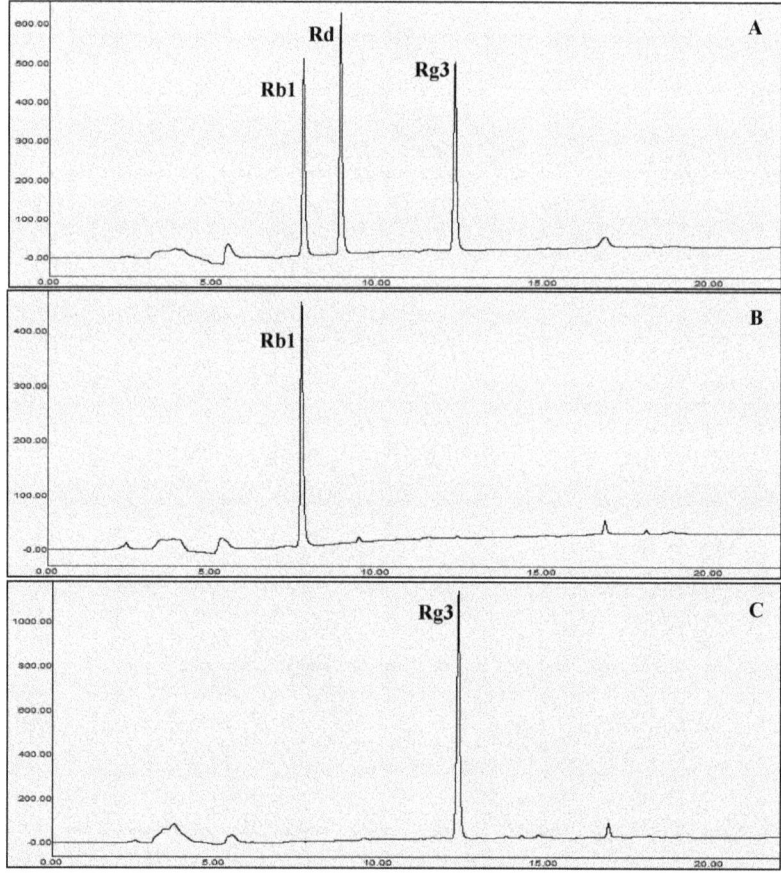

Figure 7. HPLC analysis of the transformation of Rb1 to Rg3(*S*) by recombinant BglL.gin-952. **A**, Ginsenoside standard; **B**, Rb1 as a starting substrate; **C**, Rg3(*S*) production after 24 h of reaction.

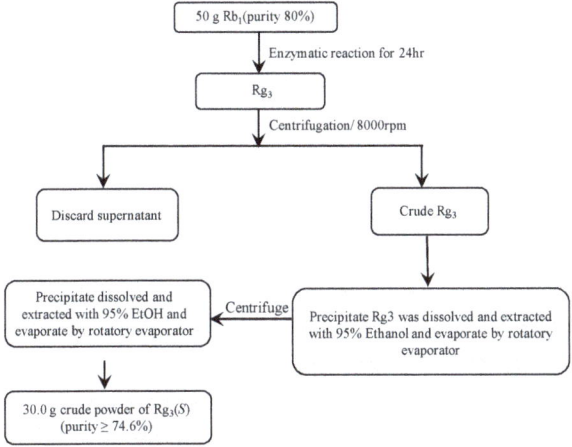

Figure 8. Gram unit production of ginsenoside Rg3(S) from ginsenoside Rb1.

3.7. Comparision of Rg3(S) Production between Bacterial Cell Fermentation and the Recombinat Enzyme Bgll.Gin952

In the comparative analysis of ginsenosude Rg3(S) production, the PPD-mix (Rb1, Rc, and Rd) was dissolved in MRS medium for cell fermentation and in sodium phosphate buffer (pH 7.0) for the recombinant BglL.gin-952. Ginsenoside fermentation and the enzymatic reactions commenced at a final concentration of 5 mg/mL (total, 5 g/L). The samples were incubated at 30 °C for whole-cell fermentation and 37 °C for the enzymatic reactions. The results indicated that the production of Rg3(S) using whole bacterial strain cells was 1.1 g with 53.1% purity after 72 h of incubation and 3.0 g after 24 h for the enzymatic reactions, as shown in Table S8.

4. Discussion

In oriental herbal medicinal plants, red ginseng is a very popular health-promoting food but contains only approximately 1% of the minor ginsenoside Rg3(S) based on its dry weight. Although Rg3(S) has strong anticancer, antimetastatic, and anti-obesity effects, the lack of selective mass-production technology has slowed down its commercial use. To scale-up the production of Rg3(S), several researchers have aimed to accomplish biotransformation of major ginsenosides to minor ginsenosides using microorganisms and recombinant enzymes in laboratory settings; however, these researchers only characterized the basic functions of the microorganism and recombinant enzymes separately from the mass production aspects [31–33]. As a result, all of the previous studies focused on the conversion of major ginsenosides into minor ginsenosides using derived glycoside hydrolases from host organisms that are not recognized as safe, with most attempts unsuccessful in obtaining the gram unit production of Rg3(S). Recently, Li et al. [31] succeeded in converting the major ginsenoside Rb1 to the minor ginsenosides Rg3 and C-K using an expression system of GRAS host organisms (*Lactococcus lactis*), but their findings were still limited to a laboratory-level production of Rg3(S).

Upon selecting appropriate experimental organisms for β-glucosidase gene, we found a food-grade bacteria for the edible production of Rg3(S) through fermentation of PPD-mix (Rb1 an Rd)-type major ginsenosides. Rg3(S) is well-known for its strong pharmacological effects, but only a few studies focused on the edible production of Rg3(S) using the GRAS host organism or recombinant enzymes [31], and none of the previous studies managed to produce the gram unit of Rg3(S) using the derived glycoside hydrolases from GRAS host organisms. Some researchers tried to use heat acid treatment for the gram unit production of Rg3(S), but did not succeed due to certain side reactions and the byproduction of various minor ginsenosides, such as Rg3(R), Rg5, and Rk1 [30].

Thus, our preliminary data demonstrated that *L. ginsenosidimutans* was suitable for the enriched, gram unit production of edible ginsenoside Rg3(S) from PPD-mix-type ginsenosides (Rb1 and Rd). The DNA sequence of BglL.gin-952 was obtained from the complete genome sequenced *L. ginsenosidimutans* EMML 3041^T., showing that BglL.gin-952 is homologous to glycoside hydrolase family 3 based on its amino acid sequence similarities to the glycoside hydrolases (or β-glucosidases) from *Lactobacillus salsicarnum* (82.5%, GenBank accession no. MQS44673.1), *Lactobacillus* sp. 256–3 (82.4%, GenBank accession no. WP 125704743.1), and *Lactobacillus*. sp M1575 (73.2%, WP 125710781.1). The β-glucosidases have been mainly characterized in glycosyl hydrolase families 1, 3, and 51 (GH1, GH3, and GH51), which usually form in closely related subfamilies with a varied range of activities. Previous research showed that some β-glucosidases of these families may have good hydrolysis specificity to only glucosides or glucosides attached to other monomers, such as β-galactosides, fucosides, β-xylosides, and β-mannosides [34]. Furthermore, some researchers demonstrated that the β-glucosidases belonging to GH3 have various types of ginsenoside-hydrolyzing pathways compared to glycoside hydrolase family 1 and family 51 (GH1 and GH51). The characterized β-glucosides in family 1 and family 51 enable the transformation of major ginsenoside Rb1 → Rd, while the β-glucosides belonging to glycoside hydrolase family 3 convert major ginsenoside Rb1 → Gyp-XVII → Gyp-LXXV [35] and Rb1→ Rd → Rg3(S) [33]. Thus, the glycoside hydrolases belonging to family 3 have better potential to make various kinds of minor ginsenosides from major ginsenosides.

As a glycoside hydrolase family 3 enzyme, BglL.gin-952 showed promising ginsenoside-transforming abilities. Furthermore, 12 novel glycoside hydrolases were identified through complete genome sequencing of *L. ginsenosidimutans* EMML 3041^T (Table 1 and Table S3), which is a presumptive circular chromosome of 2,590,556 base pairs with a G + C content of 36.71%. The online web server of multilocus sequence typing showed 87 characterized and uncharacterized species-specific genes. Based on complete genome annotation, the 10.38% of this genome is made up of carbohydrate transport and metabolism gene clusters, including β-glucoside and cellobiose operons. Moreover, among 12 glycoside hydrolases (as discussed in Section 2.5), seven genes were cloned and expressed in *E. coli* BL21 (DE3). All seven clones were positive for the substrate metabolism (*p*NPG), however, only one gene (BglL.gin-952) was positive ginsenoside conversion (Table S4). BglL.gin-952 belongs to subfamily 5 of GH3 and was responsible for the gram unit production of Rg3(S) from the major ginsenosides Rb1 and Rd. The optimum reaction condition for BglLgin-952 was 55 °C at a pH of 7.5. During conversion, BglL.gin-952 efficiently hydrolyzed the glucose attached to the C3 and C6 positions.

5. Conclusions

To the best of our knowledge, this is the first study in which 30 g of Rg3(S) (with 74.3% chromatography purity) was produced from 50 g of Rb1 in one step using a novel recombinant glucoside hydrolase, namely, BglLgin-952. Thus, BglL.gin-952 could play a pivotal role in the large-scale production of ginsensoide Rg3(S) at an industrial level. Furthermore, our pilot data showed that the enriched production of Rg3(S) using a GRAS host and a recombinant enzyme could enhance the health benefits of *Panax ginseng* in either fermented foods or bioconversion processes and pharmaceutical industries. Additionally, the brief description of the complete genome analysis of *L. ginsenosidimutans* provided in this study may be of use in future studies.

Supplementary Materials: The following are available online at http://www.mdpi.com/2218-273X/10/2/288/s1, **Figure S1** Growth profile of L. ginsenosidimutans in MRS and three food grade media [Based Food Grade (BFG), Food Grade-I (FG-I) and Food Grade-II (FG-II)]. Growth curves were performed in triplicate and the average of those measurements is displayed in the graph above; **Figure S2.** Show the conversion of PPD-mix type major ginsenoside (Rb1and Rd) to Rg3(S) by *Lac. ginsenosidimutans* EMML 3041^T; **Figure S3** Graphical map of the chromosome of Lactobacillus ginsenosidimutans EMML 3041^T. From outside to the center: Genes on the forward strand (colored by COG categories), genes on the reverse strand (colored by COG categories), RNA genes (tRNAs, green; rRNAs, red; other RNAs, black), and GC content and GC skew. And the orthologous proteins of Lactobacillus ginsenosidimutans EMML 3041^T and distribution of proteins in different KEG/COG categories are plotted. Y-axis represents the number of genes/proteins and X-axis represents the KEG/COG categories; **Figure S4.** SDS page analyses of purified BglL.gin-952. Lane 1, Protein marker; Len 2, Induced BglL.gin-952; Lane 3, purified BglL.gin-952; **Figure S5.** TLC analysis shows the time course conversion of ginsenoside Rb1 to Rg3(S) by BglL.gin-952. S, ginsenosides standards; **Table S1.** Anticancer activities of ginsenoside Rg3; **Table S2.** Show the composition of MRS (Difco), Basel Food Grade medium (BFG), Food Grade medium I and Food Grade medium II. All ingredients were used as g/L; **Table S3.** Identification of glycoside hydrolases from the whole genome sequence of L. ginsenosidimutans EMML 3041^T; **Table S4.** Show the hydrolytic activities of seven glycoside hydrolase clones of L. ginsenosidimutans EMML 3041^T for various sugar substrates. 1, α-glucosidase-556; 2, β-glucosidase-484; 3, β-glucosidase-902; 4, β-glucosidase-952; 5, α-galactosidase-556; 6, α-galactosidase-319; 7, β-galactosidase-629. ++, strong positive (98.0 ± 1.2 %); +, positive (87.0 ± 3.1 %); w, weak positive (63.0 ± 2.2 %); –, negative; **Table S5.** Show the different sugar substrate used for the BglL.gin-952; **Table S6.** Total gene count and their function; **Table S7.** The total housekeeping gene identified in the whole genome sequenced L. ginsenosidimutans EMML 3041^T; **Table S8.** Show the production of Rg3(S) using the *Lac. ginsenosidimutans* EMML 3041^T and recombinant BglLgin-952.

Author Contributions: Conceived and designed the experiments: M.Z.S., S.S., W.-T.I. Performed the experiments: M.Z.S., W.-T.I. Analyzed the data: M.Z.S., S.S., W.-T.I., H.Y.P. Wrote the paper: M.Z.S., W.-T.I. All authors have read and agreed to the published version of the manuscript.

Funding: This work was supported by a grant from the National Institute of Biological Resources (NIBR202018101), funded by the Ministry of Environment (MOE) of the Republic of Korea, and by Korea Research Fellowship (KRF) Program through the National Research Foundation of Korea (NRF) funded by the Ministry of Science and ICT (project no. 2019H1D3A1A02070958).

Conflicts of Interest: The authors declare no conflict of interest.

References

1. Jia, L.; Zhao, Y. Current evaluation of the millennium phytomedicine-ginseng (I): Etymology, pharmacognosy, phytochemistry, market and regulations. *Curr. Med. Chem.* **2009**, *16*, 2475–2484. [CrossRef] [PubMed]
2. Li, W.; Zhang, M.; Gu, J.; Meng, Z.-J.; Zhao, L.-C.; Zheng, Y.-N.; Chen, L.; Yang, G.-L. Hypoglycemic effect of protopanaxadiol-type ginsenosides and compound K on Type 2 Diabetes mice induced by High-Fat Diet combining with Streptozotocin via suppression of hepatic gluconeogenesis. *Fitoterapia* **2012**, *83*, 192–198. [CrossRef] [PubMed]
3. Siddiqi, M.H.; Siddiqi, M.Z.; Ahn, S.; Kim, Y.-J.; Yang, D.C. Ginsenoside Rh1 induces mouse osteoblast growth and differentiation through the bone morphogenetic protein 2/runt-related gene 2 signalling pathway. *J. Pharm. Pharmacol.* **2014**, *66*, 1763–1773. [CrossRef]
4. Siddiqi, M.Z.; Siddiqi, M.H.; Kim, Y.-J.; Jin, Y.; Huq, A.; Yang, D.-C. Effect of Fermented Red Ginseng Extract Enriched in Ginsenoside Rg3 on the Differentiation and Mineralization of Preosteoblastic MC3T3-E1 Cells. *J. Med. Food* **2015**, *18*, 542–548. [CrossRef] [PubMed]
5. Wong, A.S.T.; Che, C.-M.; Leung, K.-W. Recent advances in ginseng as cancer therapeutics: A functional and mechanistic overview. *Nat. Prod. Rep.* **2015**, *32*, 256–272. [CrossRef] [PubMed]
6. Baatar, D.; Siddiqi, M.Z.; Im, W.T.; Khaliq, N.U.; Hwang, S.G. Anti-Inflammatory Effect of Ginsenoside Rh2-Mix on Lipopolysaccharide-Stimulated RAW 264.7 Murine Macrophage Cells. *J. Med. Food* **2018**, *21*, 951–960. [CrossRef] [PubMed]
7. Siddiqi, M.Z.; Shafi, S.M.; Choi, K.D.; Im, W.-T.; Aslam, Z. *Sphingobacterium jejuense* sp. nov., with ginsenoside-converting activity, isolated from compost. *Int. J. Syst. Evol. Microbiol.* **2016**, *66*, 4433–4439. [CrossRef]
8. An, D.S.; Cui, C.H.; Siddiqi, M.Z.; Yu, H.S.; Jin, F.X.; Kim, S.G.; Im, W.T. Gram-Scale Production of Ginsenoside F1 Using a Recombinant Bacterial β-Glucosidase. *J. Microbiol. Biotechnol.* **2017**, *27*, 1559–1565. [CrossRef]
9. Christensen, L.P. Ginsenosides chemistry, biosynthesis, analysis, and potential health effects. *Adv. Food Nutr. Res.* **2009**, *55*, 1–99.
10. Jia, L.; Zhao, Y.; Liang, X.-J. Current evaluation of the millennium phytomedicine- ginseng (II): Collected chemical entities, modern pharmacology, and clinical applications emanated from traditional Chinese medicine. *Curr. Med. Chem.* **2009**, *16*, 2924–2942. [CrossRef]
11. Mochizuki, M.; Yoo, Y.; Matsuzawa, K.; Sato, K.; Saiki, I.; Tonooka, S.; Samukawa, K.; Azuma, I. Inhibitory Effect of Tumor Metastasis in Mice by Saponins, Ginsenoside-Rb2, 20(R)- and 20(S)-Ginsenoside-Rg3, of Red ginseng. *Boil. Pharm. Bull.* **1995**, *18*, 1197–1202. [CrossRef] [PubMed]

12. Keum, Y.-S.; Han, S.S.; Chun, K.-S.; Park, K.-K.; Park, J.-H.; Lee, S.K.; Surh, Y.-J. Inhibitory effects of the ginsenoside Rg3 on phorbol ester-induced cyclooxygenase-2 expression, NF-kappaB activation and tumor promotion. *Mutat. Res. Mol. Mech. Mutagen.* **2003**, *523–524*, 75–85. [CrossRef]
13. Han, B.; Park, M.; Han, Y.; Woo, L.; Sankawa, U.; Yahara, S.; Tanaka, O. Degradation of Ginseng Saponins under Mild Acidic Conditions. *Planta Medica* **1982**, *44*, 146–149. [CrossRef] [PubMed]
14. Iishi, H.; Tatsuta, M.; Baba, M.; Uehara, H.; Nakaizumi, A.; Shinkai, K.; Akedo, H.; Funai, H.; Ishiguro, S.; Kitagawa, I. Inhibition by ginsenoside Rg3 of bombesin-enhanced peritoneal metastasis of intestinal adenocarcinomas induced by azoxymethane in Wistar rats. *Clin. Exp. Metastasis* **1997**, *15*, 603–611. [CrossRef]
15. Kim, D.G.; Jung, K.H.; Lee, D.G.; Yoon, J.H.; Choi, K.S.; Kwon, H.M.; Morgan, M.J.; Howang, S.S.; Kim, Y.S. 20(S)-Ginsenoside Rg3 is a novel inhibitor of autophagy and sensitizes hepatocellular carcinoma to doxorubicin. *Oncotarget* **2014**, *5*, 4438–4451. [CrossRef]
16. Kim, H.-S.; Lee, E.-H.; Ko, S.-R.; Choi, K.-J.; Park, J.-H.; Im, N.-S. Effects of ginsenosides Rg3 and Rh2 on the proliferation of prostate cancer cells. *Arch. Pharmacal Res.* **2004**, *27*, 429–435. [CrossRef]
17. Xu, T.-M.; Xin, Y.; Cui, M.-H.; Jiang, X.; Gu, L.-P. Inhibitory effect of ginsenoside Rg3 combined with cyclophosphamide on growth and angiogenesis of ovarian cancer. *Chin. Med. J.* **2007**, *120*, 584–588. [CrossRef]
18. Tian, J.; Zhang, S.; Li, G.; Liu, Z.; Xu, B. 20(S)-ginsenoside Rg3, a neuroprotective agent, inhibits mitochondrial permeability transition pores in rat brain. *Phytotherapy Res.* **2009**, *23*, 486–491. [CrossRef]
19. In, J.G.; Kim, E.J.; Lee, B.S.; Park, M.H.; Yang, D.C. Saponin analysis and red ginseng production using the simplified method of Korean ginseng (Panax ginseng C.A. Meyer). *Korean J. Plant Res.* **2006**, *19*, 133–138.
20. Jung, H.M.; Liu, Q.M.; Kim, J.W.; Lee, S.T.; Kim, S.C.; Im, W.T. *Lactobacillus ginsenosidimutans* sp. nov., isolated from kimchi with the ability to transform ginsenosides. *Antonie van Leeuwenhoek* **2013**, *103*, 867–876. [CrossRef]
21. Sawatari, Y.; Hirano, T.; Yokota, A. Development of food grade media for the preparation of Lactobacillus plantarum starter culture. *J. Gen. Appl. Microbiol.* **2006**, *52*, 349–356. [CrossRef] [PubMed]
22. Siddiqi, M.Z.; Muhammad Shafi, S.; Im, W.T. Complete genome sequencing of *Arachidicoccus ginsenosidimutans* sp. nov., and its application for production of minor ginsenosides by finding a novel ginsenoside-transforming b-glucosidase. *RSC Adv.* **2017**, *7*, 46745. [CrossRef]
23. Thompson, J.D.; Gibson, T.J.; Plewniak, F.; Jeanmougin, F.; Higgins, D.G. The CLUSTAL_X windows interface: Flexible strategies for multiple sequence alignment aided by quality analysis tools. *Nucleic Acids Res.* **1997**, *25*, 4876–4882. [CrossRef] [PubMed]
24. Hall, T.A. Bioedit: A user-friendly biological sequence alignment editor and analysis program for Windows 95/98/NT. *Nucl. Acids Symp. Ser.* **1999**, *41*, 95–98.
25. Saitou, N.; Nei, M. The neighbor-joining method: A new method for reconstructing phylogenetic trees. *Mol. Boil. Evol.* **1987**, *4*, 406–425.
26. Tamura, K.; Stecher, G.; Peterson, D.; Filipski, A.; Kumar, S. MEGA6: Molecular Evolutionary Genetics Analysis Version 6.0. *Mol. Biol. Evol.* **2013**, *30*, 2725–2729. [CrossRef]
27. Felsenstein, J. Confidence limits on phylogenies: An approach using the bootstrap. *Evolution* **1985**, *39*, 783–791. [CrossRef]
28. Ruan, C.-C.; Zhang, H.; Zhang, L.-X.; Liu, Z.; Sun, G.-Z.; Lei, J.; Qin, Y.-X.; Zheng, Y.-N.; Li, X.; Pan, H.-Y. Biotransformation of Ginsenoside Rf to Rh1 by Recombinant β-Glucosidase. *Molecules* **2009**, *14*, 2043–2048. [CrossRef]
29. Choi, S.-H.; Shin, T.-J.; Hwang, S.-H.; Lee, B.-H.; Kang, J.-Y.; Kim, H.-J.; Oh, J.-W.; Bae, C.-S.; Lee, S.-H.; Nah, S.-Y. Differential Effects of Ginsenoside Metabolites on HERG K+ Channel Currents. *J. Ginseng Res.* **2011**, *35*, 191–199. [CrossRef]
30. Siddiqi, M.Z.; Cui, C.H.; Park, S.K.; Han, N.S.; Kim, S.C.; Im, W.T. Comparative analysis of the expression level of recombinant ginsenoside-transforming β-glucosidase in GRAS hosts and mass production of the ginsenoside Rh2-Mix. *PLoS ONE* **2017**, *12*, e0176098. [CrossRef]
31. Li, L.; Lee, S.J.; Yuan, Q.P.; Im, W.T.; Kim, S.C.; Han, N.N. Production of bioactive ginsenoside Rg3(S) and compound K using recombinant Lactococcus lactis. *J. Ginseng Res.* **2018**, *24*, 412–418. [CrossRef] [PubMed]
32. Cheng, L.-Q.; Na, J.R.; Bang, M.H.; Kim, M.K.; Yang, D.-C. Conversion of major ginsenoside Rb1 to 20(S)-ginsenoside Rg3 by Microbacterium sp. GS514. *Phytochemistry* **2008**, *69*, 218–224. [CrossRef] [PubMed]

33. Quan, L.H.; Min, J.W.; Yang, D.U.; Kim, Y.J.; Yang, D.C. Enzymatic biotransformation of ginsenoside Rb1 to 20(S)-Rg3 by recombinant bglucosidase from Microbacterium esteraromaticum. *Appl. Micro Biotech.* **2012**, *94*, 377–384. [CrossRef] [PubMed]
34. Opassiri, R.; Pomthong, B.; Onkoksoong, T.; Akiyama, T.; Esen, A.; Cairns, J.R.K. Analysis of rice glycosyl hydrolase family 1 and expression of Os4bglu12 β-glucosidase. *BMC Plant Boil.* **2006**, *6*, 33.
35. An, D.-S.; Cui, C.-H.; Lee, H.-G.; Wang, L.; Kim, S.C.; Lee, S.-T.; Jin, F.; Yu, H.; Chin, Y.-W.; Lee, H.-K.; et al. Identification and Characterization of a Novel Terrabacter ginsenosidimutans sp. nov. β-Glucosidase That Transforms Ginsenoside Rb1 into the Rare Gypenosides XVII and LXXV. *Appl. Environ. Microbiol.* **2010**, *76*, 5827–5836.

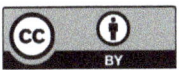

© 2020 by the authors. Licensee MDPI, Basel, Switzerland. This article is an open access article distributed under the terms and conditions of the Creative Commons Attribution (CC BY) license (http://creativecommons.org/licenses/by/4.0/).

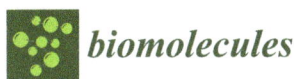

Article

A Critical Regulation of Th17 Cell Responses and Autoimmune Neuro-Inflammation by Ginsenoside Rg3

Young-Jun Park [1,†], Minkyoung Cho [1,*,†], Garam Choi [1,2], Hyeongjin Na [1,2] and Yeonseok Chung [1,2,*]

[1] Laboratory of Immune Regulation, Research Institute of Pharmaceutical Sciences, College of Pharmacy, Seoul National University, Seoul 08826, Korea; flavah00@gmail.com (Y.-J.P.); grhappy@snu.ac.kr (G.C.); hyeongjinna@snu.ac.kr (H.N.)
[2] Brain Korea 21 Program, College of Pharmacy, Seoul National University, Seoul 08826, Korea
* Correspondence: mkcho84@snu.ac.kr (M.C.); yeonseok@snu.ac.kr (Y.C.); Tel.: +82-2-880-7874 (M.C. & Y.C.); Fax: +82-2-872-1795 (M.C. & Y.C.)
† These authors contributed equally to this work.

Received: 6 December 2019; Accepted: 7 January 2020; Published: 10 January 2020

Abstract: Among diverse helper T-cell subsets, Th17 cells appear to be pathogenic in diverse autoimmune diseases, and thus, targeting Th17 cells could be beneficial for the treatment of the diseases in humans. Ginsenoside Rg3 is one of the most potent components in Korean Red Ginseng (KRG; *Panax ginseng* Meyer) in ameliorating inflammatory responses. However, the role of Rg3 in Th17 cells and Th17-mediated autoimmunity is unclear. We found that Rg3 significantly inhibited the differentiation of Th17 cells from naïve precursors in a dendritic cell (DC)–T co-culture system. While Rg3 minimally affected the secretion of IL-6, TNFα, and IL-12p40 from DCs, it significantly hampered the expression of IL-17A and RORγt in T cells in a T-cell-intrinsic manner. Moreover, Rg3 alleviated the onset and severity of experimental autoimmune encephalomyelitis (EAE), induced by transferring myelin oligodendrocyte glycoprotein (MOG)-reactive T cells. Our findings demonstrate that Rg3 inhibited Th17 differentiation and Th17-mediated neuro-inflammation, suggesting Rg3 as a potential candidate for resolving Th17-related autoimmune diseases.

Keywords: Rg3; Th17; RORγt; EAE

1. Introduction

Due to their immunomodulatory functions, several herbal medicines have been used for the treatment of immunological disorders [1]. Among them, Korean Red Ginseng (KRG) has been traditionally prescribed for various diseases, although the exact mechanisms by which KRG mitigates the severity of diseases remain unclear [2]. Recent advances in understanding the pharmacological components of KRG shed light on identifying a variety of bioactive ingredients, such as ginsenosides, polysaccharides, phytosterols, peptides, polyacetylenic alcohols, and fatty acids, that prevent and eradicate diabetes, tumors, ulcers, aging, and depression [3–6].

It has been suggested that ginsenosides are among the most potent biologically active constituents of KRG [7]. More than 100 types of ginsenosides are present, stratified by the differential polarity attributed to their chemical backbones [8]. Interestingly, numerous studies have reported that anti-inflammatory effects are common features of a myriad of ginsenosides [2,9]. For example, enhanced Rg3, one of the major ginsenosides present in KRG, inhibits IFNγ-producing helper CD4[+] T cells (Th1) that prevalently expand in the conditions of excessive inflammation [10]. Rg3 also promotes immunosuppressive M2 macrophage polarization, which can resolve self-destructive immune responses [11]. Moreover, increasing numbers of recent studies demonstrate that ginsenosides can ameliorate the disease severity in animal models of multiple sclerosis, Crohn's disease, and rheumatoid arthritis, suggesting that ginsenosides modulate autoimmune responses in vivo [1].

Autoimmune diseases are caused by unnecessarily aggressive autoreactive CD4$^+$ T-cell responses that attack self-tissue and/or self-antigen. Among diverse CD4$^+$ T-cell subsets, IL-17A-producing CD4$^+$ T cells (Th17) provide protection against extracellular pathogens and fungi, but also exert detrimental roles in mediating tissue inflammation in autoimmune diseases [12,13]. Indeed, antagonistic antibodies to IL-17A or IL-17RA have shown a clinical benefit in patients with psoriasis [14]. The differentiation of Th17 cells is induced by IL-6 and TGFβ, which activate STAT3 and subsequently induce RORγt [15–17]. Recently, two independent studies have demonstrated that KRG can inhibit Th17 cell differentiation by hampering STAT3 activation, leading to the amelioration of collagen-induced arthritis and alloantigen-induced inflammation [18,19]. Our previous study also suggested a role of Rg3 in T-cell differentiation [10], indicating a possible role of ginsenosides in T-cell-mediated immune disorders.

In the present study, we aimed to investigate whether ginsenoside Rg3 modulated Th17 differentiation and Th17-mediated experimental autoimmune encephalomyelitis (EAE), in an animal model for human multiple sclerosis. By using multiple in vitro T-cell culture systems, we found that Rg3 inhibited Th17 cell differentiation in a T-cell-intrinsic manner. Moreover, Rg3 alleviated the incidence and severity of EAE in vivo.

2. Materials and Methods

2.1. Ethics Statement

All animal experiments were approved by the Institutional Animal Care and Use Committee of Seoul National University (IACUC protocol #: SNU-170120-1) and were conducted in accordance with guidelines of Seoul National University for the care and use of laboratory animals.

2.2. Mice and EAE Model

Six-week-old C57BL/6 female mice were purchased from Orient Bio (Gyeonggi, Korea). For T-cell-transfer EAE, mice were immunized with 300 μg myelin oligodendrocyte glycoprotein peptide (MOG$_{35-55}$) peptide emulsified in complete freund's adjuvant (CFA) with heat-inactivated *Mycobacterium tuberculosis*. Seven days after immunization, cells from draining lymph nodes were isolated and cultured with 20 μg/mL MOG$_{35-55}$ and IL-23 (20 ng/mL) (PeproTech, Rocky Hill, NJ, USA). On day five post in vitro stimulation, cells were harvested and enriched with CD4$^+$ T cells by using magnetic beads. The enriched CD4$^+$ T cells (2×10^6 cells/mouse) were transferred into mice followed by immunization with MOG$_{35-55}$ in CFA (s.c.) and subsequent pertussis toxin (PT) (i.p.) injection, and the clinical severity for EAE pathology was monitored daily as previously mentioned [20].

2.3. Bone-Marrow-Derived Dendritic Cells (BMDCs) Generation

Bone marrow cells obtained from C57BL/6 mice were cultured in PRMI1640 supplemented with 10% FBS, 55 μM 2-mercaptoethanol, penicillin/streptomycin at 1×10^6 cells/mL (All from Gibco, Grand Island, NY, USA), and recombinant mouse GM-CSF (10 ng/mL) (PeproTech, Rocky Hill, NJ, USA). Twenty-four hours later, floating cells were transferred into new plates. Fresh medium was added every other day. On day seven, cells were recovered and CD11c$^+$ cells were isolated using magnetic beads, and the sorted CD11c$^+$ DCs were used in further studies.

2.4. In Vitro Th17 Cell Differentiation

Naïve CD4$^+$ T cells (CD44^{low}CD62L^{high}CD25$^-$) were isolated from wild-type mice using a cell sorter (BD BioScience, San Jose, CA, USA). For DC-mediated Th17 cell differentiation, BMDCs were co-cultured with naive CD4$^+$ T cells in the presence of anti-CD3ε (0.3 μg/mL) antibody (145-2C11,

BioXcell, NH, USA), TGFβ (1.5 ng/mL) (PeproTech, Rocky Hill, NJ, USA), and LPS (100 ng/mL) (Sigma, Seoul, Korea) for 96 h. For DC-free Th17 cell differentiation, anti-CD3ε (1 µg/mL) and anti-CD28 (1 µg/mL) (37.51, BioXcell, West Lebanon, NH, USA) were pre-coated in a 96-well flat-bottom plate overnight at 4 °C. After washing the plate with cold PBS three times, 1×10^5 naïve $CD4^+$ T cells were stimulated with IL-6 (10 ng/mL) and TGFβ (1.5 ng/mL) (PeproTech, Rocky Hill, NJ, USA) for 96 h. For Rg3 (LKT Labs, Saint Paul, MN, USA; dissolved in DMSO) treatment, various concentrations (9.37, 18.75, and 37.5 µg/mL) were added at the beginning of in vitro culture.

2.5. ELISA

IL-6, 12p40, IL-17A, and TNFα in the culture supernatants of LPS-stimulated BMDCs or T cells stimulated under Th17-skewing conditions were quantified by ELISA according to the manufacturer's instructions (eBioscience, San Diego, CA, USA).

2.6. Real-Time RT-PCR

Total RNA from cells was isolated by TRIzol reagent (Ambion, Austin, TX, USA) and cDNA was synthesized with a cDNA Synthesis kit (Thermo Fisher Scientific Inc., Waltham, MA, USA). Relative gene expression levels were evaluated using SYBR Green (Bio-Rad, Philadelphia, PA, USA) on ABI 7500 Fast Real-Time PCR Systems (Applied Biosystems, Singapore). Target genes were normalized to the *Hprt* level in each sample. Primer sets for genes were synthesized at Cosmogenetech (Seoul, Korea): *Il6* (sense, 5'- TCG GAG GCT AAA TTA CAC ATG TTC T -3', antisense, 5'- GCA TCA TCG TTG TTC ATA CAA TCA -3'), *Il12b* (sense, 5'- AAA CCA GAC CCG CCC AAG AAC -3', antisense, 5'- AAA AAG CCA ACC AAG CAG AAG ACA G -3'), *Il17a* (sense, 5'- CTC CAG AAG GCC CTC AGA CTA C -3', antisense, 5'- GGG TCT TCA TTG CGG TGG -3'), *Il22* (sense, 5'- CAT GCA GGA GGT GGT ACC TT -3', antisense, 5'- CAG ACG CAA GCA TTT CTC AG -3'), *Rorc* (sense, 5'-CCG CTG AGA GGG CTT CAC -3', antisense, 5'- TGC AGG AGT AGG CCA CAT TAC A -3'),*Tnfa* (sense, 5'- ATG AGA AGT TCC CAA ATG GCC -3', antisense, 5'- TCC ACT TGG TGG TTC GCT ACG -3'), *Hprt* (sense, 5'- GGT TAA GCA GTA CAG CCC CAA AAT -3', antisense, 5'- ATA GGC ACA TAG TGC AAA TCA AAA GTC -3').

2.7. Flow Cytometry Analysis

For intracellular cytokine staining, cells were incubated for 3 h with 100 ng/mL of PMA and 1 µM of ionomycin (all from Sigma-Aldrich, Saint Louis, MO, USA), brefeldin A, and monensin (all from eBioscience, San Diego, CA, USA). After washing cells with cold PBS containing 1.5% FBS, cells were stained with APC-Cy7-conjugated anti-CD45.2 mAb and PE/Cy7-conjugated anti-CD4 mAb (eBioscience, San Diego, CA, USA) for surface staining. Cells were then washed and stained with PerCp-Cy5.5-conjugated anti-IFNγ mAb, APC-conjugated anti-IL-17 mAb (all from BioLegend, San Diego, CA, USA) and PE-conjugated anti-RORγt mAb (eBioscience, San Diego, CA, USA) after incubation with fixation/permeabilization buffer (eBioscience, San Diego, CA, USA) for 30 min at 4 °C. Cells were analyzed by LSR III flow cytometer (BD Bioscience, San Jose, CA, USA). Data were analyzed with FlowJo (TreeStar, Ashland, OR, USA).

2.8. Statistical Analysis

All experiments were performed more than three times. Statistical analysis was conducted with mean ± SEM by unpaired two-tailed Student's *t*-test with GraphPad Prism 5.0 (GraphPad Software Inc., San Diego, CA, USA).

3. Results

3.1. Rg3 Minimally Affects the Production of Th17-Promoting Cytokines from DCs

Our previous study showed that KRG extract and enhanced Rg3 suppressed pro-inflammatory cytokines production by LPS-stimulated DCs [10]. Moreover, KRG extract has been shown to inhibit Th17-cell differentiation in the presence of cyclosporine in vitro [18]. Hence, as a first step to determine the potential role of Rg3 in Th17 cell differentiation, we asked if Rg3 impacts the production of Th17-promoting cytokines, including IL-6, TNFα, and IL-12/IL-23p40 from DCs upon LPS treatment [21]. We generated bone-marrow derived DCs (BMDCs) and stimulated them with LPS for 12 h in the presence or absence of Rg3 (Figure 1A). DMSO was used as a vehicle control since Rg3 was dissolved in DMSO. We observed that, although Rg3 treatment slightly increased the transcript level of *Tnfa*, it had little effect on the level of TNFα production by the BMDCs (Figure 1B). Similarly, treatment with Rg3 had little effect on the transcript levels of *Il12b* and *Il6* as well as on the protein levels of IL-12p40 and IL-6 (Figure 1C,D). Thus, Rg3 treatment played only a minor role in the induction of pro-Th17 cytokines from DCs in this experimental setting.

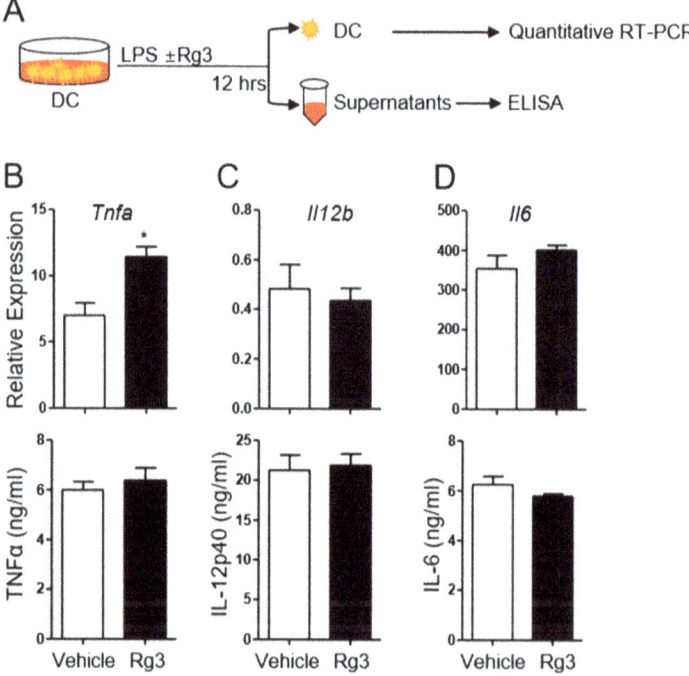

Figure 1. Effects of Rg3 treatment on the production of pro-inflammatory cytokines from LPS-stimulated bone-marrow-derived dendritic cells (BMDCs). (**A**) Experimental scheme. BMDCs were treated with LPS in the presence of DMSO (vehicle) or 37.5 μg/mL Rg3. After 12 h, the transcript and protein levels of indicated cytokines in BMDCs were measured by quantitative RT-PCR and ELISA (**B–D**). Data are mean ± SEM and represent three independent experiments. * $p < 0.05$.

3.2. Rg3 Inhibits Th17 Cell Differentiation in a T-Cell-Intrinsic Manner

To determine if Rg3 impacts Th17 cell differentiation, we employed a well-established DC-mediated Th17 cell differentiation system in which IL-17A-producing CD4[+] T cells are induced by stimulating naïve CD4[+] T cells with soluble anti-CD3, LPS, and TGFβ in the presence of BMDCs for four days [22] (Figure 2A). We observed about 10–13% of IL-17A[+] cells by day four. However, upon treatment with

Rg3, the frequency of IL-17A-producing Th17 cells was significantly decreased in a dose-dependent manner (Figure 2B). Accordingly, the production of IL-17A in the culture supernatant was significantly diminished by Rg3 treatment (Figure 2C). These results demonstrate that Rg3 can suppress the differentiation of Th17 cells from naïve precursors in vitro.

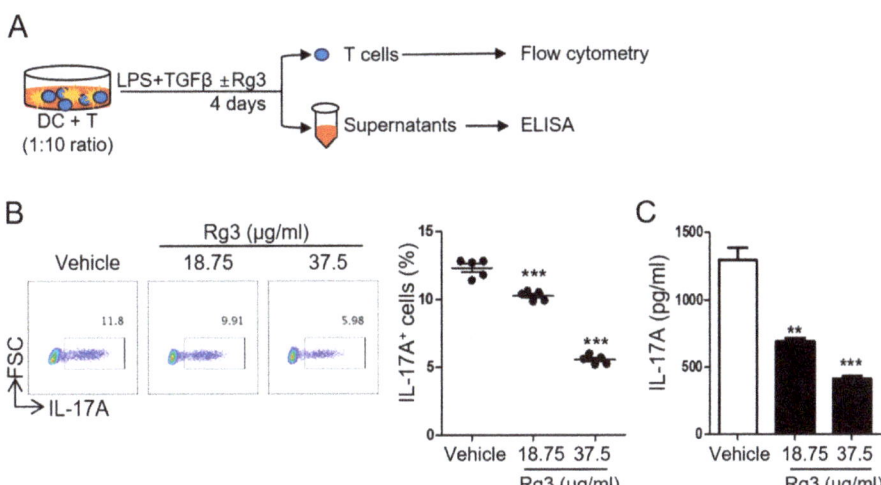

Figure 2. Rg3 inhibited DC-mediated Th17 differentiation. (**A**) Experimental scheme. Naïve CD4$^+$ T cells were incubated with LPS-stimulated BMDCs in the presence of soluble anti-CD3 and 1.5 ng/mL TGFβ. DMSO (vehicle) or indicated doses of Rg3 (18.75 or 37.5 µg/mL) was added at the beginning of cell culture. The frequency of IL-17A$^+$CD4$^+$ T cells and the level of IL-17A were determined by FACS (**B**) and ELISA (**C**), respectively. Data are mean ± SEM and represent three independent experiments. ** $p < 0.01$, *** $p < 0.001$ in comparison with the vehicle-treated group.

Since Rg3 treatment itself resulted in little change in the production of IL-6, IL-12/IL-23p40, and TNFα from BMDCs (Figure 1), we hypothesized that Rg3 might inhibit Th17 cell differentiation by acting on T cells rather than on DCs. To address the T-cell-modulatory effect of Rg3 during Th17 cell differentiation, we employed a DC-free Th17 cell differentiation system in which naïve CD4$^+$ T cells were stimulated with plate-bound anti-CD3 and anti-CD28 antibodies in the presence of IL-6 and TGFβ for 4 days [22] (Figure 3A). Consistent with the observation in the DC-mediated Th17 cell differentiation system, we observed that the addition of Rg3 remarkably reduced the frequency of IL-17A-producing T cells and the production of IL-17A in the DC-free Th17 cell differentiation system (Figure 3B,C). Moreover, the transcript levels of Th17-cell-associated genes including *Il17a*, *Il21*, *Il22*, and *Rorc* in the T cells were all diminished by Rg3 (Figure 3D). These results together indicate that Rg3 inhibits Th17 cell differentiation by directly acting on CD4$^+$ T cells rather than on DCs.

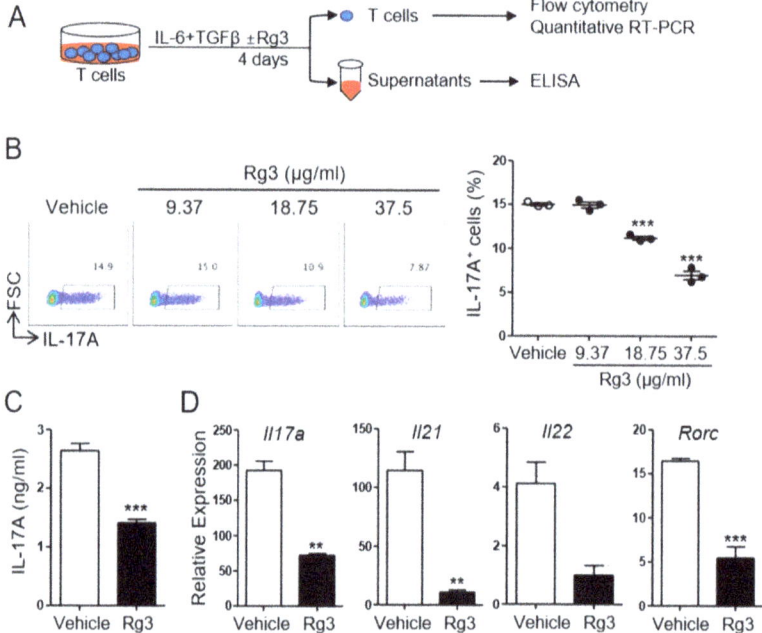

Figure 3. Rg3 inhibited Th17 differentiation in a T-cell-intrinsic manner. (**A**) Experimental scheme. Naïve CD4$^+$ T cells were stimulated with pre-coated anti-CD3 and CD28 in the presence of 10 ng/mL IL-6 and 1.5 ng/mL TGFβ. DMSO (vehicle) or indicated doses of Rg3 (18.75 or 37.5 μg/mL) was added at the beginning cell culture. The frequency of IL-17A$^+$CD4$^+$ T cells and the level of IL-17A were determined by FACS. (**B**) The amount of IL-17A and the transcript levels of indicated genes were measured by ELISA and quantitative RT-PCR, respectively (**C,D**). The concentration of Rg3 in (**C**) and (**D**) was 37.5 μg/mL. Data represent mean ± SEM and represent three independent experiments. *** $p < 0.001$ in comparison with the vehicle-treated group.

3.3. Rg3 Inhibits RORγt Expression in CD4$^+$ T Cells during Th17 Cell Differentiation

Among pro-inflammatory cytokines secreted by DCs, IL-6 is critical for Th17 differentiation [23]. Our data demonstrated that Rg3 had little role in the production of IL-6 from DCs while inhibiting Th17 cell differentiation in the presence of IL-6 and TGFβ. Thus, we hypothesized that Rg3 modulates Th17 cell differentiation by regulating signals within the T cell itself. In the presence of TGFβ (1.5 ng/mL), IL-6 induces the expression of orphan nuclear receptor RORγt in a STAT3-dependent manner, which acts as the master transcription factor Th17 cell commitment [16]. To examine if Rg3 impacts the expression of RORγt in T cells, we stimulated naïve CD4$^+$ T cells in the DC-free Th17-skewing condition with increasing doses of IL-6. Compared with 10 ng/mL of IL-6, 20 or 40 ng/mL of IL-6 induced an increase in IL-17A$^+$ T cells up to ~40%. However, the same treatment resulted in ~10% of IL-17A$^+$ T cells in the presence of Rg3 (Figure 4A). We observed a similar pattern in the frequency of IL-17A$^+$ RORγt$^+$ T cells (Figure 4B), suggesting a possible role of Rg3 in regulating RORγt expression in T cells. As shown in Figure 4C, stimulation with 10 ng/mL of IL-6 and TGFβ (1.5 ng/mL) induced the expression of RORγt in over 80% of CD4$^+$ T cells. However, the addition of Rg3 significantly hampered the expression of RORγt in CD4$^+$ T cells. Increasing IL-6 failed to restore the diminished RORγt in CD4$^+$ T cells (Figure 4C). Thus, these results strongly suggest that Rg3 inhibits Th17 cell differentiation by hampering RORγt expression in CD4$^+$ T cells.

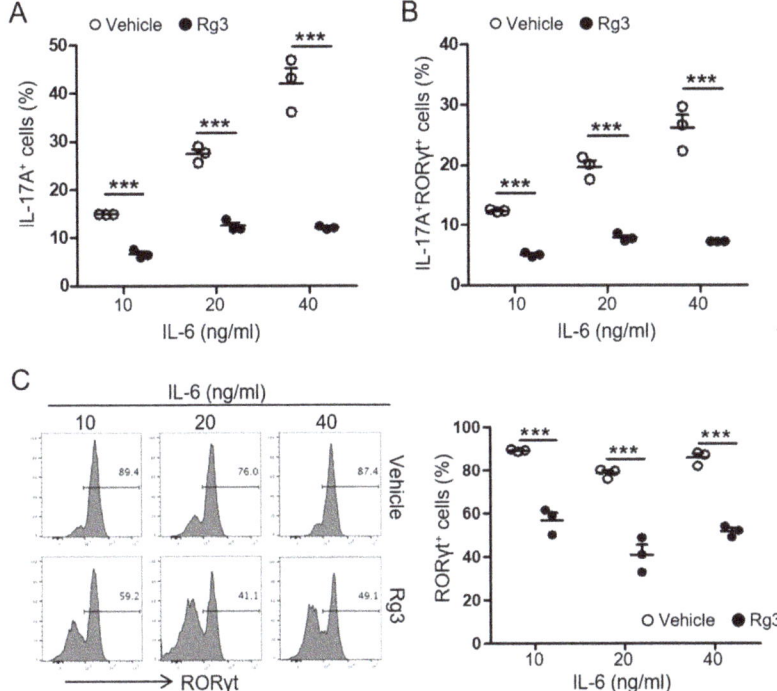

Figure 4. Rg3 diminished RORγt expression in T cells during Th17 differentiation. Naïve CD4$^+$ T cells were stimulated with pre-coated anti-CD3 and CD28 in the presence of 1.5 ng/mL TGFβ and indicated concentrations of IL-6. DMSO (vehicle) or Rg3 (37.5 μg/mL) was added at the beginning of the cell culture. The frequency of IL-17A$^+$ (**A**) and IL-17A$^+$RORγt$^+$ (**B**) CD4$^+$ T cells was measured by FACS. (**C**) The histogram of RORγt$^+$ expression in CD4$^+$ T cells is shown. Experiments were conducted three times. Data represent mean ± SEM. *** $p < 0.001$ in comparison with the vehicle-treated group.

3.4. Rg3 Attenuates the Reactivation of Autoreactive Th17 Cells and Experimental Autoimmune Encephalomyelitis Induced by MOG-Reactive CD4$^+$ T-Cell Transfer

Inhibition of Th17 cell differentiation and RORγt expression by Rg3 treatment in vitro prompted us to examine if Rg3 also inhibits the reactivation of Th17 cells generated in vivo. Stimulation of the lymphoid cells from myelin oligodendrocyte glycoprotein peptide (MOG$_{35-55}$)-immunized mice with MOG in the presence of IL-23 is known to reactivate and expand MOG-specific Th17 cells [24]. When we employed this experimental model (Figure 5A), we observed that ~40% of the CD4$^+$ T cells expressed IL-17A and ~60% expressed IFNγ (Figure 5B), indicating that MOG-specific pathogenic Th17 cells were reactivated and expanded upon restimulation. By contrast, the addition of Rg3 during the restimulation step significantly diminished the frequency of IFNγ$^-$IL-17A$^+$ as well as that of IFNγ$^+$IL-17A$^+$ T cells (Figure 5B). Rg3 treatment slightly increased the frequency of IFNγ$^+$IL-17A$^-$ population; however, the overall frequency of IFNγ-producer was diminished due to a remarkable reduction in the frequency of IFNγ$^+$IL-17A$^+$ cells (vehicle vs. Rg3; 62.37 ± 1.90 vs. 45.70 ± 0.98, $p = 0.0015$). Thus, Rg3 hampered the reactivation and ex vivo expansion of MOG-reactive Th17 cells.

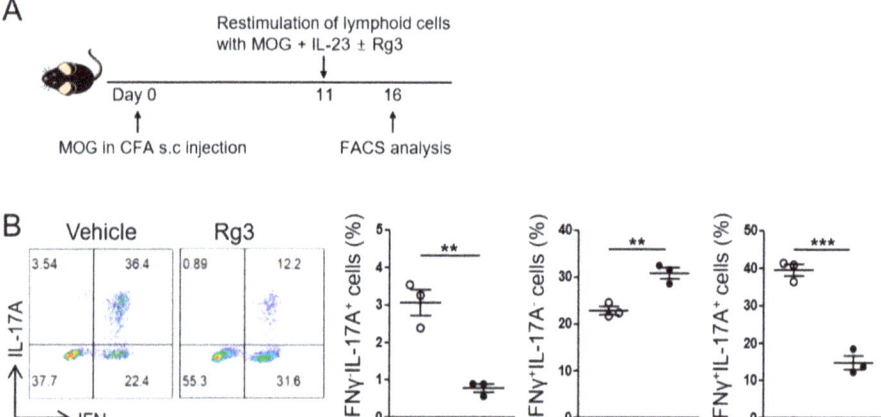

Figure 5. Rg3 inhibited the expansion of myelin oligodendrocyte glycoprotein (MOG)-reactive Th17 cells. (**A**) Experimental scheme. Mice were immunized s.c. with MOG in CFA. Seven days later, the lymphoid cells from the draining lymph nodes (LNs) were harvested and restimulated with MOG and IL-23 in the presence of DMSO (vehicle) or Rg3 (37.5 µg/mL) for 5 days. (**B**) The expression of IL-17A and IFNγ in CD4$^+$ T cells were examined by FACS. Data shown are mean ± SEM and represent one from two independent experiments. ** $p < 0.01$, *** $p < 0.001$ in comparison with the vehicle-treated group.

MOG-reactive Th17 cells are known to induce autoimmune neuroinflammation, and IL-17A has been proposed as a promising target for the treatment of multiple sclerosis (MS) [25]. Thus, we next tested whether Rg3 can ameliorate the severity of experimental autoimmune encephalomyelitis (EAE) in a mouse disease model for MS, induced by a transfer of MOG-reactive Th17 cells. Adoptive transfer of MOG-reactive ex vivo expanded Th17 cells (CD45.1$^{+/+}$) is known to induce EAE (Figure 6A) [24]. As depicted in Figure 6B,C, recipients of Rg3-treated CD4$^+$ T cells were more resistant to EAE induction concomitant with lesser weight loss, compared with the recipients of vehicle-treated CD4$^+$ T cells. Accordingly, the clinical score was significantly lower in the former (Figure 6D), indicating that Rg3 treatment rendered MOG-specific autoreactive Th17 cells to be less pathogenic in inducing neuro-inflammation. Analysis of donor T cells harvested from the central nervous system (CNS) tissues showed that Rg3-treated CD4$^+$ T cells exhibited a lower frequency of IL-17A$^+$ population than vehicle-treated T cells (Figure 6E). Similarly, the IL-17A$^+$ frequency among donor T cells was reduced in the draining inguinal lymph nodes (iLNs) of the former group (Figure 6F). In contrast, the frequency of IFN-γ$^+$ cells among donor T cells in the CNS as well as in the iLNs was comparable between the two groups (Figure 6E,F). Together, these data suggest that Rg3 inhibits the reactivation of autoreactive Th17 cells rather than Th1 cells, leading to a diminished autoimmune neuro-inflammation associated with reduced Th17 cells in CNS tissues.

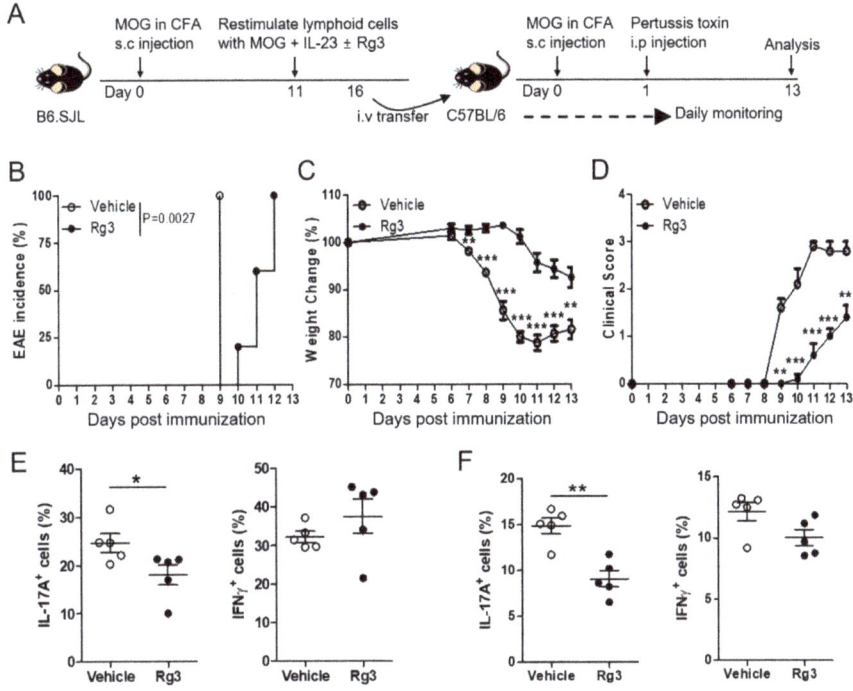

Figure 6. Rg3 decreases autoimmune neuro-inflammation induced by adoptive transfer of MOG-reactive CD4$^+$ T cells. (**A**) Experimental scheme of passive experimental autoimmune encephalomyelitis (EAE), induction. (**B–D**) EAE incidence, % weight change, and clinical score were monitored daily. The levels of IL-17A and IFNγ in CD4$^+$ T cells were examined in the CNS (**E**) and the inguinal LN (**F**) on day 13 after EAE induction. Data shown are mean ± SEM and represent two independent experiments. * $p < 0.05$, ** $p < 0.01$, *** $p < 0.001$ in comparison with the vehicle-treated group.

4. Discussion

While the immunomodulatory effects of KRG extract (KRGE) are well documented, the immuno-pharmacological effects of each component within the extracts are less clear. In this regard, ginsenoside Rg3 has been proposed to be immuno-modulatory based on the observation that Rg3-enhanced KRGE ameliorates various inflammatory diseases in animal models, including T-cell-mediated autoimmune diseases [2,4,10,18]. Among diverse helper T-cell subsets, Th17 cells appear to be critically pathogenic immune cells in autoimmune tissue inflammation, including psoriasis and multiple sclerosis. Therefore, in the present study, we aimed to investigate the role of Rg3 in Th17 cell differentiation and Th17-mediated autoimmune diseases by using animal models. Our in vitro studies revealed that Rg3 played only a minor role in the production of Th17-promoting cytokines IL-6, IL-12/23p40 and TNFα from DCs. Instead, Rg3 significantly inhibited the induction of RORγt expression in CD4$^+$ T cells and therefore hampered the differentiation of Th17 cells from naïve precursors. Moreover, Rg3 appeared to inhibit the expansion of autoreactive MOG-specific Th17 cells during ex vivo restimulation with a cognate peptide, and thus also ameliorated the incidence and severity of EAE in the recipient mice. Thus, our findings suggest an anti-inflammatory mechanism by which Rg3 ameliorates autoimmune inflammation via inhibiting RORγt expression of CD4$^+$ T cells during Th17 cell differentiation.

RORγt, a master transcription factor for Th17, is regulated by a complex regulatory circuit [26], but whether Rg3 intervenes with the RORγt expression has not been identified. Activation of STAT3 upon IL-6 signaling with concomitant TGFβ signaling induces RORγt expression [17]. Moreover, IL-23 further expands and stabilizes Th17 cells via STAT3. In this respect, it is noteworthy that Rg3 represses STAT3 phosphorylation in tumor cells by decreasing the hexokinase 2 level [27]. We observed that the transcript level of *Il21* in T cells stimulated with IL-6 and TGFβ was reduced by Rg3. IL-21 is known to be induced by IL-6 via STAT3 during Th17 cell differentiation [28]. Thus, it is feasible to hypothesize that Rg3 inhibits RORγt expression by suppressing STAT3 activation in T cells upon IL-6 and IL-23 signaling. Alternatively, it is possible that STAT5, a negative regulator of RORγt, was involved in the Th17 reduction by Rg3, given that ginseng can up-regulate STAT5 phosphorylation in cyclosporine-treated splenocytes poised to Treg differentiation [18]. It has also been delineated that natural ligands stemming from endogenous cholesterol metabolism can either promote or inhibit RORγt function by directly interacting with its binding sites [29]. Ursolic acid is one of the most well-characterized RORγt antagonists, which ameliorates EAE and allergic asthma [30,31]. Since Rg3 has a tetracyclic triterpenoid saponin structure [14], a homologue of the ursolic acid, Rg3 might belong to the specific RORγt antagonists as well. Further studies are required to dissect the direct molecular target(s) of Rg3 in developing Th17 cells and to elucidate the molecular mechanisms by which Rg3 regulates Th17 cell differentiation and expansion.

Several studies including our own showed that KRGE can modulate the production of innate cytokines from DCs and macrophages [10,11]. LPS stimulation induced the production of several Th17-promoting cytokines including IL-6, IL-23, TNFα, and IL-1β. The observed minor role of Rg3 in regulating the production of these cytokines from DCs suggests that other components within KRGE have DC-regulatory functions. The diminished RORγt expression by Rg3 treatment in T cells raises the possible role of Rg3 in regulating the functions of RORγt-expressing innate immune cells including type 3 innate lymphoid cells (ILC3) and LTi cells. Since these cells are known to play a crucial role in mucosal homeostasis and lymphoid tissue generation [32,33], it will be important to determine the potential role of Rg3 in these innate RORγt-expressing cells. Antibodies against IL-17A or IL-17RA are proven to be effective in the treatment of psoriasis in humans [34,35]. Thus, it will be of interest to investigate if Rg3 can ameliorate other autoimmune tissue inflammation, such as psoriasis.

In summary, the results of the present study indicate that Rg3 negatively regulates RORγt expression in CD4$^+$ T cells, subsequently hindering Th17 cell differentiation and Th17-mediated neuro-inflammation. These findings are novel because they attest to the fact that ginsenoside Rg3 is the active constituent of KRG extract that can inhibit the differentiation of Th17 cells and Th17-cell-mediated autoimmunity. Our findings may provide a rationale for developing Rg3 as a potential candidate for the treatment of autoimmune disorders driven by Th17 cells.

Author Contributions: Conceptualization, Y.C. and M.C.; Funding acquisition, Y.C.; Investigation, M.C. and Y.-J.P.; Original Draft Preparation, Y.-J.P. and M.C.; Review & Editing, Y.C.; Supervision, M.C. and Y.C.; Methodology, G.C. and H.N. All authors have read and agreed to the published version of the manuscript.

Funding: This work was supported by the grant from the Korean Society of Ginseng funded by Korea Ginseng Cooperation (YC).

Acknowledgments: We thank Chris Daehong Kim (Seoul National University) for proof-reading the manuscript.

Conflicts of Interest: The authors declare no conflict of interest.

References

1. Lee, J.-I.; Park, K.S.; Cho, I.-H. Panax ginseng: A candidate herbal medicine for autoimmune disease. *J Ginseng Res.* **2019**, *43*, 342–348. [CrossRef] [PubMed]
2. Kim, J.H.; Yi, Y.-S.; Kim, M.-Y.; Cho, J.Y. Role of ginsenosides, the main active components of Panax ginseng, in inflammatory responses and diseases. *J. Ginseng Res.* **2017**, *41*, 435–443. [CrossRef] [PubMed]
3. Helms, S. Cancer prevention and therapeutics: Panax ginseng. *Altern. Med. Rev.* **2004**, *9*, 259–274. [PubMed]
4. Hong, B.N.; Ji, M.G.; Kang, T.H. The efficacy of red ginseng in type 1 and type 2 diabetes in animals. *Evid. Based Complement. Alternat. Med.* **2013**, *2013*, 593181. [CrossRef] [PubMed]

5. Jeong, C.-S. Effect of butanol fraction of Panax ginseng head on gastric lesion and ulcer. *Arch. Pharm. Res.* **2002**, *25*, 61–66. [CrossRef]
6. Attele, A.S.; Wu, J.A.; Yuan, C.-S. Ginseng pharmacology: Multiple constituents and multiple actions. *Biochem. Pharmacol.* **1999**, *58*, 1685–1693. [CrossRef]
7. Yi, Y.-S. Ameliorative effects of ginseng and ginsenosides on rheumatic diseases. *J. Ginseng Res.* **2019**, *43*, 335–341. [CrossRef]
8. Liu, C.-X.; Xiao, P.-G. Recent advances on ginseng research in China. *J. Ethnopharmacol.* **1992**, *36*, 27–38.
9. Lee, S.-Y.; Jeong, J.-J.; Eun, S.-H.; Kim, D.-H. Anti-inflammatory effects of ginsenoside Rg1 and its metabolites ginsenoside Rh1 and 20(S)-protopanaxatriol in mice with TNBS-induced colitis. *Eur. J. Pharmacol.* **2015**, *762*, 333–343. [CrossRef]
10. Cho, M.; Choi, G.; Shim, I.; Chung, Y. Enhanced Rg3 negatively regulates Th1 cell responses. *J. Ginseng Res.* **2019**, *43*, 49–57. [CrossRef]
11. Kang, S.; Park, S.-J.; Lee, A.-Y.; Huang, J.; Chung, H.-Y.; Im, D.-S. Ginsenoside Rg3 promotes inflammation resolution through M2 macrophage polarization. *J. Ginseng Res.* **2018**, *42*, 68–74. [CrossRef] [PubMed]
12. Stockinger, B.; Omenetti, S. The dichotomous nature of T helper 17 cells. *Nat. Rev. Immunol.* **2017**, *17*, 535–544. [CrossRef] [PubMed]
13. Muranski, P.; Restifo, N.P. Essentials of Th17 cell commitment and plasticity. *Blood* **2013**, *121*, 2402–2414. [CrossRef] [PubMed]
14. Mohanan, P.; Subramaniyam, S.; Mathiyalagan, R.; Yang, D.-C. Molecular signaling of ginsenosides Rb1, Rg1, and Rg3 and their mode of actions. *J. Ginseng Res.* **2018**, *42*, 123–132. [CrossRef] [PubMed]
15. Mangan, P.R.; Harrington, L.E.; O'Quinn, D.B.; Helms, W.S.; Bullard, D.C.; Elson, C.O.; Hatton, R.D.; Wahl, S.M.; Schloeb, T.R.; Weaver, C.T. Transforming growth factor-beta induces development of the T(H)17 lineage. *Nature* **2006**, *441*, 231–234. [CrossRef] [PubMed]
16. Ivanov, I.I.; McKenzie, B.S.; Zhou, L.; Tadokoro, C.E.; Lepelley, A.; Lafaille, J.J.; Cua, D.J.; Littman, D.R. The orphan nuclear receptor RORgammat directs the differentiation program of proinflammatory IL-17+ T helper cells. *Cell* **2006**, *126*, 1121–1133. [CrossRef]
17. Yang, X.O.; Panopoulos, A.D.; Nurieva, R.; Chang, S.H.; Wang, D.; Watowich, S.S.; Dong, C. STAT3 regulates cytokine-mediated generation of inflammatory helper T cells. *J. Biol. Chem.* **2007**, *282*, 9358–9363. [CrossRef]
18. Heo, S.B.; Lim, S.W.; Jhun, J.Y.; Cho, M.L.; Chung, B.H.; Yang, C.W. Immunological benefits by ginseng through reciprocal regulation of Th17 and Treg cells during cyclosporine-induced immunosuppression. *J. Ginseng Res.* **2016**, *40*, 18–27. [CrossRef]
19. Jhun, J.; Lee, J.; Byun, J.-K.; Kim, E.-K.; Woo, J.-W.; Lee, J.-H.; Kwok, S.-K.; Ju, J.-H.; Park, K.-S.; Kim, H.-Y.; et al. Red ginseng extract ameliorates autoimmune arthritis via regulation of STAT3 pathway, Th17/Treg balance, and osteoclastogenesis in mice and human. *Mediat. Inflamm.* **2014**, *2014*, 351856. [CrossRef]
20. Wanke, F.; Moos, S.; Croxford, A.L.; Heinen, A.P.; Gräf, S.; Kalt, B.; Tischner, D.; Zhang, J.; Christen, I.; Bruttger, J.; et al. EBI2 Is Highly Expressed in Multiple Sclerosis Lesions and Promotes Early CNS Migration of Encephalitogenic CD4 T Cells. *Cell Rep.* **2017**, *18*, 1270–1284. [CrossRef]
21. Veldhoen, M.; Hocking, R.J.; Atkins, C.J.; Locksley, R.M.; Stockinger, B. TGFbeta in the context of an inflammatory cytokine milieu supports de novo differentiation of IL-17-producing T cells. *Immunity* **2006**, *24*, 179–189. [CrossRef] [PubMed]
22. Lim, H.; Kim, Y.U.; Sun, H.; Lee, J.H.; Reynolds, J.M.; Hanabuchi, S.; Wu, H.; Teng, B.-B.; Chung, Y. Proatherogenic conditions promote autoimmune T helper 17 cell responses in vivo. *Immunity* **2014**, *40*, 153–165. [CrossRef] [PubMed]
23. Quintana, F.J. Old dog, new tricks: IL-6 cluster signaling promotes pathogenic TH17 cell differentiation. *Nat. Immunol.* **2016**, *18*, 8–10. [CrossRef] [PubMed]
24. Chung, Y.; Chang, S.H.; Martinez, G.J.; Yang, X.O.; Nurieva, R.; Kang, H.S.; Ma, L.; Watowich, S.S.; Jetten, A.M.; Tian, Q.; et al. Critical regulation of early Th17 cell differentiation by interleukin-1 signaling. *Immunity* **2009**, *30*, 576–587. [CrossRef]
25. Kim, B.-S.; Park, Y.-J.; Chung, Y. Targeting IL-17 in autoimmunity and inflammation. *Arch. Pharm. Res.* **2016**, *39*, 1537–1547. [CrossRef]
26. Ciofani, M.; Madar, A.; Galan, C.; Sellars, M.; Mace, K.; Pauli, F.; Agarwal, A.; Huang, W.; Parkurst, C.N.; Muratet, M.; et al. A validated regulatory network for Th17 cell specification. *Cell* **2012**, *151*, 289–303. [CrossRef]

27. Li, J.; Liu, T.; Zhao, L.; Chen, W.; Hou, H.; Ye, Z.; Li, X. Ginsenoside 20(S)Rg3 inhibits the Warburg effect through STAT3 pathways in ovarian cancer cells. *Int. J. Oncol.* **2015**, *46*, 775–781. [CrossRef]
28. Nurieva, R.; Yang, X.O.; Martinez, G.; Zhang, Y.; Panopoulos, A.D.; Ma, L.; Schluns, K.; Tian, Q.; Watowich, S.S.; Jetten, A.M.; et al. Essential autocrine regulation by IL-21 in the generation of inflammatory T cells. *Nature* **2007**, *448*, 480–483. [CrossRef]
29. Santori, F.R.; Huang, P.; van de Pavert, S.A.; Douglass, E.F., Jr.; Leaver, D.J.; Haubrich, B.A.; Keber, R.; Lorbek, G.; Konijn, T.; Rosales, B.N.; et al. Identification of natural RORgamma ligands that regulate the development of lymphoid cells. *Cell Metab.* **2015**, *21*, 286–298. [CrossRef]
30. Xu, T.; Wang, X.; Zhong, B.; Nurieva, R.I.; Ding, S.; Dong, C. Ursolic acid suppresses interleukin-17 (IL-17) production by selectively antagonizing the function of RORgamma t protein. *J. Biol. Chem.* **2011**, *286*, 22707–22710. [CrossRef]
31. Na, H.; Lim, H.; Choi, G.; Kim, B.-K.; Kim, S.-H.; Chang, Y.-S.; Nurieva, R.; Dong, C.; Chang, S.H.; Chung, Y. Concomitant suppression of TH2 and TH17 cell responses in allergic asthma by targeting retinoic acid receptor-related orphan receptor gammat. *J. Allergy Clin. Immunol.* **2018**, *141*, 2061–2073. [CrossRef] [PubMed]
32. Sonnenberg, G.F.; Artis, D. Innate lymphoid cells in the initiation, regulation and resolution of inflammation. *Nat. Med.* **2015**, *21*, 698–708. [CrossRef] [PubMed]
33. Cherrier, M.; Eberl, G. The development of LTi cells. *Curr. Opin. Immunol.* **2012**, *24*, 178–183. [CrossRef] [PubMed]
34. Dyring-Andersen, B.; Skov, L.; Zachariae, C. Targeting IL-17 with ixekizumab in patients with psoriasis. *Immunotherapy* **2015**, *7*, 957–966. [CrossRef]
35. Farahnik, B.; Beroukhim, K.; Abrouk, M.; Nakamura, M.; Zhu, T.H.; Singh, R.; Lee, K.; Bhutani, T.; Koo, J. Brodalumab for the Treatment of Psoriasis: A Review of Phase III Trials. *Dermatol. Ther.* **2016**, *6*, 111–124. [CrossRef]

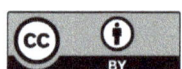

© 2020 by the authors. Licensee MDPI, Basel, Switzerland. This article is an open access article distributed under the terms and conditions of the Creative Commons Attribution (CC BY) license (http://creativecommons.org/licenses/by/4.0/).

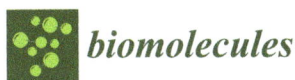

Article

Molecular Insight into Stereoselective ADME Characteristics of C20-24 Epimeric Epoxides of Protopanaxadiol by Docking Analysis

Wenna Guo [1], Zhiyong Li [1], Meng Yuan [1], Geng Chen [2], Qiao Li [1], Hui Xu [1,*] and Xin Yang [2,*]

[1] School of Pharmacy, Key Laboratory of Molecular Pharmacology and Drug Evaluation (Yantai University), Ministry of Education, Collaborative Innovation Center of Advanced Drug Delivery System and Biotech Drugs in Universities of Shandong, Yantai University, Yantai 264000, China; guowenna1@126.com (W.G.); lzhy0818@126.com (Z.L.); sjuiop@163.com (M.Y.); chloeleeq@126.com (Q.L.)
[2] School of Chemistry and Chemical Engineering, Yantai University, Yantai 264000, China; Cgeng163@163.com
* Correspondence: xuhui@ytu.edu.cn (H.X.); yangx@ytu.edu.cn (X.Y.); Tel.: +86-535-670-6066 (H.X.); +86-535-690-2063 (X.Y.)

Received: 6 December 2019; Accepted: 1 January 2020; Published: 9 January 2020

Abstract: Chirality is a common phenomenon, and it is meaningful to explore interactions between stereoselective bio-macromolecules and chiral small molecules with preclinical and clinical significance. Protopanaxadiol-type ginsenosides are main effective ingredients in ginseng and are prone to biotransformation into a pair of ocotillol C20-24 epoxide epimers, namely, (20*S*,24*S*)-epoxy-dammarane-3,12,25-triol (24*S*-PDQ) and (20*S*,24*R*)-epoxy dammarane-3,12,25-triol (24*R*-PDQ) that display stereoselective fate in vivo. However, possible molecular mechanisms involved are still unclear. The present study aimed to investigate stereoselective ADME (absorption, distribution, metabolism and excretion) characteristics of PDQ epimers based on molecular docking analysis of their interaction with some vital proteins responsible for drug disposal. Homology modeling was performed to obtain 3D-structure of the human isoenzyme UGT1A8, while calculation of docking score and binding free energy and ligand–protein interaction pattern analysis were achieved by using the Schrödinger package. Stereoselective interaction was found for both UGT1A8 and CYP3A4, demonstrating that 24*S*-PDQ was more susceptible to glucuronidation, whereas 24*R*-PDQ was more prone to oxidation catalyzed by CYP3A4. However, both epimers displayed similarly strong interaction with P-gp, a protein with energy-dependent drug-pump function, suggesting an effect of the dammarane skeleton but not C-24 stereo-configuration. These findings provide an insight into stereo-selectivity of ginsenosides, as well as a support the rational development of ginseng products.

Keywords: ocotillol type ginsenoside epimers; stereoselective ADME characteristics; molecular docking analysis; homology modeling; molecular interaction

1. Introduction

Natural biomolecules with rich diversity in chemical structure are important resources for modern drug discovery [1]. Ginsenoside is a class of triterpenoid saponins abundant in ginseng that has been reputed as the king of medicinal herbs and used as a tonic, prophylactic and restorative agent in traditional medicine for thousands of years [2]. Up to date, over 150 natural ginsenosides have been identified and classified along with different aglycones into two major types of oleanane and dammarane, among which the latter is generally sorted into three subgroups as protopanaxadiol (PPD), protopanaxatriol (PPT) and ocotillol [3–5]. The difference in spatial orientation of C-20 hydroxyl further yields a pair of epimers for each, and those in fresh ginseng are usually of the 20*S*-configuration, while processed ginseng products, such as red ginseng, contain both 20*R*- and 20*S*-epimeric forms [6,7].

Pharmacokinetic studies have demonstrated very limited oral bioavailability (<5%) of ginsenosides, for which poor oral absorption and extensive metabolism may be mainly responsible, thus, the aglycone is an actual effective motif through the hydrolysis of sugar moieties by gastric acid or microorganisms in the stomach or enteric canal [8]. Such is the case with the most abundant ginsenoside Rb that can be easily converted into more pharmaceutically potent minor ginsenosides such as Rg3, Rh2 and PPD [9,10]. The aglycone PPD is prone to further oxygenation in vivo to produce intermediate metabolites, a pair of ocotillol-type epimeric C20-24 epoxides (Figure 1), namely (20S,24S)-epoxy-dammarane-3β, 12β, 25-triol (24S-PDQ) and its 24R- epimer [4,11,12].

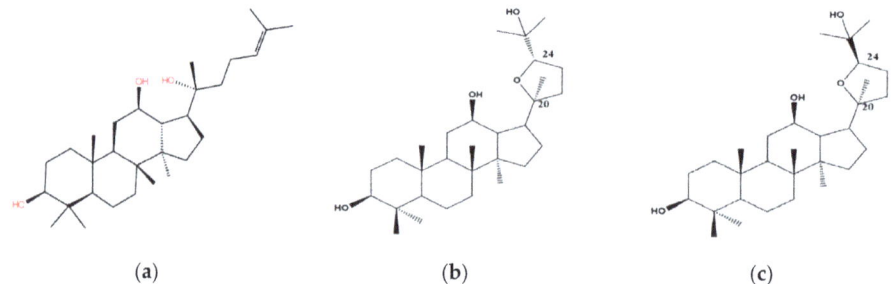

Figure 1. Chemical structure of (**a**) 20S-PPD; (**b**) 24S-PDQ; (**c**) 24R-PDQ.

The different stereochemistry of PDQ epimers leads to significant stereoselectivities in both pharmacological effects and ADME properties. More concretely, 24R-epimer was found to be equipotent with PPD in terms of attenuating myocardial ischemic injury induced by isoproterenol and hence contribute to overall therapeutic effect of PPD, while 24S-PDQ orally administered at an equal dosage had no such effect [13]. In contrast to the 24R-epimer, 24S-PDQ displayed a higher apparent formation rate from PPD along with a lower elimination rate by phase I metabolism enzymes [14]. Based on assay of in vivo biliary excretion, it was found that 24S-PDQ was more preferential to be metabolized into glucuronide conjugates than the 24R-epimer, whereas CYP3A4 was confirmed as the predominant isoform responsible for rapid oxygenation metabolism of 24R-epimer in human liver microsomes [14,15]. However, to the best of our knowledge, the molecular mechanisms underlying such stereoselective ADME fate of PDQ epimers are still unclear yet.

Our present work aimed to investigate possible mechanisms involved in stereoselective ADME properties of PDQ epimers by molecular docking, which has been demonstrated as an invaluable tool in structural molecular biology and computer-assisted drug design to predict the predominant ligand–protein binding modes for virtual screening on large libraries of compounds and exact three-dimensional (3-D) structures of proteins [16]. The findings would give some insights into stereoselective biological effects of these epimeric intermediate metabolites of naturally abundant ginsenosides and, thus, help to better understand potential mechanisms responsible for clinical efficacy and safety of ginseng products.

2. Materials and Methods

2.1. Selection of ADME-Related Protein Targets

Three types of enzymes were selected as target proteins for molecular docking analysis of stereoselective ADME properties, which included P-glycoprotein (P-gp, PDB ID: 5KOY), the cytochrome P450 (CYP) isoform 3A4 (PDB ID: 1W0F) and UDP-glucuronosyltransferase (UGT) isoform 1A8 (accession ID: Q9HAW9). According to the available results from both in vitro and in vivo experiments [14,17,18], the three target proteins are mainly involved in disposition of PDQ epimers and other ginsenosides such as absorption, phase I redox metabolism and phase II conjugation.

2.2. Homology Modeling and Model Validation of UGT1A8

The homology modeling approach in the aid of Maestro (v 10.1, Schrödinger, LLC, New York, NY, 2015) was adopted to predict 3-D structure of the target protein human UGT1A8 for molecular docking analysis since it is not available until now. Firstly, the primary amino acid sequence was retrieved as a target from the NCBI database with an accession number of Q9HAW9 and downloaded as a FAST ALL format file. Then BLAST (the program Basic Local Alignment Search Tool) was performed to find the best homologous sequence with known 3-D structure as template according to the alignment with target by pairwise comparison using BLOSUM62 matrix (Belhesda, LLC, Rockville, MA, USA). Based on the optimal template, homology model was generated with the automated protein structure homology-modeling server Prime Module using a default model. The homology model included copying backbone atom coordinates for aligned regions and side chains of conserved residues, loop modeling and optimization of side chains, building insertions and closing deletion in the alignment. After secondary structure predictions using the Prime module for alignment, the model was subjected to check for any missing side chain and all-atom ab initio energy minimization for refinement, as well as validation according to Ramachandran plot and calculation of RMSD (root-mean-square deviation) by using the Proteins program and Protein Structure Alignment panel, respectively.

2.3. Protein Preparation and Optimization

The 3-D structure of UGT1A8 was generated by using Maestro (v 10.1, Schrödinger, LLC, New York, NY, USA, 2015) according to the aligned sequence of the homology model. For the target proteins P-gp and CYP3A4 that have known crystal structures of protein-ligand complexes collected in Protein Data Bank (PDB), the 3-D structures with high resolution and good ligand similarity to the small molecules were selected for further docking. Then optimization of all the three proteins was performed by using Protein Preparation Wizard of Master, including hydrogen bonding network optimization via H-bond assignment section, restrained minimization by adding hydrogen atoms or filling missing side chains, and energy minimization-based refinement via harmonic penalty constraints. After hydrogen addition and removal of water molecules and ligands bound to the complex, the energy-minimized structures of target proteins were finally obtained by using OPLS2005 force field.

2.4. Ligands Preparation and Optimization

The PDQ epimers shown in Figure 1 were used as target ligands for docking study. After edited by the 2-D Sketcher option in Maestro (version 10.1) and converted into 3-D structure, the ligands were subjected to refinement in LigPrep module for energy optimization by using the OPLS2005 force field. Then molecular ionization yielded possible states at a target pH value of 7.0 ± 2.0, and the Epik module was performed to generate ligand conformation with the lowest energy, which was used as starting point for further docking experiments.

2.5. Binding Site Selection

The structural property, such as active site of target protein, is an important factor for ligand-receptor interaction. Sitemap is a useful module in the Schrödinger suite for binding site identification by characterizing the receptor and ligand regions and hydrophobic interaction forces [19]. According to large-scale verification tests, Sitemap is able to identify binding site bound to ligand molecule with fairly high accuracy (>96%) [20]. Therefore, Sitemap was used to predict optimal binding sites for the proteins UGT1A8 and P-gp, since their active sites ligand for ligand binding are unknown yet. For CYP3A4, the heme pocket has been determined as the active site [21], which thus was selected to investigate ligand binding.

2.6. Molecular Docking

All the ligand–protein docking studies were performed with the Glide module within Schrödinger (version 6.7) by using the standard precision (SP) mode that is generally efficient and accurate for most of the targets [22,23]. The molecular mechanics energies combined with the generalized Born and surface area continuum solvation (MM/GBSA) method, one of the popular approaches to estimate free energy of the binding of small ligands to biological macromolecules [24], was used via distance-dependent electrostatic treatment with OPLS2005 force field set to 1000 iterations at the maximum in Prime. The optimal ligand conformations for docking were screened via Emodel module in light of the GlideScore, a mixture of interaction energy and parameter-based penalty functions that roughly represents binding free energy (ΔG_{bind}) [25]. The ΔG_{bind} that permits accurate analysis of contribution from each residue by decomposing ligand–protein interaction into different terms [26,27] was calculated to quantitatively assess and rank the ligand–protein binding modes. The docking results were clustered for further analysis, including binding type, the residues involved and some empirical scoring function. Both statistics of GlideScore and ΔG_{bind} were obtained according to triplicate docking analyses with various conformations of the ligand-receptor complexes, and the results were presented as the mean ± standard deviation (SD).

3. Results

3.1. Homology Modeling and Validation of UGT1A8

Glucuronidation mediated by UGTs is of major importance in the conjugation and subsequent elimination of potentially toxic xenobiotics and endogenous compounds, and more than 35% of phase II drug metabolism is catalyzed by UGT isoforms [28]. To date, nineteen human UGT isoforms have been identified and categorized into three major subfamilies as UGT1A, 2A and 2B according to the sequence homology. It has been demonstrated that the isoenzyme UGT1A8 mainly catalyzes glucuronidation in the intestine and has great potential to influence the pharmacokinetics and biological effects of oral drugs and xenobiotics [29–32]. The study based on determination of bile excretion in rats further revealed that 24S-PDQ was more prone to glucuronidation than its 24R-epimer [14]. Therefore, it is worthwhile to investigate ligand–protein binding mode between PDQ epimers and UGT1A8 involved in their stereoselective glucuronidation.

Homology modeling was carried out for further molecular docking analysis since no relevant data of exact 3-D structure of human UGT1A8 has been reported so far. At first, a primary amino acid sequence (accession ID: Q9HAW9) with 399 amino acids was obtained as the target for modeling by BLAST homology searching. Then the crystal structure of macrolide glycosyltransferase was screened from PDB (ID: 2IYA) as the best template for modeling. The protein 2IYA displayed a sequence homology above 37% and the similarity to UGT1A8 could be reach up to 33% (Figure 2), indicating a reliable template for homology modeling in view of the rule of thumb that a sequence homology of 30% or above is adequate [27].

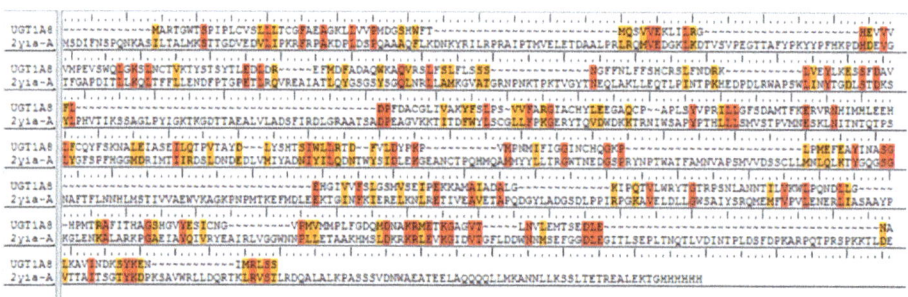

Figure 2. Sequence alignment between UGT1A8 query sequence and the template amino acid sequence of 2IYA. All the identical residues were highlighted in red color, and those similar residues in orange color respectively.

Model validation to check any potential error or deviation from the normal protein is of the utmost importance for further structure-based docking study [33,34]. The alignment score of 0.023 and RMSD value of 0.753 Å (Figure 3a) indicated a good alignment of multiple amino acid sequences between the template protein of 2IYA and homology model of UGT1A8, as well as the reasonability of the obtained homology model. The Ramachandran plot (Figure 3b) generated by Maestro software further shows phi–psi torsion angles for all residues in the structure, among which 96.99% were in the favorable or allowed regions and more than 90% of the backbone dihedral angles resided in the favorable region (in red), whereas the residues in the disallowed region (in white) made up a significantly low share (3.01%).

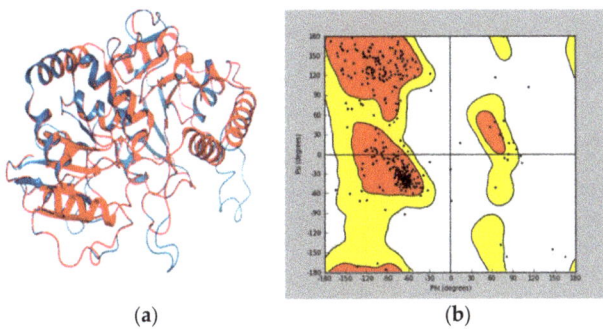

(a)   (b)

Figure 3. Homology model validation. (a) RMSD between the template (in blue) and target protein (in red). (b) Ramachandran (phi/psi) plot. Red: favorable region; yellow: allowed region; white: disallowed region.

The 3-D structure of the active site in UGT1A8 was established according to the homology model since it is of the utmost importance for protein-ligand interaction [35]. The active site prediction was performed by using Sitemap. The shade region in Figure 4a shows a 3-D map of the active site within the homologous model protein with the hydrophobic region in red, the acceptor region in blue and the ligand region in yellow, respectively. Figure 4b further illustrates that the ligand–protein interaction occurred in this active region, where all the residues involved resided in the favorable region, while those located in the disallowed regions were far from the active sites and produced little or no effect on UGT1A8 binding with PDQ epimers. All these findings clearly demonstrated structure rationality of the homology model of UGT1A8 with satisfactory geometry and stereo-chemistry for docking studies.

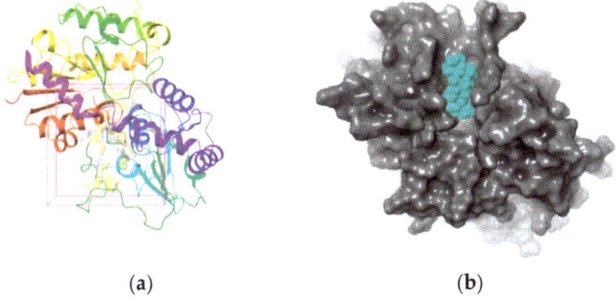

(a)   (b)

Figure 4. (a) Three-dimensional structure of active site within the homology model of UGT1A8 (region in the shadow). Stripe structure: the homology model of UGT1A8; Red: the hydrophobic region; blue: the acceptor region; yellow: the ligand region. (b) 3-D map of interaction between PDQ and UGT1A8. Gray region: UGT1A8; blue region: PDQ.

3.2. Stereoselective Interaction Between PDQ Epimers and UGT1A8

The homology model of UGT1A8 was used as a receptor for molecular docking analysis of the interaction with PDQ epimers. As shown in Table 1, both the docking score and ΔG_{bind} were negative for each interaction, suggesting stable ligand–protein complexes of both epimers. More concretely, the docking score and ΔG_{bind} were −(4.268 ± 0.174), −(49.89 ± 2.06) kcal/mol for 24*S*-PDQ, and −(3.794 ± 0.208), −(45.11 ± 1.58) kcal/mol for 24*R*-epimer respectively, suggesting significant differences between the two epimers in interaction with the target protein UGT1A8. In contrast to 24*R*-PDQ, the 24*S*-epimer showed a much higher docking score and ΔG_{bind} value, indicating a higher affinity of 24*S*-PDQ with the conjugation isoenzyme of UGT1A8. According to the previously reported in vivo study in rats, the two epimers at the same intravenous dosage indeed displayed stereoselective biliary excretion, and the biliary excretion ratio of 24*S*-PDQ glucuronide was more than 28-fold higher than that of 24*R*-epimer glucuronide [14]. Thus, it is supposed that 24*S*-PDQ, but not 24*R*-epimer, is prone to rapid in vivo glucuronidation, which may be mainly attributed to its high affinity with the UGT isoform of 1A8.

Table 1. Molecular docking statistics for interaction between PDQ epimers and various proteins [1].

Protein-Ligand Interaction		Docking Score	ΔG_{bind} [2]	Residues for Hydrogen Bonding
UGT1A8	24*S*-PDQ	−(4.268 ± 0.174)	−(49.89 ± 2.06)	Gly274, Asp356, Glu377
	24*R*-epimer	−(3.794 ± 0.208)	−(45.11 ± 1.58)	Gly274, Asn276, Glu288
CYP3A4	24*S*-PDQ	−(5.737 ± 1.350)	−(54.95 ± 5.27)	/
	24*R*-epimer	−(7.162 ± 0.0395)	−(61.65 ± 0.572)	Glu374
P-gp	24*S*-PDQ	−(5.636 ± 0.0326)	−(42.73 ± 0.577)	/
	24*R*-epimer	−(5.879 ± 0.380)	−(40.73 ± 0.774)	/

[1.] Glide module within Schrödinger (version 6.7, LLC, New York, NY, USA, 2015) was performed, and the data of docking score and binding free energy were presented as mean ± SD of triplicate docking analyses with various conformations. [2.] ΔG_{bind} represents the binding free energy in kcal/mol calculated using the Prime/MM-GBSA protocol.

The differentiation between PDQ epimers in their interaction with UGT1A8 was further expounded according to 2-D mappings from molecular docking analysis. Both epimers were anchored to the target protein mainly by hydrogen bonding and hydrophobic interaction, and the electrostatic attraction and van der Waals force could also be observed (Figure 5). Moreover, the stereochemical difference in C-24 indeed caused significantly different interaction patterns, especially the hydrophobic interactions. Both epimers formed three hydrogen bonds with UGT1A8 and showed similar hydrogen bond interactions. For 24*S*-PDQ, the hydroxyl groups at C-3, C-12 and C-25 formed hydrogen bonds via the residues Asp356, Gly274 and Glu377, respectively. Whereas the 24*R*-epimer formed hydrogen bonds via the C-12 and C-25 hydroxyl groups with the residues Glu288 and Gly274, and the third hydrogen bond was observed between the residue Asn276 and the oxygen atom in tetrahydrofuran, but not the C-3 hydroxyl group.

Meanwhile, the PDQ epimers also showed difference in hydrophobic interaction with UGT1A8 (Figure 5a-2, b-2). Although both involved the same residues such as Asn276, Asn355, Asp356 and Asn381, the total number of residues involved was 15 for 24*S*-PDQ, but only 7 for its 24*R*- epimer (including Cys277, Phe287 and Ala289), which contributed to relatively stronger interaction between UGT1A8 and 24*S*-PDQ and was mostly responsible for glucuronidation preferentiality of this 24*S*-epimer. Based on these findings, it thus could be assumed that UGT1A8 may be a major isoenzyme mediating 24*S*-PDQ conjugation with glucuronic acid and the C-24 stereochemistry plays a great role in distinguishing glucuronidation metabolism of PDQ epimers.

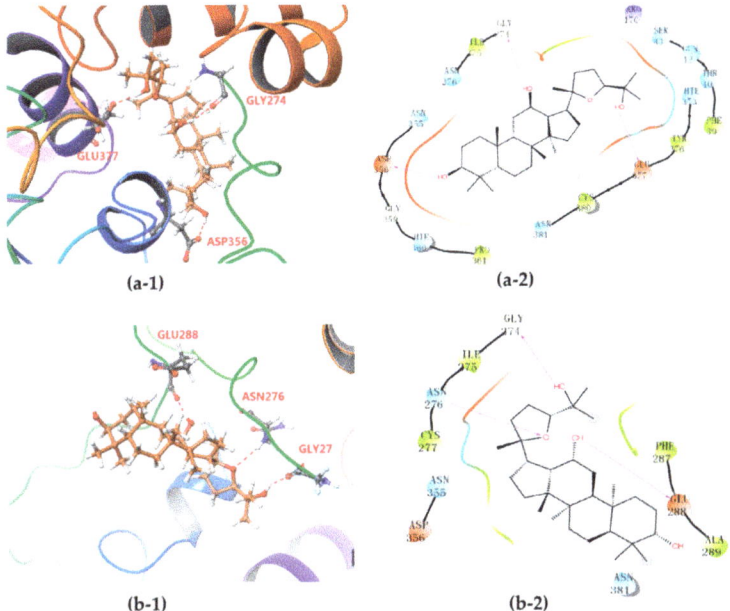

Figure 5. 3-D (**1**) and 2-D (**2**) diagrams illustrating the molecular interaction of 24*S*-PDQ (**a**) and 24*R*-epimer (**b**) with the modeled UGT1A8. (**1**) The ball-stick structure: PDQ; the cartoon stucture: UGT1A8. (**2**) Purple arrow: hydrogen bond; red: charged (negative); purple: charged (positive); white: glycine; green: hydrophobic; blue: polar.

3.3. Stereoselective Interaction between PDQ Epimers and CYP3A4

The cytochrome P450 superfamily (CYP) is a group of mono-oxygenases participating in the metabolism of both endogenous and exogenous substances, among which CYP3A is the most abundant subtype in human liver. By using chemical inhibition in human liver microsomes and recombinant human P450 isotype determination, previous studies have manifested that CYP3A4 is the major isoform responsible for difference in oxidative metabolism of PDQ epimers [12]. Herein, human CYP3A4 was used as a target protein to investigate stereoselective redox metabolism of PDQ epimers.

CYP3A4 is the most abundant xenobiotic-metabolizing cytochrome P450 isoform that contains a heme co-factor as the active site. A number of researches have clearly demonstrated the broad substrate specificity of the CYP3A4 molecule, as well as the promiscuity of ligand binding in the CYP3A4 heme pocket [21]. CYP3A4 is known to bind different sizes of compounds such as metyrapone (226Da), progesterone (314Da), bromocriptine (655Da) and cyclosporine (1203Da). Intriguingly, metyrapone bound via a pyridine nitrogen to heme iron, while progesterone did not locate in the active heme pocket but was observed on a peripheral site of the CYP3A4 molecule [36]. Taking into consideration that the molecular structure of the tetracyclic triterpenoid PDQ epimers is similar to the natural steroid hormone progesterone, the X-ray crystal structure containing the progesterone with the PDB ID of 1W0F thus was chosen for molecular docking analysis in the present study.

As shown in Table 1, the docking score and ΔG_{bind} value were $-(5.737 \pm 1.35)$ and $-(54.95 \pm 5.27)$ kcal/mol for 24*S*-PDQ, and $-(7.162 \pm 0.040)$ and $-(61.65 \pm 0.57)$ kcal/mol for 24*R*-epimer, respectively. Such negative and high values also demonstrated that both epimers could spontaneously form thermodynamically stable complexes with CYP3A4. The difference further indicated considerable differentiation in interaction with the protein CYP3A4 that was closely related to the different C-24 stereochemistry. In contrast to the 24*S*- epimer, 24*R*-PDQ showed higher docking score and ΔG_{bind} value, suggesting a stronger affinity to CYP3A4.

The 2-D plots clearly illustrate the difference in the interaction mode (Figure 6). Intriguingly, the heme co-factor of CYP3A4 only formed Fe-S coordination with the residue Cys442, but no coordination was observed with the ligand molecule of either 24S- or 24R-PDQ, which was highly consistent with the ligand binding modes of CYP3A4 previously reported [21]. More concretely, both epimers were found on a peripheral site of the CYP3A4 molecule mainly via a hydrogen bond and hydrophobic interaction. Most of the amino acid residues involved in hydrophobic interaction were identical for the two epimers, such as Phe57, Arg105, Arg106, Ser119, Ile120, Arg212, Phe215, Phe304, Ala305, Thr309, Ile369, Ala370, Arg372, Leu373 and Glu374. However, a significant difference between two epimers could be found in hydrogen bonding mode. Although 24S-PDQ did not form any hydrogen bond with CYP3A4, the 24R- epimer formed a hydrogen bond via C3-OH with the residue Glu374, which thus caused relatively stronger interaction between CYP3A4 and 24R-PDQ and was responsible for the differences in docking score and ΔG_{bind} value. This finding provided a new evidence for promiscuity of ligand binding in the CYP3A4 heme pocket [21,36], and also demonstrated the great effect of C-24 stereochemistry on how PDQ epimers interact with CYP3A4, also proved that 24R-PDQ was more prone to in vivo oxidation catalyzed by CYP3A4 [12].

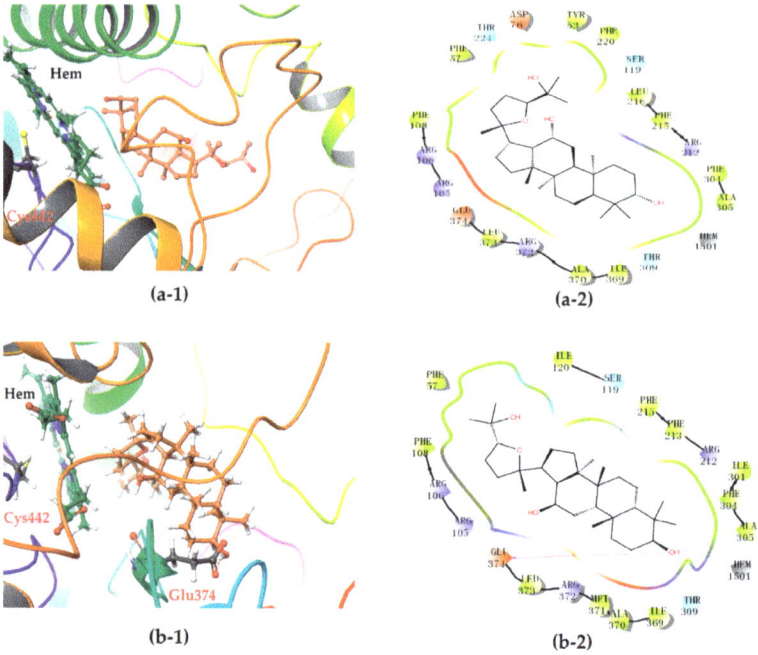

Figure 6. 3-D (**1**) and 2-D (**2**) diagrams illustrating the molecular interaction of 24S-PDQ (**a**) and 24R-epimer (**b**) with the CYP3A4. (**1**) The ball-stick structure: PDQ; the cartoon stucture: CYP3A4. (**2**) Purple arrow: hydrogen bond; red: charged (negative); purple: charged (positive); white: glycine; green: hydrophobic; blue: polar.

3.4. Stereoselective Interaction between PDQ Epimers and P-gp

P-gp is a well-known protein with energy-dependent drug-pump function that shows significant effect on drug fate in vivo [37]. The research work of Zhang et al. revealed the differential regulations of P-gp by ginsenoside Rh2 epimers in vivo, which provided new evidence of the chiral characteristics of this protein and was helpful to elucidate the stereoselective P-gp regulation mechanism of ginsenoside epimers from a pharmacokinetic view [17]. Interestingly, it was further reported that both 24S- and 24R-PDQ, which share the same dammarane skeleton, could be distinguished by P-gp and had similar inhibitory effects on P-gp by decreasing efflux of digoxin across Caco-2 cell monolayers [38]. P-gp thus was selected as a target protein in our present study for ligand–protein interaction analysis to investigate possible molecular mechanism responsible for such inhibitory effect of PDQ epimers on this stereoselective biomacromolecule P-gp, and the X-ray crystal structure with an ID of 5KOY in PDB was selected for molecular docking.

The molecular docking analysis revealed docking score and ΔG_{bind} value of $-(5.636 \pm 0.033)$ and $-(42.73 \pm 0.58)$ kcal/mol for 24S-PDQ, and $-(5.879 \pm 0.380)$ and $-(40.73 \pm 0.77)$ kcal/mol for 24R-PDQ, respectively (Table 1). Such high and similar values demonstrated that both epimers could spontaneously form stable complexes with P-gp, and these octillol type molecules may both be potent P-gp inhibitors with similarly high affinity to P-gp, which was not affected by the difference in C-24 stereochemistry.

Further interactions mode analysis by using 2-D mappings (Figure 7) clearly demonstrated that PDQ epimers could form stable complexes with P-gp primarily through hydrophobic interaction, but not any hydrogen bond, which was very different from their interactions with the protein molecules UGT1A8 or CYP3A4. More concretely, the hydrophobic binding pockets in P-gp were almost the same for embedding 24S- and 24R-PDQ, which mainly consisted of residues such as Leu857, Ile860, Val861, Ile864, Ala865, Gly868, Met945, Ser948, Tyr949, Cys952, Phe974, Val978, Ala981, Met982, Gly985 and Ser989. This result provided an additional evidence for similar P-gp inhibition potency of PQD epimers from the viewpoint of similar hydrophobic interaction with the P-gp molecule. The previously reported studies based on Western blot analyses demonstrated such a structure–activity relationship, i.e., that PDQ epimers and 20S-Rh2 shared the same dammarane skeleton as the pharmacophore responsible for P-gp inhibiting activity, while the ocotillol side chain and C-24 stereo-configuration of PDQ epimers had no effect on the expression of P-gp in Caco-2 cells [38]. The findings from in silico molecular docking analysis were highly consistent with those from in vitro cell-based assays and brought a further insight into molecular mechanism of P-gp inhibiting activity of gesenosides.

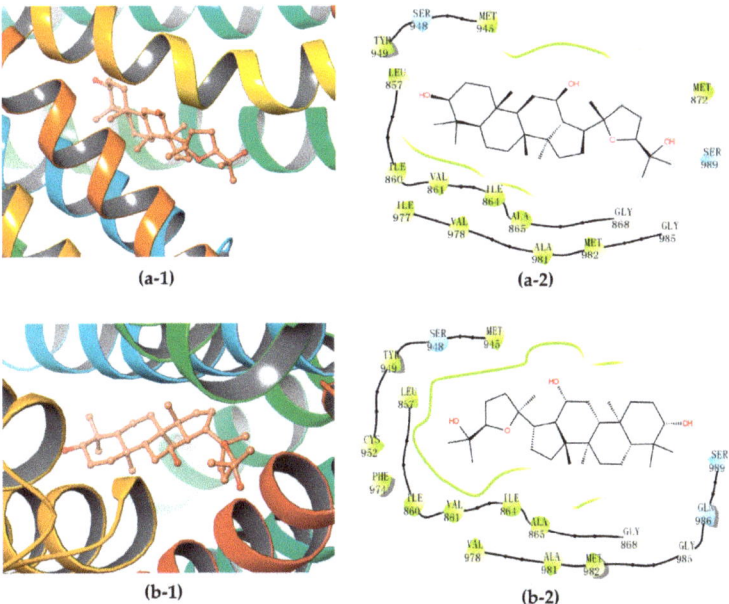

Figure 7. 3D (**1**) and 2D (**2**) diagrams illustrating the molecular interaction of 24S-PDQ (**a**) and 24R-epimer (**b**) with the P-gp. (**1**) The ball-stick structure: verapamil; the cartoon stuctures: P-gp. (**2**) White: glycine; green: hydrophobic; blue: polar.

4. Conclusions

Chirality is a common phenomenon and exploring interaction between biomacromolecules and chiral small molecules has preclinical and clinical significance. Natural protopanaxadiol-type ginsenosides are usually present in 20S-configuration and prone to oxidation into a pair of chiral ocotillol-type C20-24 epoxides, 24S-/24R-PDQ epimers. Several previous studies have revealed their stereoselective fates in vivo. Our present work brought some new insight into the molecular mechanism involved in stereoselective ADME characteristics of PDQ epimers by performing molecular docking analysis of their stereoselective interaction with those vital bio-macromolecules involved in drug disposal such as UGT1A8, CYP3A4 and P-gp. The findings were in good agreement with those cell/animal-based experimental observations and provided new evidence for stereoselectivity of structurally diverse gesenosides from the viewpoint of ligand–protein interactions.

Author Contributions: Conceptualization, W.G. and M.Y.; Data curation, W.G.; Formal analysis, W.G. and Q.L.; Funding acquisition, H.X.; Investigation, W.G.; Methodology, W.G. and Z.L.; Project administration, H.X.; Software, G.C.; Supervision, X.Y.; Validation, Z.L. and G.C.; Visualization, W.G.; Writing—original draft, W.G.; Writing—review & editing, Z.L. and M.Y. All authors have read and agreed to the published version of the manuscript.

Funding: This research was funded by Natural Science Foundation of Shandong Province (No. ZR2017MH061, ZR2019MB054), and the Key Research and Development Project of Shandong Province (No. 2018GSF119010).

Conflicts of Interest: The authors declare no conflict of interest. The funders had no role in the design of the study; in the collection, analyses, or interpretation of data; in the writing of the manuscript, or in the decision to publish the results.

References

1. Chen, Y.; De, B.K.C.; Kirchmair, J. Data resources for the computer-guided discovery of bioactive natural products. *J. Chem. Inf. Model.* **2017**, *57*, 9. [CrossRef] [PubMed]
2. Lee, C.H.; Kim, J.H. A review on the medicinal potentials of ginseng and ginsenosides on cardiovascular diseases. *J. Ginseng Res.* **2014**, *38*, 161–166. [CrossRef]
3. Kim, Y.J.; Zhang, D.; Yang, D.C. Biosynthesis and biotechnological production of ginsenosides. *Biotechnol. Adv.* **2015**, *33*, 717–735. [CrossRef] [PubMed]
4. Liu, J.; Xu, Y.R.; Yang, J.J.; Wang, W.Z.; Zhang, J.Q.; Zhang, R.M.; Meng, Q.G. Discovery, semisynthesis, biological activities, and metabolism of ocotillol-type saponins. *J. Ginseng Res.* **2017**, *41*, 373–378. [CrossRef] [PubMed]
5. Yang, Q.W.; Wang, N.; Zhang, J.; Chen, G.; Xu, H.; Meng, Q.G.; Du, Y.; Yang, X.; Fan, H.Y. In vitro and in silico evaluation of stereoselective effect of ginsenoside isomers on platelet p2y12 receptor. *Phytomedicine* **2019**, *64*, 152899. [CrossRef] [PubMed]
6. Shin, B.K.; Kwon, S.W.; Park, J.H. Chemical diversity of ginseng saponins from Panax ginseng. *J. Ginseng Res.* **2015**, *39*, 287–298. [CrossRef]
7. Wu, W.; Sun, L.; Zhang, Z.; Guo, Y.Y.; Liu, S.Y. Profiling and multivariate statistical analysis of Panax ginseng based on ultra-high-performance liquid chromatography coupled with quadrupole-time-of-flight mass spectrometry. *J. Pharm. Biomed. Anal.* **2015**, *107*, 141–150. [CrossRef]
8. Wang, W.Y.; Ni, Y.Y.; Wang, L.; Che, X.; Liu, W.H.; Meng, Q.G. Stereoselective oxidation metabolism of 20(S)–protopanaxatriol in human liver microsomes and in rats. *Xenobiotica* **2015**, *45*, 385–395. [CrossRef]
9. Yang, Z.; Gao, S.; Wang, J.R.; Yin, T.J.; Teng, Y.; Wu, B.J.; You, M.; Jiang, Z.H.; Hu, M. Enhancement of oral bioavailability of 20(S)-ginsenoside Rh2 through improved understanding of its absorption and efflux mechanisms. *Drug Metab. Dispos.* **2011**, *39*, 1866–1872. [CrossRef]
10. Kim, H.; Kim, J.H.; Lee, P.Y.; Bae, K.H.; Cho, S.; Park, B.C.; Shin, H.; Park, S.G. Ginsenoside Rb1 is transformed into Rd and Rh2 by microbacterium trichothecenolyticum. *J. Microbiol. Biotechnol.* **2013**, *23*, 1802–1805. [CrossRef]
11. Meng, Q.G.; Tan, W.J.; Hou, G.G.; Zhang, X.Y.; Hu, X.Y.; Yang, F.; Bai, G.J.; Zhu, W.W.; Cai, Y.; Bi, Y. Synthesis and structural characterization of two epimers driven from 20(S)–protopanaxadiol. *J. Mol. Struct.* **2013**, *51*, 1054–1055. [CrossRef]

12. Chiu, N.T.C.; Guns, E.S.T.; Hans, A.; William, J.; Subrata, D. Identification of human cytochrome P450 enzymes involved in the hepatic and intestinal biotransformation of 20(S)–protopanaxadiol. *Biopharm. Drug Dispos.* **2014**, *35*, 104–118. [CrossRef] [PubMed]
13. Wang, T.; Meng, Q.G.; Zhang, J.F.; Bi, Y.; Jiang, N.C. Study on the structure-function relationship of 20(S)-panaxadiol and its epimeric derivatives in myocardial injury induced by isoproterenol. *Fitoterapia* **2010**, *81*, 783–787. [CrossRef]
14. Wang, W.; Wang, L.; Wu, X.; Xu, L.; Meng, Q.; Liu, W. Stereoselective formation and metabolism of 20(S)–protopanaxadiol ocotillol type epimers in vivo and in vitro. *Chirality* **2015**, *27*, 170–176. [CrossRef] [PubMed]
15. Wang, W.Y.; Shao, Y.; Ma, S.; Wu, X.; Meng, Q.G. Determination of 20(S)–protopanaxadiol ocotillol type epimers in rat plasma by liquid chromatography tandem mass spectrometry. *J. Chromatogr. B Analyt. Technol. Biomed. Life Sci.* **2012**, *3*, 887–888. [CrossRef]
16. Morris, G.M.; Limwilby, M. Molecular docking. *Methods Mol. Biol.* **2008**, *443*, 365–382.
17. Zhang, J.; Zhou, F.; Niu, F.; Lu, M.; Wu, X.; Sun, J.; Wang, G. Stereoselective regulations of P-glycoprotein by ginsenoside Rh2 epimers and the potential mechanisms from the view of pharmacokinetics. *PLoS ONE* **2012**, *7*, e35768. [CrossRef]
18. Kim, D.; Yu, F.Z.; Min, J.S.; Park, J.B.; Bae, S.H.; Yoon, K.D.; Chin, Y.W.; Oh, E.; Bae, S.K. In vitro stereoselective inhibition of ginsenosides toward UDP-glucuronosyltransferase (UGT) isoforms. *Toxicol. Lett.* **2016**, *259*, 1–10. [CrossRef]
19. Halgren, T.A. Identifying and characterizing binding sites and assessing druggability. *J. Chem. Inf. Model.* **2009**, *49*, 377–389. [CrossRef]
20. Halgren, T.A. New method for fast and accurate binding-site identification and analysis. *Chem. Biol. Drug Des.* **2007**, *69*, 146–148. [CrossRef]
21. Ohkura, K.; Kawaguchi, Y.; Watanabe, Y.; Masubuchi, Y.; Hori, H. Flexible structure of cytochrome p450: Promiscuity of ligand binding in the cyp3a4 heme pocket. *Anticancer Res.* **2009**, *29*, 935–942. [PubMed]
22. Friesner, R.A.; Banks, J.L.; Murphy, R.B.; Halgren, T.A.; Klicic, J.J.; Mainz, D.T.; Repasky, M.P.; Knoll, E.H.; Mee, S.; Perry, J.K.; et al. Glide: A new approach for rapid, accurate docking and scoring. 1. Method and assessment of docking accuracy. *J. Med. Chem.* **2004**, *47*, 1739–1749. [CrossRef] [PubMed]
23. Park, K.; Cho, A.E. Using reverse docking to identify potential targets for ginsenosides. *J. Ginseng Res.* **2017**, *41*, 534–539. [CrossRef]
24. Genheden, S.; Ryde, U. The MM/PBSA and MM/GBSA methods to estimate ligand-binding affinities. *Expert Opin. Drug Discov.* **2015**, *10*, 449–461. [CrossRef]
25. Halgren, T.A.; Murphy, R.B.; Friesner, R.A.; Beard, H.S.; Frye, L.L.; Pollard, W.T.; Banks, J.L. Glide: A new approach for rapid, accurate docking and scoring. 2. Enrichment factors in database screening. *J. Med. Chem.* **2004**, *47*, 1750–1759. [CrossRef]
26. Friesner, R.A.; Murphy, R.B.; Repasky, M.P.; Frye, L.L.; Greenwood, J.R.; Halgren, T.A.; Sanschagrin, P.C.; Mainz, D.T. Extra precision glide: Docking and scoring incorporating a model of hydrophobic enclosure for protein-ligand complexes. *J. Med. Chem.* **2006**, *49*, 6177–6196. [CrossRef]
27. Kumar, D.H.; Barch, H.P.; Buolamwini, J.K. Homology modeling of human concentrative nucleoside transporters (hCNTs) and validation by virtual screening and experimental testing to identify novel hCNT1 inhibitors. *Drug Des.* **2017**, *146*, 6. [CrossRef]
28. Kiang, T.K.; Ensom, M.H.; Chang, T.K. UDP-glucuronosyltransferases and clinical drug-drug interactions. *Pharmacol. Ther.* **2005**, *106*, 97–132. [CrossRef]
29. Oda, S.; Fukami, T.; Yokoi, T.; Nakajima, M. A comprehensive review of UDP-glucuronosyltransferase and esterases for drug development. *Drug Metab. Pharmacokinet.* **2015**, *30*, 30–51. [CrossRef] [PubMed]
30. Ohno, S.; Nakajin, S. Determination of mRNA expression of human UDP-glucuronosyltransferases and application for localization in various human tissues by real-time reverse transcriptase-polymerase chain reaction. *Drug Metab. Dispos.* **2009**, *37*, 32–40. [CrossRef] [PubMed]
31. Strassburg, C.P.; Manns, M.P.; Tukey, R.H. Expression of the UDP-glucuronosyltransferase 1A locus in human colon. Identification and characterization of the novel extrahepatic UGT1A8. *J. Biol. Chem.* **1998**, *273*, 8719–8726. [CrossRef] [PubMed]

32. Fang, Z.Z.; Cao, Y.F.; Hu, C.M.; Hong, M.; Sun, X.Y.; Ge, G.B.; Liu, Y.; Zhang, Y.Y.; Yang, L.; Sun, H.Z. Structure-inhibition relationship of ginsenosides towards UDP-glucuronosyltransferases (UGTs). *Toxicol. Appl. Pharmacol.* **2013**, *267*, 149–154. [CrossRef] [PubMed]
33. Bohnuud, T.; Luo, L.; Wodak, S.J.; Bonvin, A.M.; Weng, Z.; Vajda, S.; Schueler-Furman, O.; Kozakov, D. A benchmark testing ground for integrating homology modeling and protein docking. *Proteins* **2016**, *85*, 10–16. [CrossRef] [PubMed]
34. Silva, R.C.D.; Siqueira, A.S.; Lima, A.R.J.; Lima, A.D.M.; Santos, A.S.; Aguiar, D.C.F.; Gonçalves, E.C. In silico characterization of a cyanobacterial plant-type isoaspartyl aminopeptidase/asparaginase. *J. Mol. Model.* **2018**, *24*, 108. [CrossRef]
35. Geoffrey, M.; Matthew, B.; Cadd, V.A.; Chaddock, J.A.; Acharya, K.R. Structure and activity of a functional derivative of Clostridium botulinum neurotoxin B. *J. Struct. Biol.* **2011**, *174*, 52–57.
36. Williams, P.A.; Cosme, J.; Vinkovic, D.M.; Ward, A.; Jhoti, H. Crystal structures of human cytochrome p450 3a4 bound to metyrapone and progesterone. *Science* **2004**, *305*, 683–686. [CrossRef]
37. Engidawork, E.; Roberts, J.C.; Hardmeier, R.; Scheper, R.J.; Lubec, G. Expression of the multidrug resistance P glycoprotein (Pgp) and multidrug resistance associated protein (MRP1) in down syndrome brains. *J. Neural. Transm. Suppl.* **2001**, *61*, 35–45.
38. Wang, W.Y.; Wu, X.M.; Wang, L.; Meng, Q.G.; Liu, W.H. Stereoselective property of 20(S)–protopanaxadiol ocotillol type epimers affects its absorption and also the inhibition of P-glycoprotein. *PLoS ONE* **2014**, *9*, e98887. [CrossRef]

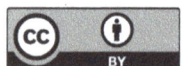

© 2020 by the authors. Licensee MDPI, Basel, Switzerland. This article is an open access article distributed under the terms and conditions of the Creative Commons Attribution (CC BY) license (http://creativecommons.org/licenses/by/4.0/).

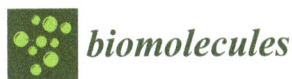

Review

Panax ginseng Pharmacopuncture: Current Status of the Research and Future Challenges

In-Seon Lee [1], Ki Sung Kang [2,*] and Song-Yi Kim [2,*]

1. Acupuncture and Meridian Science Research Center, College of Korean Medicine, Kyung Hee University, Seoul 02453, Korea; islee4u@gmail.com
2. College of Korean Medicine, Gachon University, Seongnam 13120, Korea
* Correspondence: kkang@gachon.ac.kr (K.S.K.); songyi@gachon.ac.kr (S.-Y.K.); Tel.: +82-31-750-5402 (K.S.K.); +82-31-750-8826 (S.-Y.K.)

Received: 16 November 2019; Accepted: 14 December 2019; Published: 25 December 2019

Abstract: Despite the increasing use of ginseng pharmacopuncture in clinical practice, evidence of its physiological effects, safety, and clinical outcomes is insufficient. The purpose of this review is to summarize previous studies and suggest future challenges for the clinical use of ginseng pharmacopuncture. We systematically searched clinical and animal studies that applied ginseng pharmacopuncture and reviewed the manufacturing processes of ginseng pharmacopuncture solution, safety, physiological responses, and clinical effects. Intravenous or point injection of the ginseng pharmacopuncture solution made by distillation extraction has been commonly used in studies. Ginseng pharmacopuncture does not show any toxicity in animals and humans, while it influenced the heart rate variability, pulse wave velocity, and protein synthesis in human subjects. In 25 case reports, patients with cancer, amyotrophic lateral sclerosis, skin wrinkles, and allergic rhinitis showed significant improvement of clinical outcomes. We found that more evidence is necessary to conclude that ginseng pharmacopuncture is safe and effective. First, the pharmacopuncture manufacturing process should be standardized on the basis of the safety and efficacy tests. Moreover, studies on the quantitative quality of the components of the solution and on the clinical comparison of various injection methods are required to improve clinical outcomes in the future.

Keywords: *Panax ginseng*; ginsenoside; wild ginseng; pharmacopuncture; safety; clinical trials

1. Introduction

The root of *Panax ginseng* C. A. Meyer (*P. ginseng*) has been widely used as a tonic in East Asian countries such as Korea, China, and Japan since ancient times to improve organ functions and increase vital energy based on traditional medicine theory and clinical experiences [1]. According to the Qi and flavor theories, the theoretical pharmacology systems in traditional Asian medicine using the property and flavor of a medicine, it is slightly warm and nourishes the Qi and Yang. Therefore, it has been used to treat the Qi deficiency state in various diseases such as chronic illness, fatigue, and weak functions or organs [2]. The major active components of *P. ginseng* are ginsenosides (also called saponins, Table 1), and their mechanisms have been primarily investigated to reveal the pharmacological effects of *P. ginseng*. Ginsenosides are classified as protopanaxadiol (e.g., ginsenoside Rb1, Table 2) or protopanaxatriol (e.g., ginsenoside Rg1, Table 3). In addition to the ginsenosides, there are essential oil components, phenol compounds, polysaccharides, alkaloids, and nitrogen compounds (Table 1). Traditionally, wild ginseng has been regarded as being more effective than cultivated ginseng. Wild ginseng contains a higher level of ginsenoside Rb1 and Rg1 than cultivated ginseng [3], and proteomic analysis revealed that wild ginseng contains higher levels of amino acids, amino acid-related enzymes and proteins, and derivatives than cultivated ginseng [4].

Table 1. Chemical constituents of Korean ginseng.

Groups	Contents	Ingredients
Saponin	Saponin (3–6%)	- PPD ginsenosides - PPT ginsenosides - Oleanane ginsenosides
Non-saponin	N-containing substances (12–15%)	- Proteins, amino acids - Peptides, nucleic acids - Alkaloids
Non-saponin	Fat-soluble components (1–2%)	- Fat, fatty acids - Essential oils - Phytosterol - Organic acids - Phenolics - Polyacetylenes - Terpenes
Non-saponin	Carbohydrates (50–60%)	- Polysaccharides - Oligosaccharides - Sugar, fiber, pectin
Others	Ash (4–6%)	- Minerals
Others	Vitamin (0.05%)	- Water-soluble vitamins

Table 2. Chemical structures of protopanaxadiol saponins.

Ginsenoside	R1	R2
ginsenoside-Ra1	- glc(2→1)glc	- glc(6→1)arap(4→1)xyl
ginsenoside-Ra2	- glc(2→1)glc	- glc(6→1)araf(2→1)xyl
ginsenoside-Ra3	- glc(2→1)glc	- glc(6→1)glc(3→1)xyl
ginsenoside-Rb1	- glc(2→1)glc	- glc(6→1)glc
ginsenoside-Rb2	- glc(2→1)glc	- glc(6→1)arap
ginsenoside-Rb3	- glc(2→1)glc	- glc(6→1)xyl
ginsenoside-Rc	- glc(2→1)glc	- glc(6→1)araf
ginsenoside-Rd	- glc(2→1)glc	- glc
ginsenoside-Rg3	- glc(2→1)glc	- H
ginsenoside-F2	- glc	- glc
ginsenoside-Rh2	- glc	- H
ginsenoside-R1	- glc(2→1)glc(6)Ac	- glc(6→1)glc
ginsenoside-Rs1	- glc(2→1)glc(6)Ac	- glc(6→1)arap
ginsenoside-Rs2	- glc(2→1)glc(6)Ac	- glc(6→1)araf
ginsenoside-Rs3	- glc(2→1)glc(6)Ac	- H
ginsenoside-Rb1	- glc(2→1)glc(6)Ma	- glc(6→1)glc
ginsenoside-Rb2	- glc(2→1)glc(6)Ma	- glc(6→1)arap
ginsenoside-Rc	- glc(2→1)glc(6)Ma	- glc(6→1)araf
ginsenoside-Rd	- glc(2→1)glc(6)Ma	- glc
ginsenoside-R4	- glc(2→1)glc	- glc(6→1)glc(6→1)xyl
ginsenoside-Fa	- glc(2→1)glc(2→1)xyl	- glc(6→1)glc
ginsenoside-X VII	- glc	- glc(6→1)glc

glc: β-D-glucopyranosyl; arap: α-L-arabinopyranosyl; araf: α-L-arabinofuranosyl; xyl: β-D-xylopyranosyl; Ac: acetyl; Ma: malonyl.

Table 3. Chemical structures of protopanaxatriol type saponins.

Ginsenoside	R1	R2
ginsenoside-Re	- glc(2→1)rha	- glc
ginsenoside-Rf	- glc(2→1)glc	- H
20-gluco-ginsenoside-Rf	- glc(2→1)glc	- glc
ginsenoside-Rg1	- glc	- glc
ginsenoside-Rg2	- glc(2→1)rha	- H
ginsenoside-Rh1	- glc	- H
ginsenoside-F1	- H	- glc
ginsenoside-F3	- H	- glc(6→1)arap
ginsenoside-F5	- H	- glc(6→1)araf
ginsenoside-R1	- glc(2→1)xyl	- glc
ginsenoside-R2	- glc(2→1)xyl	- H
ginsenoside-R3	- glc –glc(6→1)	- glc
ginsenoside-R6	- glc –glc(6→1)	- glc*

rha: α-L-rhamnopyranosyl; glc: β-D-glucopyranosyl; arap: α-L-arabinopyranosyl; xyl: β-D-xylopyranosyl; glc*: α-D-glucopyranosyl; araf: α-L-arabinofuranosyl.

Traditionally, *P. ginseng* is used in the decoction form and is decocted with boiling water for a certain number of hours and prepared as a drink [5]. More recently, ginseng concentrates, extracted using water or alcohol, are also used [6]. In addition, ginseng has been transformed into red ginseng or fermented black ginseng through steaming, repeated heating and drying, or fermentation [6,7]. In addition to oral intake of ginseng, whose clinical effects and safety have been demonstrated [8,9], ginseng has been also administered via injection (intravenous or intramuscular on either acupoints or non-acupoints), and this technique is called pharmacopuncture.

Pharmacopuncture is a relatively new acupuncture therapy in Traditional Korean Medicine (TKM) that combines acupuncture with herbal medicine [10]. Pharmacopuncture involves injection of filtered and sterilized herbal medicine extracts, which are extracted using different techniques (e.g., alcohol immersion, distillation, or pressing) depending on the herbs [11]. Thus, it simultaneously induces mechanical stimulation of acupoints and a pharmacological effect. It was originally developed under the name of 'Aqua-acupuncture' in the 1950s in China [10]. Aqua-acupuncture uses both herbal and non-herbal medicines and has been regarded as a combined therapy with traditional and Western medicine. However, pharmacopuncture in South Korea is exclusively associated with TKM, as it uses herbs that have been used in the form of other formulations (decoction, granule, etc.) and involves injection of the herbal extracts intravenously or into acupuncture points (acupoint), trigger points, or response points. The herbs and acupoints (in the case of herbal extracts injected into acupoints) are selected according to the meridian, Qi, and flavor theories, and the syndrome differentiation diagnosis protocol from TKM [2,11].

Ginseng pharmacopuncture is a typical single-herb pharmacopuncture, which contains diverse substances such as ginsenoside Rg1, ginsenoside Rb2, and phenolic compounds, and the amount of substances vary depending on the extraction methods (e.g., distilled versus ethanol extract [12]). A review of animal studies suggested that ginseng pharmacopuncture is useful in the prevention of diseases and strengthening immune response, especially in Yang insufficiency animal models induced by hydrocortisone acetate injection [13]. Furthermore, several studies have investigated the toxicity of ginseng pharmacopuncture, and its safety has been studied in animals [14,15]. On the basis of these lines of evidence, single-herb ginseng pharmacopuncture has been widely used in clinics as one of the standard TKM therapies in South Korea, while pharmacopuncture with several herbs combined (combination of various herbal extracts; e.g., Shenmai or Shenfu injections) has been more extensively used in China. Despite its wide usage in clinics, evidence is insufficient to prove whether ginseng pharmacopuncture therapy significantly improves the clinical outcomes and risk of adverse events (AEs) in patients.

In this study, we restrictively defined ginseng as the root of *Panax ginseng C. A. Meyer*, and our aim was to provide a comprehensive review of the clinical application of *P. ginseng* pharmacopuncture, which we referred to as 'ginseng pharmacopuncture', including its safety, physiological, and clinical responses. To achieve this goal, we (1) provided an overview of the physiological responses to and side effects of ginseng pharmacopuncture in animals or humans (patients and healthy participants), and (2) systematically reviewed previous clinical trials using ginseng pharmacopuncture in patients with various diseases. Lastly, we emphasized that more basic and clinical studies are needed to confirm the effects and safety of ginseng pharmacopuncture, and suggested future directions for developing ginseng pharmacopuncture as a safe and effective treatment for patients seeking TKM therapies.

2. Materials and Methods

2.1. Search Strategy

We used a systematic search strategy following the preferred reporting items for systematic reviews and meta-analyses (PRISMA) guidelines for systematic reviews. Electronic searches of articles were conducted from their inception to January 2018, without language restrictions in PubMed, the Research Information Sharing Service (RISS), the Korean Studies Information Service System (KISS), KoreaMed, and the China National Knowledge Infrastructure (CNKI). The search terms used were "ginseng" including *Panax ginseng* Radix, *Panax ginseng*, ginseng radix, or red ginseng; and "pharmacopuncture", including aqua acupuncture, herbal/herb acupuncture, point-injection, or yakchim. "Red ginseng", which is the most common processed type of *P. ginseng*, was added as a search term. Furthermore, a secondary search was performed by screening the reference lists of articles that met the inclusion criteria.

2.2. Study Selection, Data Extraction, and Data Analysis

Three categories of studies were included in the search strategy if they evaluated pharmacopuncture using *Panax ginseng C. A. Meyer* roots as follows: (1) preclinical trial in animals, (2) study of physiological responses in human subjects, and (3) clinical trial in patients to identify the clinical effects of ginseng pharmacopuncture.

We followed the process of systematic literature review. First, searched articles were screened on the basis of the title and abstract before the full text was assessed. Second, articles identified as duplicates or non-original studies such as reviews, opinions, or protocols were removed. Third, publications that did not meet our definition of ginseng pharmacopuncture (single-herb ginseng administered via intravenous or intramuscular injection), studies that used pharmacopuncture consisting multiple herbs, and articles not written in English, Chinese, or Korean were excluded. The included studies were classified as animal studies, studies on the physiological responses of healthy participants, or clinical trials in patients. After the selection of the articles to be analyzed, we extracted data from the included clinical trials by using a predefined form that contained the following items presented in a separate table: manufacturing process of pharmacopuncture solution and characteristics of participants (e.g., age, sex, disorder or symptoms), intervention details (injection site, volume of injection, number and duration of treatment and co-intervention), and clinical outcomes. Results of animal studies and physiological responses are summarized narratively in the manuscript.

3. Results

3.1. The Manufacturing Process of the Ginseng Pharmacopuncture Solution

Distillation extraction, alcohol immersion, the combined method of distillation and alcohol immersion, compression, and dilution methods are used for the manufacture of pharmacopuncture solution [2,11]. Among these methods, the ginseng pharmacopuncture solution is generally produced using the distillation method. In the included studies, ginseng plant was rinsed with clean water (in some cases, the rhizome part of the ginseng is removed) followed by distillation and/or decoction, filtering, and sterilization of the solution. Rarely, in some cases, extracts of certain active or target substances such as polysaccharides from ginseng were used to make the solution [16] (Figure 1). Recently, the Accreditation System of External Herbal Dispensaries (EHDs) was announced. The quality of pharmacopuncture should be managed according to the EHDs and clinicians and patients can verify whether the pharmacopuncture solution is produced in herbal dispensaries with an EHD certification mark [17].

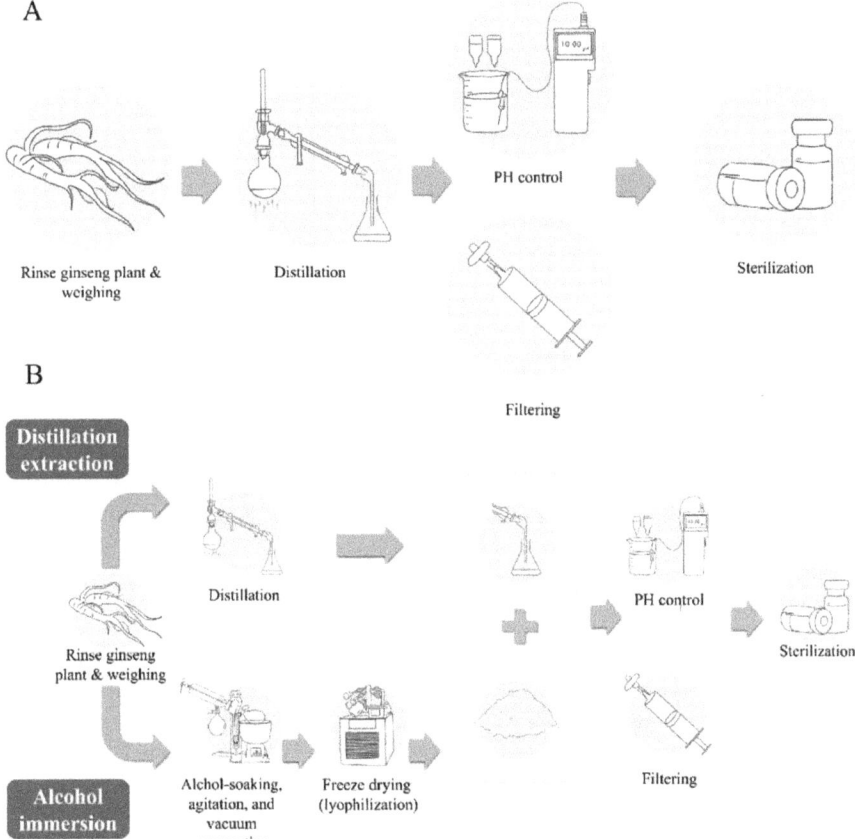

Figure 1. Manufacturing process of pharmacopuncture. (**A**) Distillation extraction; (**B**) combined method of distillation and alcohol immersion.

3.2. Physiological Response to Ginseng Pharmacopuncture in Human Subjects

In this review, 13 studies measured various physiological responses before and after receiving ginseng pharmacopuncture. In the healthy subjects, intravenous injection of wild ginseng pharmacopuncture did not change the blood pressure, pulse, temperature, respiration, and blood test indexes [18,19]. Wild ginseng pharmacopuncture injected at acupoints (ST36 and ST37) did not significantly change the acupuncture sensations as compared with other types of complex-herb pharmacopuncture (e.g., BUM pharmacopuncture made of *Calculus Bovis*, *Fel Ursi*, *Moschus*) and saline injection [20]. Another study showed that only the volume of injected solution, but not the stimulation methods (perpendicular versus transverse injection) at acupoints, affected the subjective intensity reporting of pharmacopuncture stimulation [21].

By contrast, randomized controlled trials (RCTs) showed that the sympathetic nervous system in healthy participants was activated significantly by wild ginseng pharmacopuncture injected at acupoints as compared with saline injection [22–25]. Intravenous wild ginseng pharmacopuncture decreased the mean heart rate variability (HRV) and pulse wave velocity (PWV) and increased the mean and standard deviation of normal R-R intervals and very low frequency oscillation power in patients with breast cancer [26], while it decreased the mean HRV and PWV and increased the mean normal R-R intervals in healthy volunteers [27]. Intravenous wild ginseng pharmacopuncture injection also affected pulse-related factors (e.g., increased the stability of the pulse wave) [28]. It also increased the level of proteins CR2-C3d, Ral-A, proapolipoprotein, apolipoprotein, transferrin, human hemoglobin, and vitamin D binding protein and reduced the transthyretin and antitrypsin levels in blood samples [29,30].

Current evidence suggests that ginseng pharmacopuncture may activate the sympathetic nervous system and change the protein synthesis mechanisms, while the sensory stimulation aspect (e.g., De-Qi sensation induced by needle injection at acupuncture points) may not specifically be involved in the effect of ginseng pharmacopuncture. However, the underlying mechanisms and physiological actions of ginseng pharmacopuncture have not yet been fully explained owing to insufficient evidence.

3.3. Safety Tests of Ginseng Pharmacopuncture

Several studies have tested the safety of ginseng pharmacopuncture in animals using different dosages and treatment frequencies. For example, both single administration (20 or 10 mL/kg) and repeated administration (10, 5 or 2.5 mL/kg for 4 weeks, once a day) of ginseng pharmacopuncture evoked no significant toxic responses in Sprague-Dawley rats (e.g., changes in mortality, histological observations, body weight, clinical signs, and food consumption behavior) [14,15]. In addition, pharmacopuncture using intravenous or intramuscular injection of radix ginseng (dried root of *P. ginseng*) at a single dose (0.1 0.5, or 1.0 mL/animal) did not change body weight, general condition, and hematological or biochemistry test results in rats [31,32].

In a case report, drug-induced liver injury (increased alkaline phosphatase level, white blood cells, and platelets; all indexes were outside the normal range) was suspected after intravenous wild ginseng pharmacopuncture treatment in a patient with shoulder pain, however, the causal influence of the wild ginseng pharmacopuncture treatment on the liver injury was not proven in the study [33]. In the RCT that compared the combination therapy of ginseng polysaccharides pharmacopuncture, Bupleurum pharmacopuncture, and paroxetine (pharmacopuncture group) with paroxetine monotherapy (control group), seven cases of AEs such as headache, dry mouth, or tremor were reported in the pharmacopuncture group. However, 21 cases of AEs such as diarrhea, constipation, weakness, or anorexia were reported in the control group, including nine cases of the same type of AEs as the treatment group [16].

In summary, the safety of ginseng pharmacopuncture injection has been mainly studied in animals, but more empirical investigations are necessary to prove its safety in humans.

3.4. Systematic Review of Clinical Studies

3.4.1. Search Results

Figure 2 summarizes the results of the literature search process for analysis of clinical studies. Our research strategy retrieved a total of 595 articles, 245 of which were duplicates. An additional 324 studies were discarded after screening the full text or abstract including 95 not related to pharmacopuncture, 47 not related to *P. ginseng*, 53 that used pharmacopuncture with combined herbs. Finally, 25 case reports (24 studies written in English [14,34–55] and one study in Chinese [56]) and one RCT (written in Chinese) [16] met the inclusion criteria and were incorporated in the systematic review (Figure 2 and Table 4).

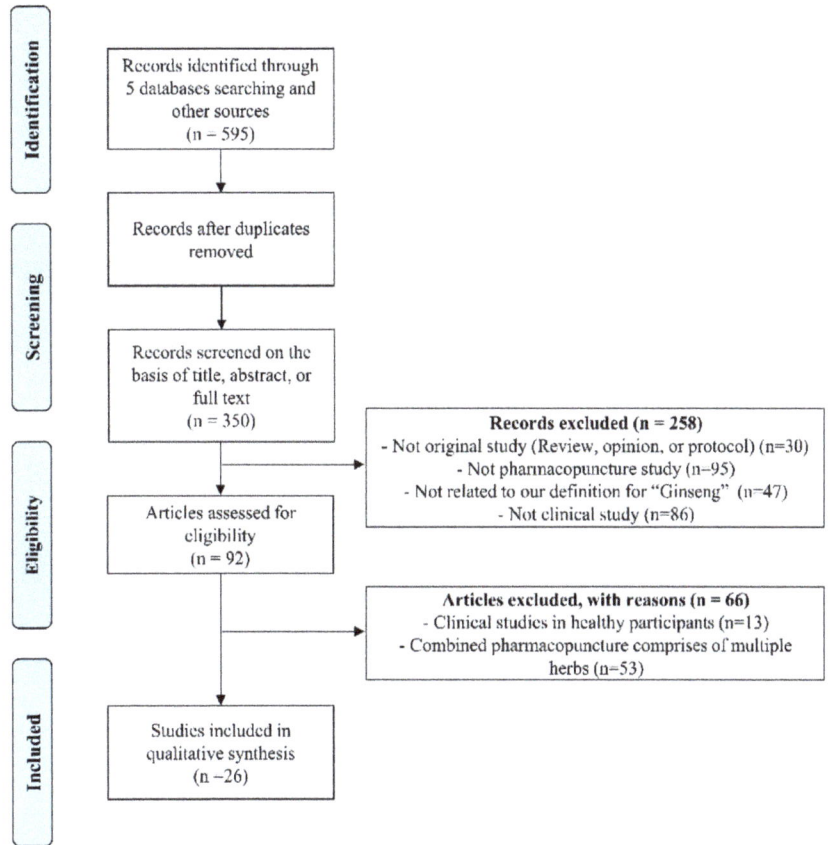

Figure 2. PRISMA flow chart for the search and selection of the included clinical trials.

Table 4. Summary of included clinical trials using (wild) ginseng pharmacopuncture in patients with various diseases.

No. Author (Year), Article Type	Disorder (Symptoms), n *, Gender, Age	Treatment (1, 2, 3 ...: Serial Treatment or Group; a, b, c ...: Combined Treatment)					Significant Results
		Pharmacopuncture		Co-Interventions			
		Herb, Location, Dose, Injection Methods	Duration, Number	Interventions	Duration, Number		
Case report/series in cancer patients							
1. Kwon (2005) [34]	Hepatocellular carcinoma, liver cirrhosis, hepatitis B+, lung metastasis (abdominal discomfort), m, 41	a. Cultivated wild ginseng, 0.5–1 cc, IV (at the points of BL13, BL18, LR14, CV12) total 4–40 cc	5 months, 5 times/week	b. Moxibustion, CV4, CV6 c. Cupping	-		CT: near elimination of the cancer cells metastasized into lungs
2. Park (2007) [37]	Squamous cell carcinoma Stage 3B (severe cough, dyspnea, shoulder discomfort), m, 58	2. Cultivated wild ginseng, 10 mL, IV 3. Cultivated wild ginseng, 10 mL, PI (LU1) 4. Cultivated wild ginseng, 10 mL, PI (LU1)	2. 54 days, 1/day 3. 6 days, 1/day 4. 28 days, -	1. Herbal medicine	-		1. CT: aggravation of cancer 2. CT: mass size increased and invaded the mediastinum after the first trial, stabilized after 54 treatments 3. Discontinue the treatment due to a slow of speech and hemiplegia (cerebral infarction) 4. CT: mass invaded the heart Deceased
3. Bang (2008) [38]	Case 1. Lung cancer (adenocarcinoma, Stage T2N3 3B, cough, phlegm), f, 68	a. Cultivated wild ginseng, 20 mL, IV	a. 8 months, 1/day	b. Herbal medication (globule, Hangamdan) c. Herbal medication (granule, decoction)	b. 3/day, 8 months		Overall decrease/maintain of cough and phlegm CT, PET-CT: stabilized mass size
	Case 2. NSCLC stage T1N2 3A, m, 64	Cultivated wild ginseng, IV	a. 5 months	-	-		Overall decrease/maintain of cough, weakness, phlegm CT, PET-CT: stabilized mass size
4. Lee (2010) [39]	Lung cancer (n = 3), colorectal cancer (n = 2), stomach cancer (n = 1), malignant mesothelioma (n = 1) (f, 1), median 56	Cultivated wild ginseng, 20 mL, IV	14 days, 1/day (1 cycle)	-	-		median survival days: 544; 1 year survival rate: 57.1%; drop out (n = 2), progressive (n = 2), stable disease (n = 3)
	Case 1: Colon cancer stage 3B, ECOG 3		2 cycles	-	-		Median survival days: 26 days; drop out
	Case 2: Mesothelioma stage 4, ECOG 3		2 cycles	-	-		Median survival days: 56 days; progressive disease; increased size and number of mass
	Case 3: NSCLC stage 4, ECOG 3		1 cycle	-	-		Median survival days: 140 days; drop out
	Case 4: Gastric carcinoma stage 4, ECOG 2, m, 55		13 cycles	-	-		Median survival days: 544 days; stable disease; no changes of stomach mass, increased liver metastasis
	Case 5: Colon cancer stage 4, ECOG 2		3 cycles	-	-		Median survival days: 596 days; progressive disease; increased rectal mass, liver and lung metastasis
	Case 6: NSCLC stage 3A, ECOG 1, m, 63		13 cycles	-	-		Median survival days: 718 days; stable disease; no changes (early)/increased mass (later)
	Case 7: NSCLC stage 3, ECOG 1, f, 67		21 cycles	-	-		Median survival days: 898 days; stable disease; slight increased mass in left lower lobe (early)/no changes (later), right adrenal gland metastasis (later)

Table 4. Cont.

No. Author (Year), Article Type	Disorder (Symptoms), n *, Gender, Age	Treatment (1, 2, 3 …: Serial Treatment or Group; a, b, c …: Combined Treatment)					Significant Results
		Pharmacopuncture		Co-Interventions			
		Herb, Location, Dose, Injection Methods	Duration, Number	Interventions	Duration, Number		
5. Lee (2011) [36]	Prostate cancer, n = 2 (f, 0), mean 52	a. Cultivated wild ginseng, 20 mL, IV	-	b. AKDH pharmacopuncture c. Sweet BV pharmacopuncture	-		
	Case 1. Prostate adenocarcinoma (T3bN0M0, fatigue, pain, nocturia, impotence), m, 51	a.	2/week	b. AKDH pharmacopuncture c. Acupuncture	-	Decreased PSA and prostate volume; prostate cancer disappeared, remain cancer in a seminal vesicle and left apex, T3bN0M0 (25 weeks) PSA maintained, no discomfort symptoms (30 months)	
	Case 2. Prostate cancer T3bN0M1c (metastasis to bone/lung, pelvic pain, knee pain, short breath, weakness, abnormal urination), m, 53	a.	5/week	c. Sweet BV pharmacopuncture d. Acupuncture e. Medication	2–3/week	Ups and downs of PSA and symptoms, stable health condition (19 months)	
	NSCLC, n = 6 (f, 5), median 67	a. Wild ginseng, 20 mL, IV b. Wild ginseng, 10 mL, P1 (LU1)	a, b. 4 weeks/cycle				
	Case 1. Adenocarcinoma stage 4, m, 64	2. b 3. a	2. 2 cycles 3. 4 cycles	1. Chemotherapy, operation	-	2. CT: tumor progressed (progressed disease) 3. normal range of blood cancer markers, tumor growth has stopped for 9 weeks, increase of mass (stable disease)	
	Case 2. Squamous cell carcinoma stage 4, m, 60	2. a	4 cycles	1. Chemotherapy, operation	-	1. tumor progressed 2. tumor growth has shown stable condition (4 weeks; stable disease); CT: slight progress	
6. Kwon (2011) [40]	Case 3. Squamous cell carcinoma stage 4, f, 62	b.	2 cycles	-	-	CT: Tumor markedly increased (progressed disease)	
	Case 4. Breathing difficulties with weight loss, m, 70	b.	1 cycle	-	-	CT: Tumor size slightly increased (stable disease)	
	Case 5. Squamous cell carcinoma stage 3A, m, 65	1. a 2. b	1. 5 cycles 2. 2 cycles	-	-	1. CT: Tumor growth showed stable condition for 20 weeks (stable disease) 2. CT: tumor size slightly increased (progressed disease)	
	Case 6. Squamous cell carcinoma stage 3B (dyspnea, hemoptysis, fever and weight loss), m, 78	a.	16 cycles	-	-	a. all cancer related symptoms and the tumor growth showed stable condition (16 months, stable disease)	
7. Kim (2011) [41]	Squamous cell lung carcinoma T2bN1, stage 2B (dyspnea, phlegm, hemoptysis, weight lose), m, 75	a. Cultivated wild ginseng, 0.5 mL, P1 (CV12, CV4, BL13)	1/day, 12 days or 2/week, 3 weeks	b. Acupuncture c. Cupping d. Moxibustion	-	Dyspnea maintained, phlegm and hemoptysis disappeared CT: decrease of mass	

Table 4. Cont.

No. Author (Year), Article Type	Disorder (Symptoms), n *, Gender, Age	Treatment (1, 2, 3 … : Serial Treatment or Group; a, b, c … : Combined Treatment)					Significant Results
		Pharmacopuncture		Co-Interventions			
		Herb, Location, Dose, Injection Methods	Duration, Number	Interventions	Duration, Number		
8. Im (2012) [42]	Colorectal cancer (metastasis in liver, lung, ovary, chest pain, insomnia), f, 47	a. Cultivated wild ginseng, 10 mL, IV	3–5/week	b. Soram pharmacopuncture; ** c. Herbal medicine d. Moxibustion e. Acupuncture	b. 1, 2, 5/day		Decreased pain (2 weeks) Decreased size of metastasized mass in lung (13 weeks) CEA, CA19-9 decreased
9. Ha (2013) [43]	Colorectal adenocarcinoma stage 4B (recurrence, metastasis in liver, spleen, lung), m, 42	a. Cultivated wild ginseng, 30 mL, IV	a. 3/week, 34 weeks	b. FOLFIRI chemotherapy	b. 12/2 weeks, 31 weeks		Recurrence of colorectal adenocarcinoma and metastasis disappeared, no adverse events reported to FOLFIRA chemotherapy
10. Han (2013) [44]	Breast cancer (recurrence, metastasis in lung, chest pain, cough, short breath, shoulder pain, excessive sweating), f, 53	a. Cultivated wild ginseng, 10 mL, IV	3/week	b. Cordyceps militaris pharmacopuncture c. Acupuncture d. Moxibustion e. Herbal medicine	3/week		Chest pain and cough disappeared (1 month) Tubercles in lung disappeared (6 weeks) PET-CT: Recurrence disappeared (30 days)
11. Yun (2013) [46]	Pancreatic cancer (abdominal pain, indigestion, post-prandial pain, abdominal inflation), f, 68	a. Cultivated wild ginseng, 20 mL, NA	3/week, 5 months	b. Medication c. Herbal medication (globule, Hangamdan; globule, Ginseng-pil) d. Acupuncture	b. 4/week c. 3/day		Decreased pain and intake of analgesics (5 months) Improvement of all symptom; CT: decreased hydrothorax and mass size (stable disease)
12. Lee (2013) [47]	NSCLC squamous cell carcinoma stage 4 (cough, dyspnoea, weakness), m, 79	a. Wild ginseng, 10 mL, IV	a. 1/week, 7 months	b. Berbal medication (globule, Soramdan) c. Cordyceps sinensis pharmacopuncture, 10 mL, IV d. Trichosanthes kirilowii pharmacopuncture, 10mL, IV	b. 2/week, 7 months c, d. 1/week, 7 months		ECOG scale maintained (4 weeks) and decreased (5 week) Tumor size decreased
13. Kang (2014) [45]	Case 1. Signet ring cell carcinoma stage 4 (abdominal pain, diarrhea, nausea, fatigue, bloating, heartburn), f, 41	a. Cultivated wild ginseng, 1 mL, subcutaneous injection (EX-B2)	a. 20 times	b. Acupuncture c. Analgesics	b. 46 days, 1/day		Reduced analgesics (10 days) Improvement of symptoms and adverse events of analgesics (sedation, nausea)
	Case 2. bronchioalveolar carcinoma, adenocarcinoma stage 4 (dizziness, nausea, vomiting, insomnia, fatigue, diarrhea, dyspnea), f, 51	a.	a. 5 times	b. Chemotherapy	-		Pain disappeared, able to perform daily activities without analgesics
	Case 3. tubulovillous adenoma, neuroendocrine carcinoma stage 4A (diarrhea, abdominal discomfort, rash, dyspnea), m, 81	a.	a. 13 times	b. Analgesics	-		Decreased pain, improved health condition, reduced analgesics Worsening of liver and kidney functions

Table 4. Cont.

No. Author (Year), Article Type	Disorder (Symptoms), n *, Gender, Age	Treatment (1, 2, 3 ...: Serial Treatment or Group; a, b, c ...: Combined Treatment)					Significant Results
		Pharmacopuncture		Co-Interventions			
		Herb, Location, Dose, Injection Methods	Duration, Number	Interventions	Duration, Number		
14. Park (2015) [48]	Case 1. Thymic cancer (fatigue, fever, anorexia, itching), f, 40	a. Wild ginseng, 1 mL, total 20 mL, subcutaneous injection (EX-B2)	a. 1/2–3 days, 4 times	-	-		Increased white blood cells Decreased erythrocyte sedimentation rate, thyroglobulin Ag level, Korean version of the Revised Piper Fatigue Scale total score
	Case 2. cervical cancer (fatigue, lower limb edema and pain, lower back pain, gait disturbance), f, 61	a. Wild ginseng, 1 mL, total 20 mL, subcutaneous injection (EX-B2)	a. 12 times	-	-		Increased total protein level, lower limb pain Decreased g-glutamyl transferase level, C-reactive protein, fatigue
15. Lee (2015) [35]	Breast cancer stage 3, f, 46	2, 3, 4-a. Wild ginseng, 10 mL, IV	all 3 times/week except 4-e: daily	1. Neoadjuvant chemotherapy, breast conservation surgery, adjuvant radiotherapy 2-b. Cordyceps sinensis 2-c. Trichosanthes kirilowii 2-d. Euonymus alatus 2-e. Astragalus membranaceus pharmacopuncture 3-b. C. sinensis 3-c. T. kirilowii 3-d. E. alatus 3-e. P. vulgaris pharmacopuncture 4-b. E. alatus 4-c. Sorum nebulizer solution 4-d. Nebulizer solution 4-e. Herbal medication (globule, Hangamdan)	-		1. nodule in right upper lung, increased 2. 15 mm lymphadenopathies in right paratracheal, interlobar hilar, and subcarinal area 3. lymph node decreased to less than 10 mm 4. no recurrence was observed
16. Kim (2015a) [49]	recurrent oligodendroglioma (hemiparesis, dysarthria, severe daily seizures, headache, drowsiness, constipation, dysuria), m, 54	a. Wild ginseng, 0.5 mL, PI (BL13)	a. 1/week	b. BV pharmacopuncture, GV20, EX-HN1, 0.2 mL c. Acupuncture d. Herbal medicine (fermented red ginseng solution)	c, d. 1/day		brain MRI: decreased tumor size (18 months) free from seizure, left-side hemiparesis was improved, symptoms disappeared (21 months) maintain the treated status without any deterioration (5 years)
17. Kim (2015b) [50]	Hepatocellular carcinoma (stage 2, cirrhosis, abdominal pain, lack of appetite, sleep disorder, fatigue, weakness), m, 57	3-a. Cultivated wild ginseng, 0.25–0.5cc, PI (BL18, CV12, ST25)	3-a. 1/day	1. Ascites puncture, albumin injection, diuretic 2. Ascites puncture 3-b. Medication 3-c. Herbal medication (globule, Hangamdan) 3-d. Acupuncture	various		1. unmanageable liver index and ascites 2. Ascites and symptoms maintained 3. symptoms relieved, abdominal circumference decreased (22 days) normal ALP (50 days) Ascites reduced (64 days) Symptoms disappeared except slight and seldom abdominal pain, increase of ALP/AST (71 days) Symptoms disappeared, normal blood test index (340 days) Ascites almost disappeared (351 days)

Table 4. Cont.

No. Author (Year), Article Type	Disorder (Symptoms), n *, Gender, Age	Treatment (1, 2, 3 …: Serial Treatment or Group; a, b, c …: Combined Treatment)					Significant Results
		Pharmacopuncture		Co-Interventions			
		Herb, Location, Dose, Injection Methods	Duration, Number	Interventions	Duration, Number		
18. Lee (2017) [51]	Right breast invasive ductal carcinoma T1N0M0 (metastases in the liver, retroperitoneum, mesentery, pelvic bones, cranium, whole-body bone, pleural effusion, back pain, jaundice, ascites), f, 45	4-a. Wild ginseng, IV or PI (acupoint)	1/day or 2 days	1. Chemotherapy (trastuzumab, paclitaxel) 2. Medication (trastuzumab, vancomycin, tazoperan) 3. Chemotherapy (trastuzumab, paclitaxel) 4-b. Herbal medication (Soramdan) 4-c. Herbal medication (Jeobgoldan)	4-b. 1/day or 3/week 4-c. 2/day		1. – 2. CT, bone scan: reduction of liver metastases, pleural effusion increased, new lesions on the sternum, ribs, acetabulum 3. find vancomycin-resistant enterococci 4-a, b, c. CT: reduction of the liver metastasis lesion, scar, contraction of the liver parenchyma PET-CT: reduction of the tumor size in the right breast, the primary site of the tumor, right axillary lymph node, liver, bone metastases
Case report/series in patients with other diseases							
19. Li (1994) [56]	Allergic rhinitis, n = 100 (f, 44), range 16–51	Panax ginseng, 4 mL, Sphenopalatine ganglion	1/week, 4–12 week	-	-		Complete symptom relief without recurrence (68%), significant symptom relief (29%), not significant results (3%)
20. Kim (2009) [52]	Case 1. Behçet's disease (canker sore, edema, chronic fatigue, drug-induced hepatitis), m, 47	a. Cultivated wild ginseng, 10 mL, IV	1–2/week	b. Acupuncture c. AKDH pharmacopuncture	-		Improvement of all symptoms
	Case 2. Drug-induced hepatitis (weakness, fatigue, low back pain, indigestion), m, 51	a. Cultivated wild ginseng, 10 mL, IV	1/week	b. Acupuncture c. AKDH pharmacopuncture	-		Improvement of symptoms, satisfied by the results
	Case 3. Hepatocirrhosis (bleeding, weakness, indigestion), m, 72	Cultivated wild ginseng, 20 mL, IV	3/week	-	-		Improvement of all symptoms, normalization of AST/ALT
21. Ryu (2010) [53]	ALS	a. Cultivated wild ginseng, 20 mL, IV	a. 1–2/2 weeks or 1/2 days	b. AKDH pharmacopuncture c. Sweet BV pharmacopuncture	b. 1–2/2 weeks or 1/2 days		Improvement of general health condition without muscle weakness (2–3 months) Slow movement, became pessimistic and depressed, slight muscle atrophy (4–5.5 months) Decrease of thigh thickness, ALS functional rating scale, ALS severity score (motor ability) (26.5 weeks)
	Case 1. ALS (myo-atrophy, tetraparesis), f, 51						
	Case 2. ALS (myo-atrophy, tetraparesis), m, 47						Increased strength of limbs and ALS functional rating scale (2–6 weeks) Increase of muscular strength, decrease of thickness of thigh/upper limbs and ALS functional rating scale (6–9 weeks)
	Case 3. ALS (myo-atrophy, tetraparesis), f, 70						Increased pain (2–3 months) Decreased low back pain, discomfort (4–5 months) Decreased weight, thickness of body, muscular strength, ALS functional rating scale, ALS severity scale

Table 4. Cont.

No. Author (Year), Article Type	Disorder (Symptoms), n *, Gender, Age	Treatment (1, 2, 3 ...: Serial Treatment or Group; a, b, c ...: Combined Treatment)				Significant Results
		Pharmacopuncture		Co-Interventions		
		Herb, Location, Dose, Injection Methods	Duration, Number	Interventions	Duration, Number	
22. Han (2012) [54]	Cervical dysplasia (genital itching, HPV 52 positive), f, 49	a. Cultivated wild ginseng, 30 mL, IV	6/week, 3 months	b. Herbal medicine c. Moxibustion		Improvement of symptoms, negative HPV 52 test
23. Lim (2014) [14]	Plexiform neurofibroma (general weakness, coldness of the hands/feet, skin rashes), f, 16	2-a. Wild ginseng, 20 mL, IV	1/2 weeks	1. Surgeries 2-b. Sweet BV, 5 mL, intracutaneous	2-b. 1/2 weeks	2. Tumor stopped growing, range of motion improved, no bones or organs affected
24. Park (2014) [55]	Acute demyelinating encephalomyelitis (paraplegia), m, 16	a. Cultivated wild ginseng, 20 mL, IV	1/week, 8 weeks	b. Acupuncture c. Moxibustion d. Herbal medicine e. Rehabilitation f. Medication	b. 2/day c. 1/day	Increased muscular strength, Improved Modified Bathel Index, Normalized muscular motor ability, Decreased pain
25. Lee (2015) [21]	Skin wrinkles, n = 23 (f, 20), mean 34	Cultivated wild ginseng, 0.5cc, PI (Ex-HN3, GB1, GB3, LI20, ST4)	2/week, 5 times	-	-	Decreased width and depth of skinfold
Randomized controlled trial in patients with other diseases						
26. Liu (2017) [16]	Depression, Intervention group: n = 51 (f, 28), range 22–54 Control group: n = 51 (f, 29), range 21–56	Intervention group: 1.a. ginseng polysaccharide, 1 mL, PI (BL15, BL20, ST36), 5/week 1.b. Bupleurum pharmacopuncture, 1 mL, PI (BL18, LR8) 1.c. paroxetine	30 days (10 days/session, 3 sessions)	Control group: 2. paroxetine (40–60 mg/day, 1–2 times/day)		Intervention group was significantly improved symptoms more than control group at 2, 4, 6 weeks after treatment (The Hamilton Depression Scale (HAMD), $p < 0.05$). Intervention group showed significantly higher total effective rate (98%) than control group (82%). Intervention group reported significantly lower adverse events (7 cases) than control group (21cases).

* Number of samples is omitted in the case of a single subject case study; ** *Astragalus propinquus*, *Curcuma zedoaria* pharmacopuncture. AKDH: ascending kidney water and descending heart fire; ALS: amyotrophic lateral sclerosis; ALT: alanine amino transferase; AST: aspartate transaminase; BL: bladder meridian; BV: bee venom; CT: computed tomography scan; CV: conception vessel meridian; ECOG: Eastern Cooperative Oncology Group scale; EX-B2: extra back 2nd line acupoint; EX-HN: extra head/neck acupoint; f: female; FOLFIRI: chemotherapy made up of folinic acid, fluorouracil, and irinotecan; GB: gallbladder meridian; IV: intravenous injection; n: number of samples; LI: large intestine meridian; LR: liver meridian; LU: lung meridian; MRI: magnetic resonance imaging; NSCLC: non-small-cell lung carcinoma; PET: positron emission tomography; PI: point injection; PSA: prostate specific antigen; ST: stomach meridian.

3.4.2. Participants and Settings

Twenty-four studies were conducted in Korea, and two studies were conducted in China [16,56]. Among the case reports, 18 used wild ginseng pharmacopuncture in patients with cancer [lung cancer (*n* = 17, patients); hepatocellular carcinoma, prostate cancer, colorectal cancer, or pancreatic cancer (*n* = 2, respectively); cervical cancer, thymus cancer, breast cancer, Signet ring cell carcinoma, bronchioloalveolar carcinoma, or tubulovillous adenoma (*n* = 1, respectively)] [34–51]. One hundred patients with rhinitis [56], 23 with skin wrinkles [21], three with amyotrophic lateral sclerosis (ALS) [53], and one with Behçet's disease, hepatitis, hepatocirrhosis [52], cervical dysplasia [54], neurofibroma [14], and acute demyelinating encephalomyelitis [55] were included in the systematic review. A RCT included 102 patients with depression and compared the effect and AEs of combined therapy composed of ginseng polysaccharides pharmacopuncture, Bupleurum pharmacopuncture, and paroxetine with those of paroxetine-only treatment [16].

3.4.3. Ginseng Pharmacopuncture Interventions

Among the 26 included studies, seven used wild ginseng pharmacopuncture [14,35,40,47–49,51], one study used ginseng polysaccharides pharmacopuncture [16], and 18 used cultivated ginseng pharmacopuncture.

Four studies [21,39,48,56] applied ginseng pharmacopuncture alone, and the others used various co-interventions such as antidepressants, anticancer drugs, analgesics, herbal medication, chemotherapy, cupping, moxibustion, acupuncture, diuretics, rehabilitation, surgery, and pharmacopuncture using other herbs. Fifteen studies involved pharmacopuncture performed intravenously, 10 involved injections in acupoints (three studies used both intravenous and acupoint injections [34,37,40]), and one involved injection into the sphenopalatine ganglion [56] (Figure 3). Injection methods were not clearly described in one study [46].

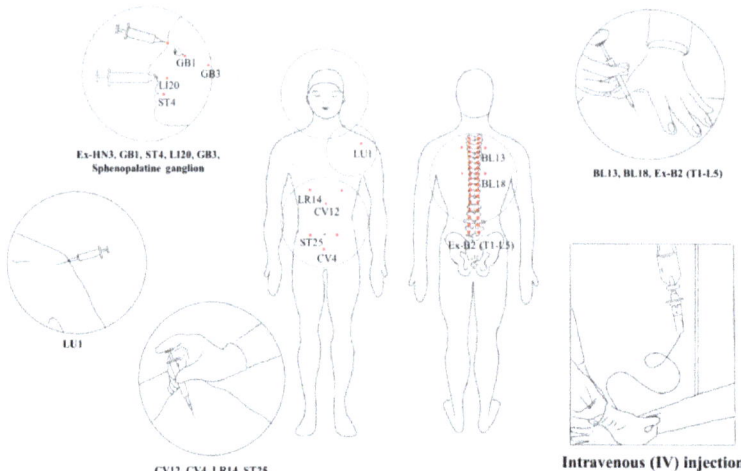

Figure 3. Intravenous and acupoint injections of pharmacopuncture. The area inside the circle means the acupoint injection site or each acupuncture point.

3.4.4. Outcome Measures

Clinical outcomes were classified into three categories as follows: objective measurement (e.g., tumor size in patients with cancer measured using computed tomography, blood test results, and intake of analgesics), subjective reporting of symptom changes, and reports of side effects or death. Ginseng pharmacopuncture improved the objective clinical outcomes in patients with skin wrinkles (width and depth), cervical dysplasia, cancer (in 13 of 18 studies), and amyotrophic lateral sclerosis. The stabilized tumor size in the patients with cancer was reported in two studies. Subjective improvements of symptoms were reported in patients with allergic rhinitis, Behçet's disease, drug-induced hepatitis, acute demyelinating encephalomyelitis, depression (one RCT), and cancer (11 of 18 studies). Four studies reported the aggravation of diseases such as increase in tumor mass size, metastasis to other organs, and death (one patient) after the treatment session.

3.4.5. Changes in Clinical Outcomes: Examples from Case Reports

To investigate changes in clinical outcomes by treatment session, we summarized two case reports that reported symptoms and clinical indexes over time. Ryu et al. [53] reported three clinical cases of ALS (Figure 4A). In Case 1, combined therapy of three different pharmacopunctures showed the improved general condition after 2–3 months of treatment; however, symptoms and muscular activity were aggravated after 6–7 months of treatment. In Case 2, muscular strength increased after 6–9 weeks of treatment, although the circumference of the limbs decreased. The subject also reported subjective improvement of general condition. In Case 3, pain fluctuated over time, and some symptoms were relieved such as low back pain and discomfort, while muscular strength was decreased. Kim et al. [50] reported a single case of hepatocellular carcinoma, and subjective symptoms (abdominal pain, sleep disorder, and loss of appetite) and ascites were reduced by the combined therapy of wild ginseng pharmacopuncture, acupuncture, and herbal medicine. The alkaline phosphatase (ALP) level returned to normal, and the subject stopped receiving other treatments except medications for hepatitis B (Figure 4B) [50]. In summary, ginseng pharmacopuncture induced improvement of symptoms might vary in each individual and also change over time.

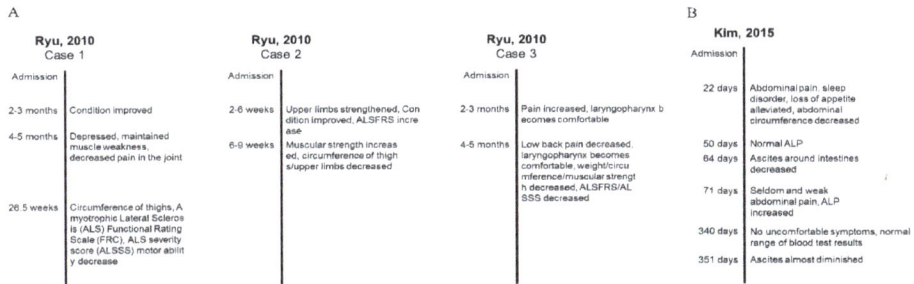

Figure 4. Examples of changes of clinical outcomes induced by ginseng pharmacopuncture over time from two case reports. (A) Changes of symptoms of three amyotrophic lateral sclerosis patients after cultivated wild ginseng pharmacopuncture. (B) Change of symptoms of a patient with hepatocellular carcinoma after cultivated wild ginseng pharmacopuncture.

4. Discussion

This study provides an overview of the current knowledge of the clinical usage and safety of the use of ginseng pharmacopuncture in place of the traditional oral intake of ginseng. To the best of our knowledge, this is the first review article that covers the clinical usage of ginseng pharmacopuncture by summarizing results of previous clinical studies as well as the toxicity test results in animals and physiological responses in humans. Based on the safety test results in animals, physiological responses to ginseng pharmacopuncture have been conducted, and ginseng pharmacopuncture has been demonstrated to significantly increase the sympathetic nervous system activities and influence protein synthesis in humans. According to the 26 clinical studies, ginseng pharmacopuncture is widely used in clinics, primarily in patients with cancer (lung cancer, hepatocellular carcinoma, prostate cancer, colorectal cancer, pancreatic cancer, cervical cancer, thymus cancer, breast cancer, etc.). In addition to cancer, ginseng pharmacopuncture has been used for the treatment of rhinitis, skin wrinkles, ALS, hepatitis, hepatocirrhosis, and depression, and it has shown significant clinical improvements in patients. Almost all studies applied ginseng pharmacopuncture intravenously, and only a few studies injected it at acupoints.

Previous studies showed the inhibitory effect of ginseng pharmacopuncture on the growth of human non-small cell lung cancer cells (NCI-H460)-induced solid tumor [57] and on the inflammation-related cytokine levels in hepatic metastatic mice model using colon carcinoma cells [58]. The results suggest that ginseng pharmacopuncture could be used in patients with cancer in combination with conventional therapies for cancer (e.g., chemotherapy) by improving the quality of life and general conditions and reducing the AEs of conventional therapies. However, the underlying mechanisms, safety, and clinical efficacy of ginseng pharmacopuncture remain controversial, which necessitates obtaining empirical data from large-scale and well-designed clinical studies.

Although the present review showed that clinical and basic research on ginseng pharmacopuncture has been carried out on many diseases, but it is still far from sufficient. As with other therapies, ginseng pharmacopuncture needs more evidence of its underlying mechanisms and safety at a fundamental level, and requires better evidence of its clinical efficacy and effectiveness from large-scale clinical studies. For example, whether the marker substances, ginsenosides (saponins), of ginseng pharmacopuncture depend on the manufacturing process is controversial. A standard method for extracting the active ingredients of ginseng for pharmacopuncture solution has not been developed, and the extracted substances vary depending on the extraction process (e.g., no index compounds were extracted in the distilled extract of ginseng while ethanol extraction successfully extracted the ginsenosides Rg1 and Rb1 [12]). Baek et al. [59] tested the marker substances of a combined ginseng pharmacopuncture solution comprising distilled extract and alcohol-extracted liquid using high-performance liquid chromatography. The combination method extracted all marker substances (ginsenosides Rg1, Rb1, and Rg3) and did not show significant toxicological changes in rats [59]. However, the clinical effects of ginseng pharmacopuncture manufactured using the combined extraction method (mixture of water-distilled solution and alcohol-extracted compound) have not been studied, while the water-distilled extracts have been mainly tested in our included clinical trials.

As only one RCT using ginseng polysaccharide extract as a pharmacopuncture solution has been reported [16], the clinical effect and safety of ginseng pharmacopuncture described in this review can be interpreted as the complex effects of multiple components in the whole-plant extracts, instead of a single compound. Studies on the pharmacokinetics of active components such as ginsenosides, polysaccharides, fatty acids, essential oils, and phenolic compounds and interactions between multiple components (e.g., a synergistic or antagonistic effect) of ginseng solutions for pharmacopuncture are necessary to demonstrate the pharmacological mechanisms of ginseng pharmacopuncture and develop the most effective solution in the future.

Moreover, among the 26 clinical trials, 15 used intravenous injections and 10 used the acupoint injection method. However, the pharmacokinetics of ginseng pharmacopuncture injected at different injection sites remain unclear. Future studies on various extraction and injection methods in terms of safety, mechanisms, and clinical effects will allow us to improve the efficacy and safety of ginseng pharmacopuncture therapy.

Although not included in this review, the ginseng-related pharmacopuncture research conducted in China often used ginseng extract in combination with various herbs. However, the different types of ginseng pharmacopuncture solution have never been compared to their clinical efficacy and safety. Therefore, clinical studies are necessary to test the effects and toxicity of the many different ginseng extraction methods and injection procedures (intravenous, intramuscular, and acupoints injection), combination of extracts from various herbs as compared with single ginseng extraction, and substance extracted solution as compared with whole plant extracted solution. Future studies should begin with testing the pharmacokinetics and pharmacological interactions of each substance in the ginseng pharmacopuncture solution and compare the substances and effects of ginseng solutions made by various extraction processes. In addition, various toxicity tests in animals and humans should be conducted. These approaches will allow us to find the best manufacturing method to produce the safest and most effective ginseng pharmacopuncture solution. The final and key challenges in the future application of the ginseng pharmacopuncture technique are proving its safety by various toxicity tests such as gene toxicity, carcinogenicity, developmental toxicity, toxicity of single or repeated administration of various doses, and efficacy in patients through a large-scale RCT with an appropriate placebo control. Although ginseng pharmacopuncture has been widely used in TKM clinics, we strongly argue that more concrete evidence is necessary for a safer and more prevalent use of the therapeutic modality in the future. Moreover, quality checks, management of the manufacturing facility, and relevant regulations are required, as pharmacopuncture techniques basically use direct intravenous or intramuscular injection of solutions in the human body.

5. Conclusions

In conclusion, although clinical trials and animal experiments showed that ginseng pharmacopuncture treatment is safe and effective for various diseases such as cancer, a higher level of evidence is still needed to confirm its safety and effects before using it widely in the clinical setting. Considering that injection of pharmacopuncture solution could be an alternative to the oral intake of herbal decoction in patients in a coma state or patients with liver damage, we believe that further studies on ginseng pharmacopuncture will bring benefits.

Author Contributions: Conceptualization, K.S.K. and S.-Y.K.; Data curation, I.-S.L. and S.-Y.K.; Methodology, S.-Y.K.; Resources, S.-Y.K.; Formal analysis, I.-S.L. and S.-Y.K.; Writing—original draft, I.-S.L.; Writing—review and editing, I.-S.L., K.S.K. and S.-Y.K. All authors have read and agreed to the published version of the manuscript.

Funding: This work was supported by the National Research Foundation of Korea (NRF) grant funded by the Korea government (MSIP; Ministry of Science, ICT & Future Planning) (No. 2017R1C1B5018164).

Acknowledgments: We thank Eunji Choi and Beop-Gyu Kim (Gachon University) for preparing the figures and paper screening assistance in this work.

Conflicts of Interest: The authors declare no conflict of interest.

References

1. Park, S.Y.; Park, J.H.; Kim, H.S.; Lee, C.Y.; Lee, H.J.; Kang, K.S.; Kim, C.E. Systems-level mechanisms of action of Panax ginseng: A network pharmacological approach. *J. Ginseng Res.* **2018**, *42*, 98–106. [CrossRef] [PubMed]
2. Nam, S.C. *Immune Pharmacopuncturology*; Meridian Medicine Publishing Company: Daejeon, Korea, 2009; pp. 1–475.
3. Jeong, H.S.; Lim, C.S.; Cha, B.C.; Choi, S.H.; Kwon, K.R. Component analysis of cultivated ginseng, cultivated wild ginseng, and wild ginseng and the change of ginsenoside components in the process of red ginseng. *J. Pharmacopunct.* **2010**, *13*, 63–77. [CrossRef]
4. Sun, H.; Liu, F.; Sun, L.; Liu, J.; Wang, M.; Chen, X.; Xu, X.; Ma, R.; Feng, K.; Jiang, R. Proteomic analysis of amino acid metabolism differences between wild and cultivated Panax ginseng. *J. Ginseng Res.* **2016**, *40*, 113–120. [CrossRef]
5. Sung, I.J.; Ghimeray, A.K.; Chang, K.J.; Park, C.H. Changes in Contents of Ginsenoside Due to Boiling Process of Panax ginseng C.A. Mayer. *Korea J. Plant Res.* **2013**, *26*, 726–730. [CrossRef]
6. Lee, S.M.; Bae, B.S.; Park, H.W.; Ahn, N.G.; Cho, B.G.; Cho, Y.L.; Kwak, Y.S. Characterization of Korean Red Ginseng (Panax ginseng Meyer): History, preparation method, and chemical composition. *J. Ginseng Res.* **2015**, *39*, 384–391. [CrossRef]
7. Park, J.Y.; Lee, D.S.; Kim, C.E.; Shin, M.S.; Seo, C.S.; Shin, H.K.; Hwang, G.S.; An, J.M.; Kim, S.N.; Kang, K.S. Effects of fermented black ginseng on wound healing mediated by angiogenesis through the mitogen-activated protein kinase pathway in human umbilical vein endothelial cells. *J. Ginseng Res.* **2018**, *42*, 524–531. [CrossRef]
8. Jin, X.; Che, D.B.; Zhang, Z.H.; Yan, H.M.; Jia, Z.Y.; Jia, X.B. Ginseng consumption and risk of cancer: A meta-analysis. *J. Ginseng Res.* **2016**, *40*, 269–277. [CrossRef]

9. Hernandez-Garcia, D.; Granado-Serrano, A.B.; Martin-Gari, M.; Naudi, A.; Serrano, J.C. Efficacy of Panax ginseng supplementation on blood lipid profile. A meta-analysis and systematic review of clinical randomized trials. *J. Ethnopharmacol.* **2019**, *243*, 112090. [CrossRef]
10. Lee, K.H.; Cho, Y.Y.; Kim, S.; Sun, S.H. History of research on pharmacopuncture in Korea. *J. Pharmacopunct.* **2016**, *19*, 101.
11. Korean Pharmacopuncture Institute. *Pharmacopuncturology-Principles and Clinical Applications*; Elsevier Korea: Seoul, Korea, 2011; pp. 76–89.
12. Lee, D.Y.; Choi, B.S.; Lee, I.H.; Kim, J.H.; Gwon, P.S. Comparison of index compounds content and antioxidative activity of Wild Ginseng Pharmacopuncture by extraction method. *Korean J. Intern. Med.* **2018**, *39*, 313–322. [CrossRef]
13. Kang, S.K.; Lee, H.J.; Park, Y.B. Experimental studies on the effect of ginseng radix aqua-acupuncture. *Int. Symp. East-West Med.* **1989**, *1989*, 61–83.
14. Lim, C.; Kwon, K.; Lee, K. Plexiform neurofibroma treated with pharmacopuncture. *J. Pharmacopunct.* **2014**, *17*, 74. [CrossRef]
15. Lee, K.; Yu, J.; Sun, S.; Kwon, K.; Lim, C. A 4-week, repeated, intravenous dose, toxicity test of mountain ginseng pharmacopuncture in sprague-dawley rats. *J. Pharmacopunct.* **2014**, *17*, 27–35. [CrossRef]
16. Liu, P. A clinical controlled trial of ginseng polysaccharide pharmacopuncture in the treatment of depressive disorder. *Neimong J. Tradit. Chin. Med.* **2017**, *36*, 103.
17. Sung, S.H.; Shin, B.C.; Park, M.J.; Kim, K.H.; Kim, J.W.; Ryu, J.Y.; Park, J.K. Current Status of Management on Pharmacopuncture in Korea through Introduction of an Accreditation System. *J. Pharmacopunct.* **2019**, *22*, 75–82.
18. Kwon, K.A. Clinical Study on the Effects of Intravenous Wild Ginseng Herbal Acupuncture on the Human Body. *J. Pharmacopunct.* **2004**, *7*, 15–26.
19. Lee, H.Y.; You, J.S.; Yook, T.H.; Hong, K.E. The Effects of Distilled Astragali Radix Herbal Acupuncture, Wild Ginseng Herbal Acupuncture and Rehmannia Glutinosa Herbal Acupuncture on Vital Sign—A Randomized, Placebo-controlled, Double-blind Clinical Trial. *J. Acupunct. Res.* **2007**, *24*, 207–217.
20. Lee, E.S.; Oh, J.Y.; Kim, Y.J.; Yu, A.M.; Jang, S.H.; Cho, H.S.; Kim, K.H.; Lee, S.D.; Kim, K.S.; Kim, E.J. The Clinical Study about Qualitative and Quantitative Characteristics of Acupuncture Sensation According to the Type of Pharmacopuncture: Study about BUM Pharmacopuncture, Mountain Ginseng Pharmacopuncture and Sciatica No. 5 Pharmacopuncture. *J. Korean Acupunct. Moxib. Soc.* **2013**, *30*, 25–39. [CrossRef]
21. Choi, Y.N.; Oh, J.Y.; Cho, H.S.; Kim, K.H.; Kim, K.S.; Lee, S.D.; Kim, E.J. Research on the Amount of Stimulus Differences According to Pharmacopuncture Injected dose and Characters Method. *Acupuncture* **2015**, *32*, 89–95. [CrossRef]
22. Roh, J.D.; Kim, L.H.; Song, B.Y.; Yook, T.H. The Effects of distilled Wild Ginseng Herbal Acupuncture on the Heart Rate Variability(HRV). *J. Pharmacopunct.* **2008**, *11*, 55–69. [CrossRef]
23. Yook, T.; Yu, J.; Lee, H.; Song, B.; Kim, L.; Roh, J.; Shin, J.; Lim, S. Comparing the effects of distilled Rehmannia glutinosa, Wild Ginseng and Astragali Radix pharmacopuncture with heart rate variability (HRV): A randomized, sham-controlled and double-blind clinical trial. *J. Acupunct. Meridian Stud.* **2009**, *2*, 239–247. [PubMed]
24. Lee, J.B. The Effects of Distilled Rehmannia Glutinosa and Wild Ginseng Pharmacopuncture CV17, CV4 on Heart Rate Variability—A Randomized and Double-Blind Clinical Trial. Ph.D. Thesis, Department of Korean Medicine Graduate School of Woosuk University, Wanju, Korea, 2012.
25. Seol, H.; Song, B.Y.; Yook, T.H. The Effects of Panax Ginseng Radix Pharmacopuncture and Zizyphi Spinosi Semen Pharmacopuncture on the Heart Rate Variability. *J. Acupunct. Res.* **2009**, *26*, 19–28.
26. Kim, G.C.; Park, S.W.; Kim, Y.S. Effect of heart rate variability, pulse wave velocity in women of breast cancer patients care by mountain cultivated ginseng pharmacopuncture. *J. Korea Inst. Orient. Med. Diagn.* **2011**, *15*, 245–260.
27. Park, S.W.; Kim, Y.S.; Hwang, W.D.; Kim, G.C. Effect of mountain cultivated ginseng pharmacopuncture on Heart Rate Variability (HRV), Pulse Wave Velocity (PWV) in middle aged women. *J. Acupunct. Res.* **2011**, *28*, 97–105.
28. Park, S.W.; Kim, Y.S.; Hwang, W.D.; Kim, G.C. Effect of pulse-wave factors in middle aged women by mountain cultivated ginseng pharmacopuncture original articles. *J. Pharmacopunct.* **2011**, *14*, 35–49. [CrossRef]

29. Lee, D.H.; Kwon, K.R. Analysis of Serum Proteom after Intravenous Injection of cultivated wild ginseng pharmacopuncture. *J. Pharmacopunct.* **2006**, *9*, 17–37.
30. Kang, T.S.; Lee, S.G.; Kwon, K.R. Analysis of Serum proteom before and after Intravenous Injection of wild ginseng herbal acupuncture. *J. Pharmacopunct.* **2004**, *7*, 5–25.
31. Yu, J.; Sun, S.; Lee, K.; Kwon, K. Single-dose Toxicity of Water-soluble Ginseng Pharmacopuncture Injected Intramuscularly in Rats. *J. Pharmacopunct.* **2015**, *18*, 76–85.
32. Yu, J.S.; Sun, S.H.; Lee, K.H.; Kwon, K.R. Intravenous Toxicity Study of Water-soluble Ginseng Pharmacopuncture in SD Rats. *J. Pharmacopunct.* **2015**, *18*, 38–44.
33. Jo, H.G.; Jung, P.S.; Kim, H.Y.; Bae, S.Y.; Jo, M.J.; Shin, J.H.; Han, S.H.; Na, J.I.; Sul, J.U.; Lee, S.Y. Case of Suspected Drug-Induced Liver Injury after Intravenous Wild Ginseng Pharmacopuncture. *J. Physiol. Pathol. Korean Med.* **2014**, *28*, 102–106. [CrossRef]
34. Kwon, K.R.; Park, C.W.; Ra, M.S.; Cho, C.K. Clinical observation of multiple metastatic cancer patient with hepatocellular carcinoma treated with cultivated wild ginseng herbal acupuncture therapy. *J. Korean Acupunct. Moxib. Soc.* **2005**, *22*, 211–217.
35. Lee, D.H.; Kim, S.S.; Seong, S.; Kim, N.; Han, J.B. Korean medicine therapy as a substitute for chemotherapy for metastatic breast cancer: A case report. *Case Rep. Oncol.* **2015**, *8*, 64–71. [CrossRef] [PubMed]
36. Lee, Y.H.; Kim, C.W.; Lee, K.H. A case report of monitoring PSA level changes in two prostate cancer patients treated with mountain ginseng pharmacopuncture and sweet bee venom along with western anticancer therapy. *J. Pharmacopunct.* **2011**, *14*, 81–88. [CrossRef]
37. Park, B.K.; Cho, C.K.; Kwon, K.R.; Yoo, H.S. A Case Report for Stage IIIB Squamous Cell Lung Carcinoma Patient Treated with Cultured Wild Ginseng Pharmacopuncture Therapy. *J. Pharmacopunct.* **2007**, *10*, 143–147. [CrossRef]
38. Bang, S.H.; Kwon, K.R.; Yoo, H.S. Two Cases of Non-Small Cell Lung Cancer Treated with Intravenous Cultivated Wild Ginseng Pharmacopuncture. *J. Pharmacopunct.* **2008**, *11*, 13–19. [CrossRef]
39. Lee, J.H.; Kwon, K.R.; Cho, C.K.; Han, S.S.R.; Yoo, H.S. Advanced cancer cases treated with cultivated wild ginseng phamacopuncture. *J. Acupunct. Meridian Stud.* **2010**, *3*, 119–124. [CrossRef]
40. Kwon, K.R.; Kim, H.; Kim, J.S.; Yoo, H.S.; Cho, C.K. Case series of non-small cell lung cancer treated with mountain Ginseng pharmacopuncture. *J. Acupunct. Meridian Stud.* **2011**, *4*, 61–68. [CrossRef]
41. Kim, K.; Choi, Y.S.; Joo, J.C.; Moon, G. A case report for lung cancer patient showing remission treated with cultivated Wild Ginseng pharmacopuncture. *J. Pharmacopunct.* **2011**, *14*, 33–37. [CrossRef]
42. Im, C.R.; Kwon, K.; Sur, Y.C.; Bang, S.H.; Kim, S.S.; Seong, S. A case of hepatic and pulmonary metastatic colorectal cancer patient treated by traditional korean therapy and XELOX chemotherapy. *J. Korean Tradit. Oncol.* **2012**, *17*, 17–25.
43. Ha, T.H.; Seong, S.; Lee, D.H.; Kim, S.S. Improved case of recurred and metastatic ascending colon cancer by combination of Oriental medical therapy and FOLFIRI chemotherapy. *J. Physiol. Pathol. Korean Med.* **2013**, *27*, 148–151.
44. Han, J.B.; Ha, T.H.; Kim, S.S.; Seong, S. Case of complete remission of breast cancer metastasized to lung treated by traditional Korean therapy. *J. Physiol. Pathol. Korean Med.* **2013**, *27*, 818–822.
45. Kang, H.J.; Yoon, J.W.; Park, J.H.; Cho, C.K.; Yoo, H.S. Cancer pain control for advanced cancer patients by using autonomic nerve pharmacopuncture. *J. Pharmacopunct.* **2014**, *17*, 62. [CrossRef] [PubMed]
46. Yun, H.; Cho, C.; Yoo, H.; Bang, S. A Case Report of Unresectable Pancreatic Carcinoma Patient for Relieving Cancer Related Pain and Improving Quality of Life by Korean Medical Treatment. *J. Korean Tradit. Oncol.* **2013**, *18*, 9–15.
47. Lee, D.H.; Seong, S.; Kim, S.S.; Han, J.B. A case of stage IV non-small cell lung cancer treated with Korean medicine therapy alone. *Case Rep. Oncol.* **2013**, *6*, 574–578. [CrossRef]
48. Park, J.H.; Jeon, H.J.; Kang, H.J.; Jeong, I.S.; Cho, C.K.; Yoo, H.S. Cancer-related fatigue in patients with advanced cancer treated with autonomic nerve pharmacopuncture. *J. Acupunct. Meridian Stud.* **2015**, *8*, 142–146. [CrossRef]
49. Kim, J.S.; Lee, H.J.; Lee, S.H.; Lee, B.H. Recurrent Oligodendroglioma Treated with Acupuncture and Pharmacopuncture. *J. Acupunct. Meridian Stud.* **2015**, *8*, 147–151. [CrossRef]
50. Kim, H.R.; Jeong, H.R.; Jang, C.Y.; Woo, C.; Ha, Y.J.; Moon, G.; Baek, D.G. Cirrhosis after liver lobectomy managed with traditional Korean medical treatment: A case report. *J. Int. Korean Med.* **2015**, *36*, 410–418.

51. Lee, D.H.; Kim, S.S.; Seong, S. A Case Report of Metastatic Breast Cancer Treated with Korean Medicine Therapy as a Substitute for Chemotherapy. *Case Rep. Oncol.* **2017**, *10*, 27–36. [CrossRef]
52. Kim, Y.J.; Park, D.I.; Kwon, K.R. Case report on the improvement of liver functions by mountain cultivated wild ginseng pharmacopuncture. *J. Pharmacopunct.* **2009**, *12*, 107–112. [CrossRef]
53. Ryu, Y.J.; Lee, K.H.; Kwon, K.R.; Lee, Y.H.; An, J.C.; Sun, S.H.; Lee, S.J. Mountain ginseng pharmacopuncture treatment on three amyotrophic lateral sclerosis patients. *J. Pharmacopunct.* **2010**, *13*, 119–128. [CrossRef]
54. Han, J.H.; Kim, S.S.; Seong, S.; Bang, S.H. A Case of Intractable Cervical Dysplasia Patient Treated with Korean Medicine for Three Months. *Korean J. Obstet. Gynecol.* **2012**, *25*, 154–160.
55. Park, J.H.; Oh, D.J.; Jang, S.H.; Hur, H.S. A Clinical Case Report on a Patient of Acute Disseminated Encephalomyelitis Using Korean Medicine. *J. Korean Med. Rehabil.* **2014**, *24*, 141–153.
56. Li, Y. Preliminary study on 100 cases of allergic rhinitis treated by ginseng pharmacopuncture on sphenopalatine ganglion. *Xinjiang Tradit. Chin. Med.* **1994**, *2*, 25–26.
57. Kwon, K.R. Anticancer effect of mountain ginseng Pharmacopuncture to the nude mouse oflung carcinoma induced by NCI-H460 human non-small cell lung cancer cells. *J. Pharmacopunct.* **2010**, *13*, 5–14. [CrossRef]
58. Cho, B.J.; Kwon, K.R. Effects of Cultivated Wild Ginseng Herbal Acupuncture to the serum cytokine on Hepatic Metastatic Model using Colon26-L5 Carcinoma Cells. *J. Pharmacopunct.* **2006**, *9*, 127–137.
59. Baek, S.H.; Lee, I.H.; Kim, M.J.; Kim, E.J.; Ha, I.H.; Lee, J.H.; Lee, J.W. Component analysis and toxicity study of combined cultivated wild ginseng pharmacopuncture. *J. Int. Korean Med.* **2015**, *36*, 189–199.

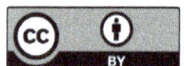

© 2019 by the authors. Licensee MDPI, Basel, Switzerland. This article is an open access article distributed under the terms and conditions of the Creative Commons Attribution (CC BY) license (http://creativecommons.org/licenses/by/4.0/).

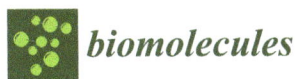

Article

HMGB1-triggered inflammation inhibition of notoginseng leaf triterpenes against cerebral ischemia and reperfusion injury via MAPK and NF-κB signaling pathways

Weijie Xie [1,2,3,4,5], Ting Zhu [1,2,3,4,5], Xi Dong [1,2,3,4,5], Fengwei Nan [1,2,3,4,5], Xiangbao Meng [1,2,3,4,5], Ping Zhou [1,2,3,4,5], Guibo Sun [1,2,3,4,5],* and Xiaobo Sun [1,2,3,4,5],*

1. Beijing Key Laboratory of Innovative Drug Discovery of Traditional Chinese Medicine (Natural Medicine) and Translational Medicine, Institute of Medicinal Plant Development, Peking Union Medical College and Chinese Academy of Medical Sciences, Beijing 100193, China; xwjginseng@126.com (W.X.); ginseng123@163.com (T.Z.); dx5212004@126.com (X.D.); pumchNFW@163.com (F.N.); xbmeng@implad.ac.cn (X.M.); zhoup0520@163.com (P.Z.)
2. Key Laboratory of Bioactive Substances and Resources Utilization of Chinese Herbal Medicine, Ministry of Education, Institute of Medicinal Plant Development, Chinese Academy of Medical Sciences & Peking Union Medical College, Beijing 100193, China
3. Key Laboratory of Efficacy Evaluation of Chinese Medicine against Glycolipid Metabolic Disorders, State Administration of Traditional Chinese Medicine, Institute of Medicinal Plant Development, Peking Union Medical College and Chinese Academy of Medical Sciences, Beijing 100193, China
4. Zhongguancun Open Laboratory of the Research and Development of Natural Medicine and Health Products, Institute of Medicinal Plant Development, Chinese Academy of Medical Sciences & Peking Union Medical College, Beijing 100193, China
5. Key Laboratory of new drug discovery based on Classic Chinese medicine prescription, Chinese Academy of Medical Sciences, Beijing 100193, China
* Correspondence: Correspondence: sunguibo@126.com (G.S.); sun_xiaobo163@163.com (X.S.); Tel.: +86-10-5783-3220 (G.S.); +86-10-5783-3013 (X.S.)

Received: 2 September 2019; Accepted: 18 September 2019; Published: 20 September 2019

Abstract: Ischemic stroke is a clinically common cerebrovascular disease whose main risks include necrosis, apoptosis and cerebral infarction, all caused by cerebral ischemia and reperfusion (I/R) injury. This process has particular significance for the treatment of stroke patients. Notoginseng leaf triterpenes (PNGL), as a valuable medicine, have been discovered to have neuroprotective effects. However, it was not confirmed that whether PNGL may possess neuroprotective effects against cerebral I/R injury. To explore the neuroprotective effects of PNGL and their underlying mechanisms, a middle cerebral artery occlusion/reperfusion (MCAO/R) model was established. In vivo results suggested that in MCAO/R model rats, PNGL pretreatment (73.0, 146, 292 mg/kg) remarkably decreased infarct volume, reduced brain water content, and improved neurological functions; moreover, PNGL (73.0, 146, 292 mg/kg) significantly alleviated blood-brain barrier (BBB) disruption and inhibited neuronal apoptosis and neuronal loss caused by cerebral I/R injury, while PNGL with a different concertation (146, 292 mg/kg) significantly reduced the concentrations of IL-6, TNF-α, IL-1 β, and HMGB1 in serums in a dose-dependent way, which indicated that inflammation inhibition could be involved in the neuroprotective effects of PNGL. The immunofluorescence and western blot analysis showed PNGL decreased HMGB1 expression, suppressed the HMGB1-triggered inflammation, and inhibited microglia activation (IBA1) in hippocampus and cortex, thus dose-dependently downregulating inflammatory cytokines including VCAM-1, MMP-9, MMP-2, and ICAM-1 concentrations in ischemic brains. Interestingly, PNGL administration (146 mg/kg) significantly downregulated the levels of p-P44/42, p-JNK1/2 and p-P38 MAPK, and also inhibited expressions of the total NF-κB and phosphorylated NF-κB in ischemic brains, which was the downstream pathway triggered by HMGB1. All of these results indicated that the protective effects of PNGL against cerebral I/R injury could be associated with inhibiting HMGB1-triggered inflammation, suppressing the activation of MAPKs and NF-κB, and thus improved cerebral I/R-induced neuropathological changes. This study may offer insight into discovering new active compounds for the treatment of ischemic stroke.

Keywords: notoginseng leaf triterpenes; HMGB1; cerebral ischemia and reperfusion injury; inflammation; MAPK; NF-κB

1. Introduction

Ischemic stroke, also known as cerebral infarction, is one of the leading causes of death with substantial morbidity and mortality worldwide. Nearly 6.2 million people die from stroke each year, and it is estimated that the lifetime risk for stroke is 8% to 10%. Ischemic stroke accounts for 85% of all strokes [1]. Ischemia causes brain infarction, however. Moreover, the subsequent reperfusion phase results in brain injury, including BBB disruption, hemorrhagic transformation, and massive brain edema, which is involved in a wide range of neuropathic alteration and processes including oxidative stress, inflammatory stress [2] and cytokine damage glutamate toxicity, Ca^{2+} overload, excessive nitric oxide synthesis, and apoptosis [1,3,4]. Although the mechanisms of cerebral ischemia and reperfusion I/R injury are complex and involve the interaction of numerous pathophysiological processes, there are accumulating evidences that inflammation and apoptosis are involved [5–8].

The high mobility group box-1 protein (HMGB1), as a nuclear DNA-binding protein and an important damage associated molecular pattern (DAMP), is released from necrotic and dying neural cells in the ischemic brain, leading to the activation of microglia and the expression of inflammatory factors in ischemic brain, and it may activate TLR 2/4 and RAGEs signaling following rapid translocation to the cytoplasm or release from dying cells after cerebral ischemia [9,10], which can promote the activation of inflammatory responses. Sequentially, the signalosome comprising inflammatory response, triggered by HMGB-1/TLR4, can stimulate nuclear factor kappa B (NF-κB) translocation. Moreover, the TRAF6–IRAK1–TAK1 complex triggers mitogen-activated protein kinase (MAPK) phosphorylation including p38, JNK, and ERK, which play key roles in inflammation [11–15]. The activated MAPKs mainly function as mediators of cellular stress by phosphorylating intracellular enzymes, transcription factors, and cytosolic proteins involved in cell survival, inflammatory mediators production, and apoptosis [16]. Accordingly, the therapeutic strategy associated with HMGB-1/TLR4 signaling might represent a promising approach to the restriction of neuro-inflammatory processes and the amelioration of cerebral stroke damage [10,17–19]. Development of an effective anti-inflammatory drug may be an efficient approach for the treatment of ischemic stroke-induced brain injury [10,16,20]. However, most of these treatments have disappointingly been found to be ineffective during the acute phase of stroke [21]. Furthermore, many anti-neuro-inflammatory drugs show poor outcomes for the treatment of ischemic stroke in clinical trials. Hence, development of new and effective neuroprotective agents for ischemic stroke is clinically significant and urgently needed.

Traditional Chinese medicines, used in China for thousands of years with high efficiency and low toxicity, have attracted great interest in recent years [22–25]. *Panax notoginseng (Burk) F. H. Chen* is a commonly used Chinese medicinal herb and plant, the roots and stems of which have been used for the treatment of cardiovascular disease in many Asian countries [22]. Current experimental evidences indicate that *panax notoginseng*, and their extracts, panax notoginseng saponins (PNS) possess many beneficial effects, such as neuroprotective, antiinflammatory, antiapoptotic [26], and anticonvulsant effects in various models [3,24,27–29]. Additionally, recent studies have demonstrated that PNS exerts protective effects against cerebral I/R injuries, which are involved in the aspects: anti-oxidant and associated apoptotic effects; anti-inflammatory or immunostimulatory-related effects on apoptosis or necrosis; neurological cell cycle, proliferation, differentiation, and regeneration; and energy metabolism and regulation of cellular ATP levels, BBB permeability, excitatory amino acids, and other processes, including the activation of nerve growth factor, excitotoxicity, and excessive Ca^{2+} influx into neurons [3,24,27–31].

It was known that PNS were mainly obtained and purified from the roots of *panax notoginseng (Burk) F. H. Chen*. However, the *panax notoginseng (Burk) F. H. Chen* stems and leaves were often ignored. Annual production of Panax notoginseng stems and leaves is over 25 million kilograms in China, but its effective utilizing rate is under 5%, so many panax notoginseng resources are wasted. In contrast, panax notoginseng stems and leaves contain high protein, crude fiber, vitamin C and carotenoids, low fat and rich mineral element, among which contents of zinc, iron and manganese are remarkably high. The contents of protein, carotenoids and vitamin C are higher than those of ordinary vegetables, thus, *panax notoginseng* stems and leaves have a higher nutritional value. Its major active ingredients in panax notoginseng stems and leaves are saponins, the chemical structure is mainly protopanaxadiol type that has functions of sedative-hypnotic action, analgesia, blood lipid regulating, anti-inflammatory/retarding the aging process. And panax notoginseng stems and leaves has been confirmed as the raw materials of production of advanced cosmetics, functional foods and common foods [31–35], which deserves further research and development into new products. Currently, notoginseng leaf friterpenes (PNGL), as the total saponins of Panax notoginseng stem and leaf, have already been shown to exert potent neuroprotective and anti-apoptotic properties. However, the beneficial effects of PNGL were rarely detected in nervous diseases, and several reports have revealed its diverse pharmacological properties and raised some speculative proposals concerning its effect mechanisms [31–33]. At present, there was no clear evidence on whether PNGL has neuroprotective effects against cerebral I/R injury.

Base on the reported neuroprotective effects of PNS against cerebral I/R injuries, we hypothesized that PNGL may have neuroprotective effects of relieving cerebral I/R injury with inhibiting HMGB1-triggered inflammation and apoptosis by regulating the MAPK and NF-κB signaling pathways. Therefore, middle cerebral artery occlusion/reperfusion (MCAO/R)-operated rats were used to explore the effects of the PNGL against cerebral ischemia stroke. In additions, our chemical researchers have found that the content of total saponins of panax notoginseng stems and leaves is 4% to 6%. Among them, monomeric saponins contained are mainly 20(s)-protopanaxadiol saponins, and contains almost no ginseng triol saponins which is the biggest difference between PNS and PNGL. As shown in Figure 1, it mainly contains ginsenoside Rb1, ginsenoside Rb2, ginsenoside Rb3, and ginsenoside Rc. Additionally, eleven batches of PNGL samples were monitored by the chemical fingerprinting assay (Supplementary Material S1).

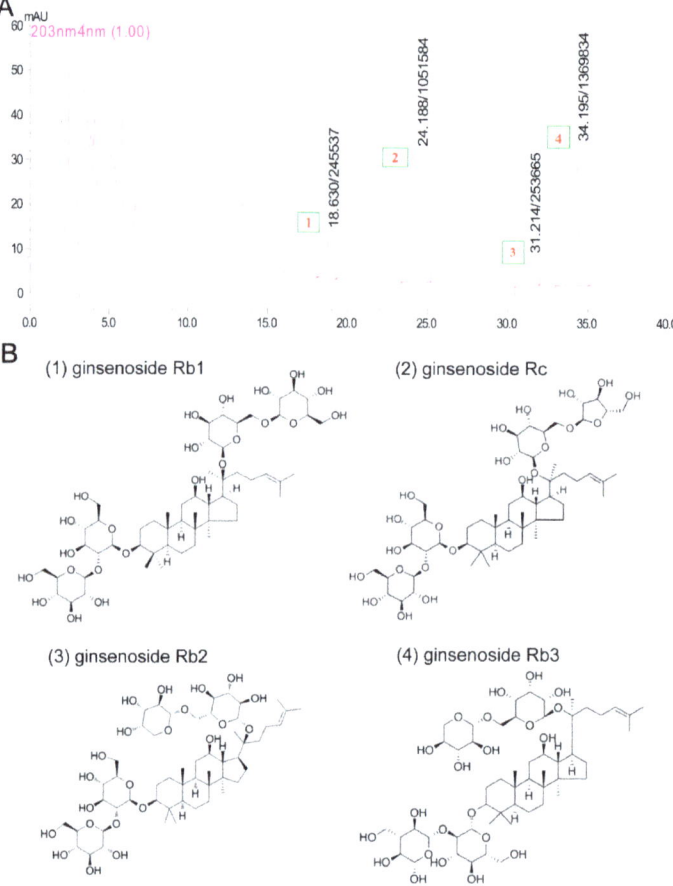

Figure 1. The chromatograms and chemical components of notoginseng leaf triterpenes (PNGL) used in experiments via the high performance liquid chromatography. (**A**) The chromatograms of PNGL samples. (**B**) Chemical component structures, mainly including ginsenoside Rb1 (No.1), ginsenoside Rb2 (No.3), ginsenoside Rb3 (No.4), and ginsenoside Rc (No.2).

2. Methods and Materials

2.1. Animals

Male Sprague Dawley (SD) rats (specific pathogen free, weighing 280–300 g) were used in this study, and they were purchased from Beijing Vital Lihua Experimental Animals Co., Ltd. Rats were housed at an ambient temperature of 20 ± 1 °C and a relative humidity of 55 ± 15% with artificial light for 12 h each day and free access to a standard laboratory chow diet and sterilized drinking water throughout the experiments. All efforts were made to minimize the number of animals used and their suffering. The study was conducted in accordance with the Declaration of Helsinki. The protocol was approved by the Laboratory Animal Ethics Committee of the Institute of Medicinal Plant Development, Peking Union Medical College, and conformed to the Guide for the Care and Use of Laboratory Animals (Permit Number: SYXK 2017-0020).

2.2. Experimental Groups and Drug Administration

Rats were divided into seven groups (10 for each group), namely, a sham-operated group, a MCAO/R model group, a 73 mg/kg dose of PNGL group, a 146 mg/kg dose of PNGL group, a 192 mg/kg dose of PNGL group, and a positive drug butylphthalide (NBP, 60 mg/kg) group and an aspirin group (ASP, 10 mg/kg), according to a random number table. The PNGL, NBP, and ASP samples were all dissolved in normal saline. Then, rats were intragastrically administered daily in a constant volume. Moreover the animals in the sham and MCAO/R groups were given an equal volume of saline water. Drug administration groups were exposed to continuous gastric administration (once per day) for 7 days before MCAO/R operations.

2.3. Transient Focal Brain Ischemia/Reperfusion Mode

As previously described [3,36], MCAO/R model was employed to induce transient focal brain ischemia/reperfusion. In brief, rats were anaesthetized with Zoletil 50 (Virbac S.A, Carros, France) via intraperitoneal injections. A silicone-coated 3/0 monofilament was introduced into the right internal carotid artery and advanced to occlude the middle cerebral artery for 2 h. Rats in sham-operated group underwent the same procedures except occluding the MCA. The temperature was maintained at 32 ± 0.1 °C until animals woke up completely.

As shown in Figure 2A, cerebral blood flow velocity of the right MCA territory (core cortex, 2 mm posterior and 6 mm lateral to the bregma) was assessed by the laser Doppler blood flow assessment (FLPI-2, Moor Instruments, Wilmington, DE). After 2 h, suture was removed to induce blood reperfusion whose flow velocity was monitored again (Figure 2B–E) at different time points (2,5,12,24 h), which contributed to improving the reliability and repeatability of the MCAO/R model.

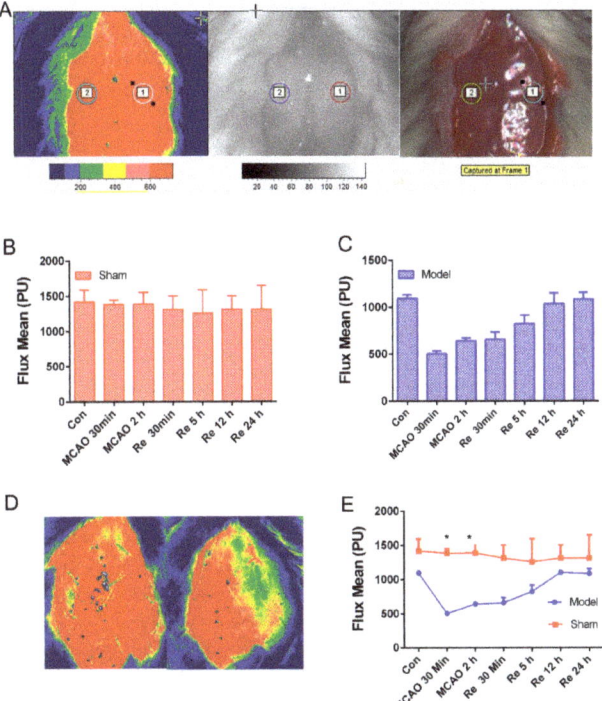

Figure 2. Cerebral blood flow assessed by the laser Doppler blood flow assessment in rats with a middle cerebral artery occlusion/reperfusion MCAO/R injury.

(**A**) The monitored place (core cortex, 2 mm posterior and 6 mm lateral to the bregma). (**B**,**C**) Flux mean value of cerebral blood flows in sham and MCAO/R group. (**D**) The images of cerebral blood flow in the sham group (left) and the model group (right). (**E**) Flux mean value at different time points. Mean values ± SEM; * $p < 0.05$, sham group versus MCAO/R group.

2.4. Measurement of Neurological Deficit

Rats were monitored by video camera after surgery, and the time of death was recorded. Neurological deficits at 22 h after MCAO were assessed using Zea Longa Scores [37–39]. Based on Longa Scores, neurological function was graded on a series of scales from 0 to 4 with higher scores indicating more severe neurologic deficits. Tests were independently performed by two investigators blinded to animal grouping.

2.5. TTC Staining

As previously described [9,10,36], 2,3,5-triphenyltetrazolium chloride (TTC, Sigma, St. Louis, MO, USA) staining was used to assess the ischemic infarction. After MCAO/R operation, rats were anaesthetized with Zoletil 50 (20 mg·kg^{-1}) via intramuscular injection (Virbac S.A, Carros, France). All brains were sliced into 2 mm sections, incubated for 20 min in a 2% solution of TTC (37 °C) temperature, and then fixed in 4% paraformaldehyde. The infarct areas on each slice were quantified by using the ImageJ 1.44p software (National Institutes of Health, Bethesda, MD, USA).

2.6. Detection of Brain Water Content

As previously described [9,10,36], a 3-mm section of the ischemic hemisphere brain was cut from the anterior pole to detect the water content in the brain tissue. The wet-dry method was applied to determine brain water content in another subgroup. An electronic scale was used to weigh the ischemic and non-ischemic hemispheres (wet weight). After the ischemic brain hemisphere was dried overnight at 105 °C in a desiccating oven, it was weighed again (dry weight), and the total brain water content was calculated according to previous reports [36].

2.7. Measurement of BBB Permeability

BBB integrity and permeability was quantitatively assessed by measuring the extravasation of Evans blue dye, which serves as a marker of albumin leakage. As previously described [36]. Evans blue (2% in saline, 4 mL/kg; Sigma-Aldrich) was administered 90 min before sacrifice followed by transcardially perfused with saline to remove the residual dye from the vessels. The hemispheres were weighed and incubated in dimethyl formamide (DMF, Sigma-Aldrich, Shanghai -Greater China Regional Headquarters, China) in 60 °C water bath overnight. After that, Evans blue content was determined in supernatants at 632 nm and expressed as microgram per gram brain. Gradient concentrations of Evans blue were used to build standard curve.

2.8. Detection of Inflammatory Cytokines in Serums and Brain Tissues from Rats

The blood samples from each groups were collected [36,40,41], and then centrifuged at 3000 rpm·min^{-1} for 20 min, the blood serums were obtained and stored at −80 °C for further measurement. Furthermore, the hippocampus and cortex tissues were rapidly removed and carefully dissected on an ice plate, frozen in liquid nitrogen and then stored at −80 °C until the assays were performed. Then, the hippocampus and cortex samples were partly weighed and homogenized by sonication in a specified amount of normal saline (100 microliters/ 10 milligrams). The homogenate was kept at 4 °C for 30 min and then centrifuged at 12,000 rpm for 3 min at 4 °C. The supernatant was collected, obtained and stored at −20 °C and then used to measure the inflammatory cytokines by using assay kits.

The protein concentration of the collected supernatants was determined via the BCA protein assay kit (CWBIO, Beijing, China). The inflammatory cytokines from the ischemic brains and the blood serums were analyzed using ELISA kits (Beijing HaiTai Tong, Da Sci Tech Ltd., Beijing, China). All experimental steps were performed according to the kit operation specifications. OD values were measured by a microplate reader.

2.9. Histopathological Examination

Giemsa staining was commonly used to revealed morphological features of injured neurons in the cerebral cortex. As previously described [9,10,36], the samples were embedded in paraffin and cut in 5-µm slices; 5-µm-thick serial coronal sections were generated and mounted on slides. The sections were stained according to the described standard protocol. Images of stained slides were acquired using a light microscope (Leica, Leica DM4000B, Wetzlar, Germany). After 24 h following MCAO/R operation, the brains were processed as above. Samples were embedded in paraffin and cut in 5-µm slices; 5-µm-thick serial coronal sections were generated and mounted on slides. After washed in cold water, the paraffin sections were stained with Giemsa staining for 20 min, rinsed with PBS, dehydrated with graded alcohol, made transparent with xylene, and fixed with neutral glue. An optical microscope was used to observe each section, and images were randomly selected for image analysis via ImageJ software (Media Cybernetics, USA).

2.10. TUNEL Staining Assay

To measure the extent of neuronal apoptosis in cerebral I/R injury, an in situ apoptosis detection kit (POD, Roche, and Mannheim, Germany) was employed to discover neuronal apoptosis caused by ischemia. A TUNEL analysis was carried out with minor modification according to the manufacturer's instructions. Firstly, the sections were installed on the slides and permeabilized by incubating them with 100 µL of 20 µg/mL proteinase K solution for 15 min. Next, the sections were incubated with 100 µL of 0.3% H_2O_2 for 5 min and incubated by equilibration buffer and terminal deoxynucleotidyl transferase to inactivate endogenous peroxidases. Then, anti-digoxigenin-peroxidase conjugates were employed to incubate the sections. Finally, the utilization of diaminobenzidine demonstrated peroxidase activity in all tissue sections, and the slices were counterstained with hematoxylin. TUNEL-positive cells were visualized by using a Leica microscope (Leica DM4000B, Germany), and images were randomly selected for image analysis via ImageJ software.

2.11. Immunofluorescence

To explore the effects of PNGL on HMGB expression and IBA1-marked microglia activation in CUMS-induced rats [42,43], immunofluorescence staining was performed as previously described [7,8,44,45]. Briefly, after the micro slides were deparaffinized, dewatered, and restored with a citrate-EDTA antigen retrieval solution (P0086, Beyotime, Shanghai, China) for 20 min at 95 °C, they were cooled down and washed with PBS three times (10 min per time), blocked with 5% goat serum albumin at room temperature for 60 min, and then incubated overnight with an anti-HMGB1 antibody (ab79823, 1:500 in dilution) and IBA1 (ab15690, 1:400 in dilution) at 4 °C. Subsequently, they were incubated with a TRITC-conjugated goat anti-rabbit IgG at a 1:100 dilution (CW0160, CWBIO, Beijing, China) and a Alexa Fluor 488-labeled goat anti-mouse IgG (P0188, Beyotime, Shanghai, China) for 2 h at room temperature, and then counterstained by DAPI (5 µg/mL) for 10 min. Images were observed using fluorescence microscopy (Leica, Germany Q9). The fluorescence intensity was evaluated by the ImageJ 1.44p software.

2.12. Western Blot Analysis

Western blotting was performed as previously reported [28,30,36,46]. Based on the manufacturer's instructions, the hippocampal and cortex tissues were weighed and homogenized using a tissue protein extraction kit (CWBIO, Shanghai, China) supplemented with 1% proteases and a phosphatase inhibitor cocktail (CWBIO, Shanghai, China), and the non-ischemia correspondent hippocampal and cortex tissues were treated as the PNGL control samples. After the homogenates were centrifuged at 12,000×g for 15 min at 4 °C, the supernatant samples including total protein proteins were collected. Then, the protein concentration in the supernatant was determined by a BCA assay (CWBIO, Shanghai, China). Finally, the protein samples (3.5 mg/mL) were diluted with 5 × SDS loading buffer (CWBIO, Shanghai, China), denatured in boiling water for 5 min, and then stored at −80 °C until use. Protein samples were loaded onto the SDS-PAGE gel (10–15%), separated electrophoretically, and transferred onto NC membranes (Millipore, Bedford, MA, USA). After blocking the nonspecific binding sites for 2 h in 5% non-fat milk and Tris-buffered saline (TBS)/Tween 20 at room temperature, the membranes were individually incubated overnight at 4 °C with the following primary antibodies: P44/42 (CST4695, 1:1000), SARK/JNK (CST9525, 1:1000), P38 (CST8690, 1:1000), p-P44/42 (CST4370, 1:1000), p-SARK/JNK (CST4668, 1:1000), p-P38 (CST4511, 1:1000), NF-κB (CST8242, 1:1000), p-NF-κB (CST3033, 1:1000), Cox2 (CST12282, 1:1000), c-Fos (ab134122, 1:5000), Caspase 9 (ab1884768, 1:1000), Cleaved Caspase 3 (ab49822, 1:500), Caspase 8 (ab25901 1:1000), IL-1β (EXP. 1:500), and β-actin (EXP0036 F, 1:2000). Then, the membrane was incubated at room temperature for 2 h with horseradish peroxidase conjugated antibodies at a 1:2000 dilution. Protein expression was detected by an enhanced chemiluminescence method and imaged by using the ChemiDoc XRS instrument (Bio-Rad, Hercules, CA, USA). To eliminate variations in protein expression, three independent experiments were performed.

2.13. Data and Statistical Analyses

Data are presented as the mean values ± standard deviation (SD) or standard error of the mean (SEM). All analyses were performed by using GraphPad Prism 8.0 statistical software (GraphPad Software, Inc., La Jolla, San Diego, CA, USA). Two-way analysis of variance (ANOVA) was used with drug (PNGL versus Vehicle) and treatment (MCAO/R vsrsus Control) as independent factors. Group differences after significant ANOVAs were measured by post hoc Bonferroni test, and $p < 0.05$ was considered statistically significant.

3. Results

3.1. PNGL Improves Neurological Functions and Attenuate Brain Swellings and Infarcts in MCAO/R Rats

To assess the neuroprotective effects of PNGL on focal brain ischemic injury, SD rats were subjected to 2 h of MCAO and 24 h of reperfusion. Extensive infarction was detected by TTC staining in the cerebral cortical and subcortical areas over a series of sections of the ipsilateral hemisphere in rats subjected to MCAO (Figure 3A), and the brain water content was examined to evaluate brain swelling in the ischemic brain (Figure 3B). Rats pretreated with PNGL (73, 146, 292 mg/kg) had significantly smaller infarcts volumes than those in the MCAO/R group (respectively, 73, * $p < 0.05$; 146, ** $p < 0.01$; 292, ** $p < 0.01$, Figure 3A,C). Moreover, there was a significant increase in brain swellings (brain water content) after 24 h of reperfusion, whereas PNGL (146, 292 mg/kg) pretreatment remarkably reduced the brain water contents (respectively, 146, * $p < 0.05$; 292, ** $p < 0.01$, Figure 3B). Furthermore, NBP (60 mg/kg) and ASP (10 mg/kg) has similar neuroprotective effects against brain swellings and infarcts with a dose-dependent way (Figure 3B,C).

Moreover, the neurological deficit scores were evaluated using the scoring criteria of Zea-Longa. Longa scores suggested that MCAO/R significantly increased neurological deficit scores in rats (## $p < 0.01$, Figure 3D). In comparison with the MCAO/R group, PNGL administration (73, 146, 292 mg/kg) resulted in a significant decrease in neurological deficit scores (respectively, 73, * $p < 0.05$; 146, ** $p < 0.01$; 292, ** $p < 0.01$, Figure 3D). A 146 and 292 mg/kg doses approximately possessed equivalent neuroprotective effects, compared with those in NBP and ASP.

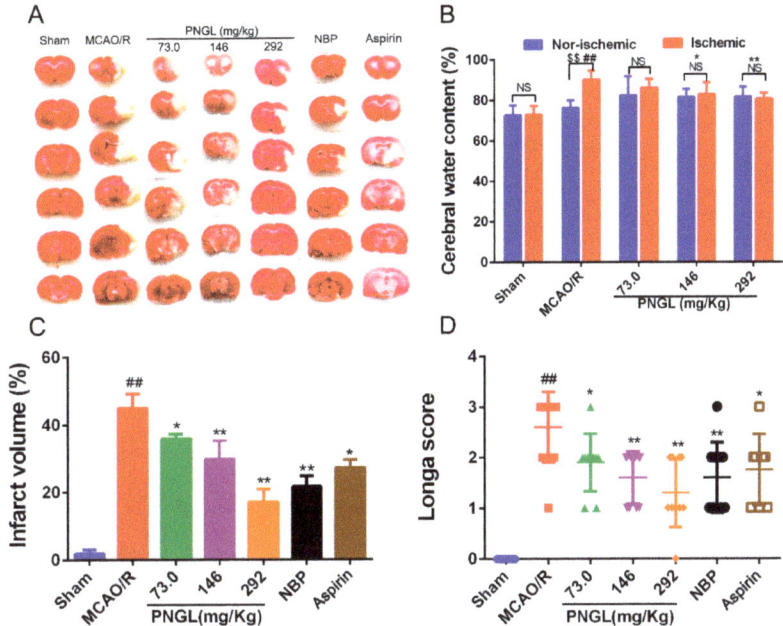

Figure 3. Effects of PNGL on infarct volume, brain water content, and neurological deficit scores in MCAO/R injury rats. PNGL improves neurological functions and attenuate brain swellings and infarcts in MCAO/R rats. (**A**) Representative images of 2, 3, 5-triphenyltetrazolium chloride -stained brain sections from the sham-operated or PNGL-treated animals collected 24 h after infarction; red tissue is healthy; white tissue is infarcted (n = 3–6 in each group). (**B**) Brain water content in ischemia hemispheres of all groups (n = 4 in each group). (**C**) Quantitative analysis of the infarct volume (n = 3 in each group). (**D**) Neurological deficit scores in all groups (n = 10 in each group). Mean values ± SD; * $p < 0.05$, ** $p < 0.01$ versus MCAO/R group; # $p < 0.05$, ## $p < 0.01$, versus sham group; \$\$$p < 0.01$, Nor-ischemic versus Ischemic; NS means no significance, Nor-ischemic versus Ischemic.

3.2. PNGL Alleviates BBB Disruption and Inflammatory Cytokines in MCAO/R Rats

Cerebral I/R injury was reported to exaggerate BBB breakdown in animal stroke models. BBB permeability in MCAO rats was evaluated via the observation of the Evans blue dye (Figure 4A,B). Results showed that Evans blue content in ipsilateral ischemic hemispheres was remarkably increased in the MCAO/R group compared with the sham group ($p < 0.01$, Figure 4A,B). PNGL (73.0, 146, 292 mg/kg) pretreatment significantly decreased the Evans blue leakage content through BBB in ipsilateral ischemic hemispheres ($p < 0.01$, Figure 4B). The non-ischemic hemispheres were not significantly different with the ischemic hemispheres ($p > 0.05$, Figure 4B).

Inflammation has been reported to be involved in the disruption of the BBB. To explore whether PNGL pretreatment could induce anti-inflammatory pattern, ELISA and specific assay kits were used to investigate the expression inflammatory cytokines in serum from MCAO rats after 24 h of reperfusion. The MCAO/R group had significantly higher concentrations of IL-6, TNF-α, IL-1β, and HMGB1 compared to the sham group ($p < 0.01$, Figure 4). In comparison with the MCAO/R group, PNGL (146, 292 mg/kg) pretreatment significantly reduced concentrations of the IL-6, TNF-α, IL-1β, and HMGB1 in the serums ($p < 0.01$, Figure 4C–F). PNGL (73 mg/kg) showed no significant differences on the IL-6, TNF-α, and HMGB1 concentrations with MCAO/R groups ($p > 0.05$, Figure 4C,D,F). Additionally, NBP (60 mg/kg) and ASP (10 mg/kg) has similar decreases in the IL-6, TNF-α, and IL-1 β, concentrations in the serums ($p > 0.05$, Figure 4). Moreover, PNGL (292 mg/kg) pretreatment significantly decreased the ICAM-1 concentration in the serums ($p < 0.01$, Supplementary Material S2A).

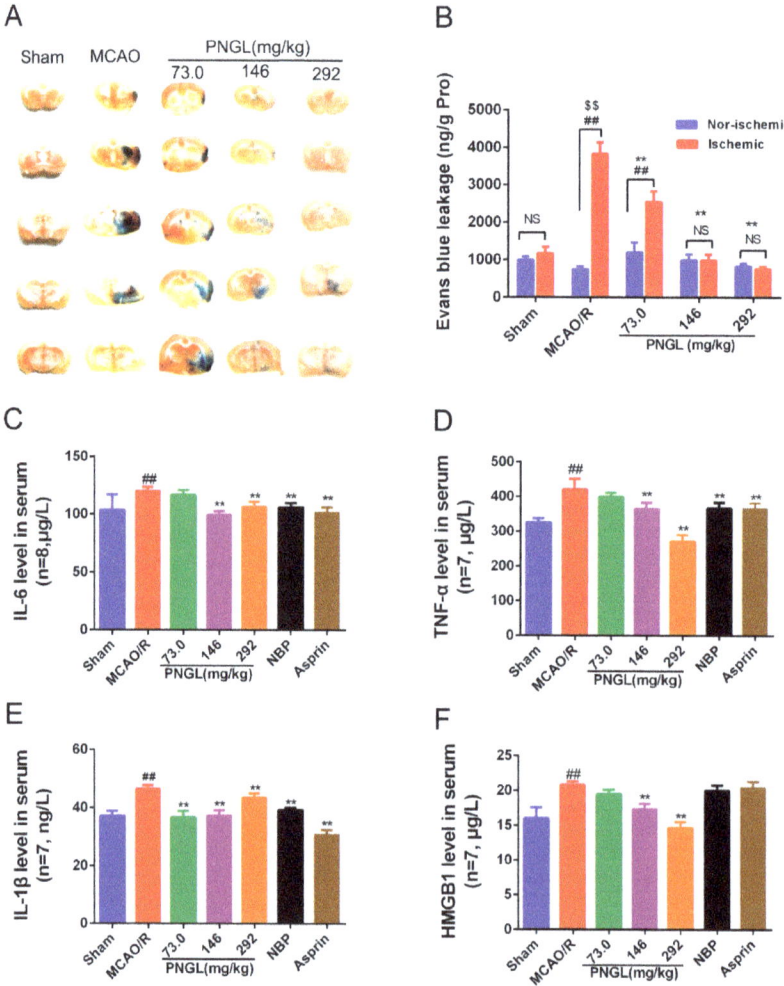

Figure 4. Effects of PNGL on BBB disruption and inflammatory cytokines in MCAO/R rats. PNGL alleviates BBB disruption and inflammatory cytokines in MCAO/R rats. (**A**) Representative images of the Evans blue dye -stained brain sections from the sham-operated or PNGL-treated animals collected 24 h after infarction (4 in each group). (**B**) The Evans blue leakage content of all groups, measured at 632 nm using spectrophotometry ($n = 5$ in each group). (**C**)–(**F**) the IL-6, TNF-α, IL-1 β, and HMGB1 concentrations, determined by ELISA and specific assay kit ($n = 7$–8 in each group). Mean values ± SD; * $p < 0.05$, ** $p < 0.01$ versus MCAO/R group; ## $p < 0.01$, versus sham group; \$\$$p < 0.01$, Nor-ischemic versus Ischemic; NS means no significance, Nor-ischemic versus Ischemic.

3.3. PNGL Decreases Neuronal Apoptosis and Loss Caused By Ischemia

The CA1 and CA3 areas of the hippocampus are commonly considered to be sensitive to ischemic injury [47–50], and so the CA1 and CA3 areas are used to monitor the neuronal apoptosis and loss. To explore the histopathological changes in the ischaemic brain hemisphere, we performed Giemsa staining. Giemsa staining revealed a change in neuron density. After MCAO/R induction, most neurons exhibited weak staining, which indicated that neurons were diffusely deteriorated, and many neurons were lost in the hippocampus neurons (Figure 5A,C, CA1, $p < 0.01$; CA3, $p < 0.001$; cortex,

$p < 0.01$). In contrast, PNGL (146, 292 mg/kg) pretreatment exhibited strong staining and possessed neurons arranged regularly in the hippocampus and cortex (Figure 5A). PNGL (292 mg/kg) presented a significant increase in neuron density (Figure 5C, $p < 0.01$). In addition, PNGL (146 mg/kg) showed similar improvements of nervous density in the hippocampus regions with significant differences (Figure 5C, $p < 0.01$), and ASP (10 mg/kg) were equivalent to those of PNGL in improving neuron density, indicating that PNGL decreases neuronal apoptosis and loss caused by CIRI.

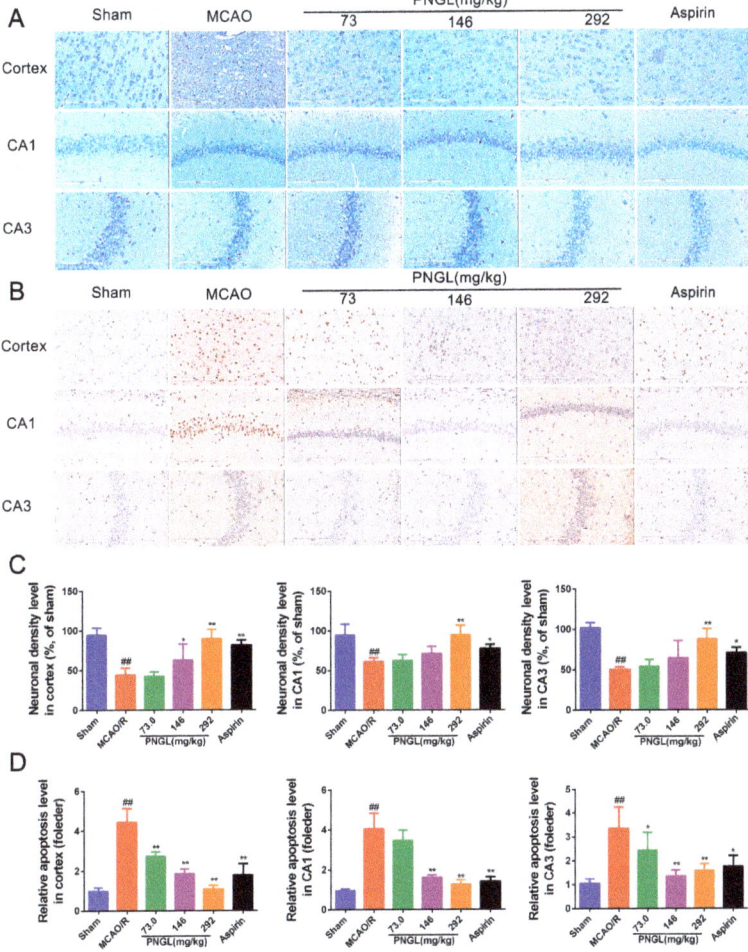

Figure 5. PNGL decreases neuronal apoptosis and neurons loss caused by ischemia. PNGL decreases neuronal apoptosis and neurons loss caused by ischemia in rats. (**A**) Representative images of Giemsa staining performed in hippocampus CA1, CA3 regions, and cortex regions from ischemic brains, measured by an in situ apoptosis detection kit. (**B**) Representative images of TUNEL assay performed in hippocampus CA1 and CA3 regions, and cortex regions. (**C**) The relative neuronal density (%, of sham) in the in hippocampus CA1 and CA3 regions, and cortex regions in all groups ($n = 4$ in each group). (**D**) The relative neuronal apoptotic rate levels in the in hippocampus CA1 and CA3 regions, and cortex regions in all groups ($n = 3$ in each group). Mean values ± SD; * $p < 0.05$, ** $p < 0.01$ versus MCAO/R group; ## $p < 0.01$, versus sham group. Scale bar, 200 μm.

Contrary to Giemsa staining, TUNEL Staining (Figure 5B,D) showed that the relative apoptosis cell levels in the model group was significantly higher than that of the sham group. PNGL (73.0, 146, 292 mg/kg) pretreatment dose dependently markedly decreased neuropathological apoptotic alterations in the brain after 24 h reperfusion following 2 h of MCAO (Figure 5D, * $p < 0.05$, ** $p < 0.01$, $p < 0.01$). Moreover, ASP (10 mg/kg) evidently inhibited the neuronal apoptosis in hippocampus CA1, CA3, and cortex regions, which nearly corresponded to PNGL (146 mg/kg).

3.4. PNGL Downregulates Inflammatory Cytokines and Inhibits Microglia Activation in Ischemic Brains

Researches exhibited that the inflammatory factors were induced not only in microglia of the CA1 region in the ischaemic hippocampus but also of the CA3 and DG regions [42,43], so the CA1 region and DG regions were further used to detect the inflammatory response [42,43,47,51,52].

To further explore neuropathological alterations of neurogenic inflammation in ischemic brains from all groups, inflammatory cytokines and microglia activation in ischemic brains were also examined after 24 h reperfusion following 2 h of MCAO. Immunofluorescent results showed that the MCAO/R model rats exhibited more IBA1-positive neurons in the ischemic hippocampus CA1, dentate gyrus (DG), and cortex regions than the sham-operated group (Figure 5A). However, PNGL (146 mg/kg) administration decreased the number of IBA1-positive neurons in the ischemic brain.

Similarly, the MCAO/R group significantly increased the inflammatory cytokines in ischemic brains than did the sham group ($p < 0.05$, Figure 6B–E), including the MMP-2, MMP-9, ICAM-1, and VCAM-1 concentrations in the hippocampus and cortex regions. In comparison with the MCAO/R group, PNGL (73.0, 146, 292 mg/kg) pretreatment dose dependently decreased the inflammatory cytokines in hippocampus and cortex regions. Additionally, PNGL (292 mg/kg) pretreatment significantly reduced the concentrations of MMP-2, MMP-9, and ICAM-1 ($p < 0.05$, Figure 6B,D,E). PNGL (146 mg/kg) pretreatment significantly decreased the VCAM-1, MMP-9, and ICAM-1 concentrations ($p < 0.05$, Figure 6B,C,E). PNGL (73 mg/kg) showed a minor decrease in the inflammatory cytokine concentrations with no significant difference. In additions, NBP (60 mg/kg) has similar decreases of the inflammatory cytokine concentrations in ischemic brains ($p < 0.01$, Figure 6 B–E).

Taken together, these results indicated that PNGL treatment effectively deceased the inflammatory cytokine concentrations, inhibited the microglia activation, and reduced the neuronal loss and apoptosis, thus improving cerebral I/R-induced neuropathological changes by inhibiting neurogenic inflammation.

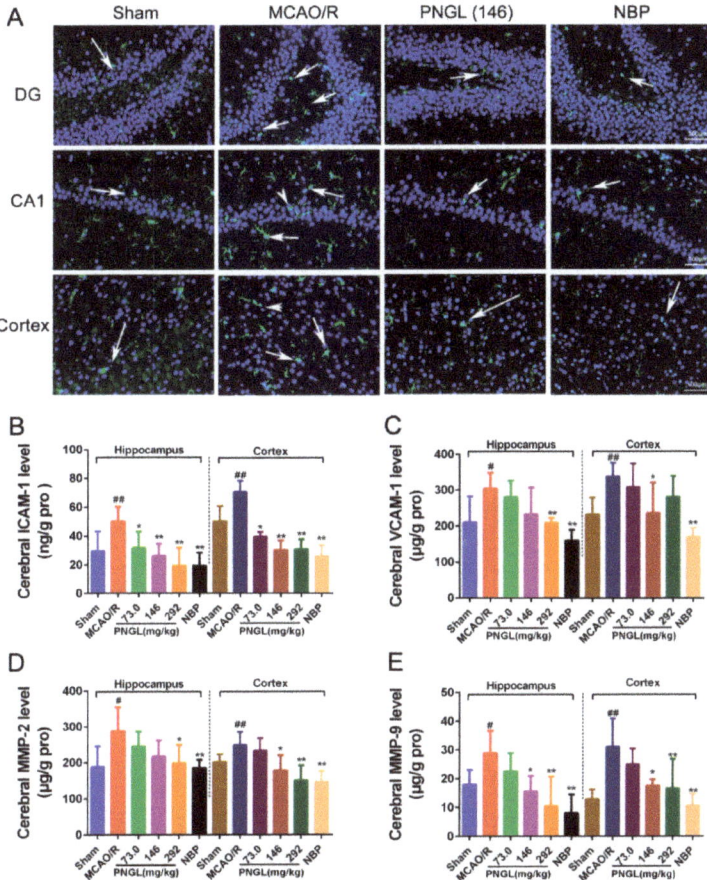

Figure 6. PNGL downregulates inflammatory cytokines and inhibits microglia activation in ischemic brains. PNGL treatment effectively deceased the inflammatory cytokine concentrations, inhibited the microglia activation, and reduced the neuronal loss and apoptosis, thus improving cerebral I/R-induced neuropathological changes by inhibiting neurogenic inflammation. (**A**) Representative images of IBA1-immunopositive microglia (green) with DAPI (blue) staining from hippocampus CA1, dentate gyrus (DG), and cortex regions in rat brains after MCAO/R injury, measured by immunofluorescence. (**B**)–(**E**) The MMP-2, MMP-9, ICAM-1, and VCAM-1 concentrations in hippocampus and cortex in rat brains after MCAO/R injury, determined by ELISA and specific as; (**F**) the IOD of IBA1-immunopositive microglia (n = 4–6 in each group). Mean values ± SD; * $p < 0.05$, ** $p < 0.01$ versus MCAO/R group; # $p < 0.05$, ## $p < 0.01$, versus sham group. Scale bar, 100 μm.

3.5. PNGL Inhibits NF-Kb Signaling Pathway

Considering that the activation of NF-κB signaling pathway is related to inflammatory reactions, we finally investigated whether PNGL can inhibit the NF-κB signaling pathway to reduce inflammatory, contributing to the attenuation of cerebral I/R injury. Hence, western blot analysis was used to examine the NF-κB and it regulated downstream Caspase 3/8/9 expression in the hippocampus and cortex regions from ischemic brains. Compared to the control group, the MCAO/R group significantly increased the expressions of the total NF-κB and phosphorylated NF-κB in the hippocampus and cortex regions from ischemic brains ($p < 0.05$, $p < 0.01$, respectively, Figure 7A,C,D). PNGL (146 mg/kg) pretreatment notably inhibited the expressions of the total NF-κB and phosphorylated NF-κB in cerebral ischemia brains ($p < 0.05$, $p < 0.01$, respectively, Figure 7B,C). Similarly, the increase expressions of its downstream caspase 3/8/9 proteins induced by MCAO/R was strikingly abrogated by PNGL pretreatment (hippocampus, $p < 0.05$; cortex, $p < 0.01$, Figure 7B,E,F). These findings suggested that PNGL inhibited the NF-κB activation, it regulated neuronal apoptosis and neuroinflammation reactions caused by CIRI. In additions, no significant change in the expression of cleaved caspase 9 was observed in hippocampus.

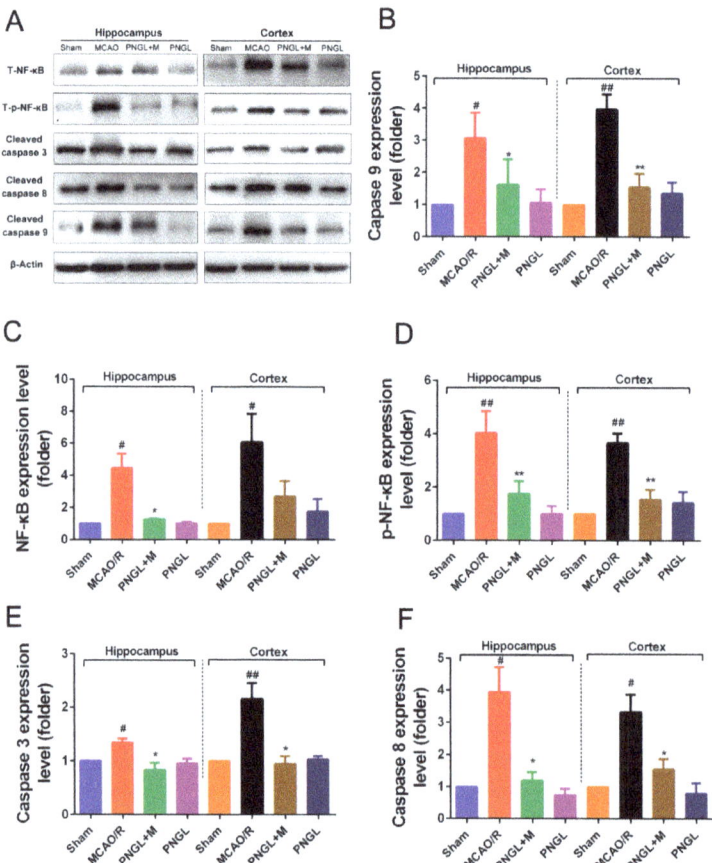

Figure 7. Effects of PNGL on the expression levels of phosphorylated NF-κB. PNGL regulated downstream Caspase 3/8/9 signaling pathway in the ischemic brain. PNGL inhibited the NF-κB activation, it regulated neuronal apoptosis and neuroinflammation reactions caused by CIRI. (**A**) The protein bands of the NF-κB regulated downstream Caspase 3/8/9 signaling pathways in the ischemic brain, which were examined by western blot analysis. (**C**) the relative NF-κB expression level; (**D**) the relative expression levels of the phosphorylated NF-κB; (**E**) (**F**) (**B**) The relative expression levels of its downstream Caspase 3/8/9, respectively, quantified and analyzed by using Gel-Pro analyzer software. Mean values ± SD ($n = 3$); Mean values ± SEM; * $p < 0.05$, ** $p < 0.01$ versus MCAO/R group; # $p < 0.05$, ## $p < 0.01$, versus sham group.

3.6. PNGL Regulates Mapks Signaling Pathway

The MAPKs signaling pathways plays a critical protective role against OGD/R and MCAO/R-induced apoptosis and inflammation. Western blot analysis at 24 h following reperfusion showed, the expression levels of total phosphorylated JNK1/2 (p-JNK1/2), phosphorylated P44/42 (p-P44/42), and phosphorylated P38 (p-P38) significantly increased in the MCAO/R model ($p < 0.01$, $p < 0.05$, $p < 0.01$, respectively, Figure 8). Comparatively, PNGL (146 mg/kg) pretreatment markedly reduced the total phosphorylation levels of the JNK1/2, P44/42 and P38 ($p < 0.01$, $p < 0.05$, $p < 0.01$, respectively, Figure 8 B–D). Additionally, the ratio between the phosphorylated and the non-phosphorylated expression levels of MAPKs showed similar results ($p < 0.01$, $p < 0.05$, $p < 0.01$, respectively, Figure 8 B–D). Moreover, no significant differences were observed in the expression of cortex p-P44/42, total P44/42, total JNK1/2, and total p38 MAPK among all experimental groups ($p > 0.05$, Supplementary Material S2B–D), indicating that PNGL may downregulate the phosphorylation levels of the MAPKs, thus decreasing neuroinflammation after ischemia by modulating innate and adaptive immunity.

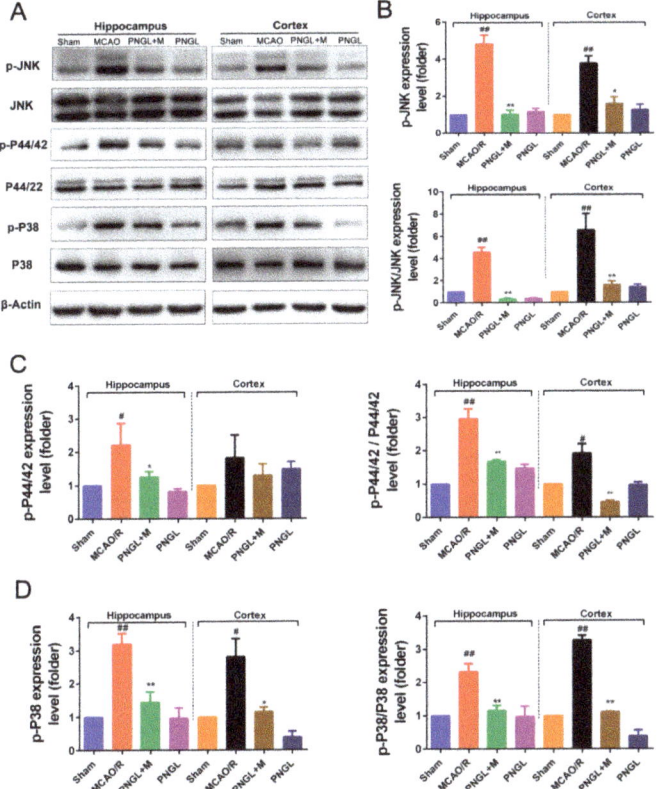

Figure 8. Effects of PNGL on the expression levels of phosphorylated P44/42, JNK1/2, and P38 of MAPKs signaling pathway in the ischemic brain. PNGL downregulated the expression levels of phosphorylated P44/42, JNK1/2, and P38 of MAPKs. (**A**) The protein bands of phospho-ERK, phospho-P38, and phospho-JNK, respectively, in the ischemic brain sections were examined by western blot analysis. (**B**)–(**D**) The relative expression levels of phosphorylated P44/42, JNK1/2, and P38, respectively, were quantified and analyzed by using Gel-Pro analyzer software. Mean values ± SEM ($n = 3$); $p < 0.05$, ** $p < 0.01$, versus MCAO/R group; # $p < 0.05$, ## $p < 0.01$ versus sham-operated group.

3.7. PNGL Inhibits HMGB1 Expression and Its HMGB1-Triggered Inflammation

It was proven that HMGB-1 triggers the NF-κB, MAPKs, STAT3, and AP-1 signaling via activating TLR4 signaling, which in turn increases innate and acquired immunity, and further heightens the post-ischemic neuroinflammation response. Accordingly, intercepting the HMGB-1/TLR4 signaling pathway is a promising therapeutic strategy for alleviating cerebral stroke injury and limiting neuroinflammation.

As shown in Figure 9, the total HMGB1 level in ischemic brain was notably upregulated in the model group compared with the sham control group ($p < 0.05$, $p < 0.01$, Figure 9A,D), which was obviously downregulated by PNGL (146 mg/kg) pretreatment in hippocampus and cortex regions ($p < 0.05$, $p < 0.01$, Figure 9A,D). Meanwhile, MCAO/R markedly increased the HMGB1-triggered inflammation protein Cox2 and IL-1β expression levels, whereas conversely PNGL (146 mg/kg) pretreatment markedly reversed the increased changes ($p < 0.05$, $p < 0.01$, Figure 9 B,C,E). Hence, our findings suggested that PNGL may decrease HMGB-1 expression in hippocampus and cortex regions and inhibit its HMGB1-triggered inflammation in ischemic brain cells.

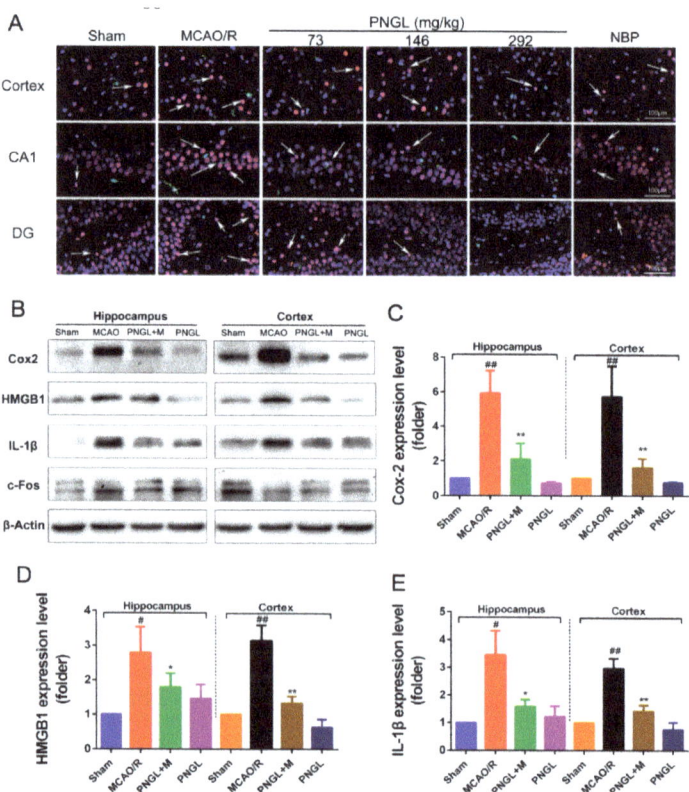

Figure 9. Effects of PNGL on HMGB1 expression and its HMGB1-triggered inflammation in ischemic brains. PNGL treatment effectively deceased the HMGB1 expression and its HMGB1-triggered inflammation, thus improving cerebral I/R-induced neuropathological changes by inhibiting neurogenic inflammation. (**A**) Representative images of HMGB1-immunopositive neurons (red) and IBA1-immunopositive microglia (green) with DAPI (blue) staining in hippocampus CA1, dentate gyrus (DG), and cortex regions in rat brains after cerebral I/R, measured by immunofluorescence; scale bar, 100 μm. (**B**) The protein bands of HMGB1, and the HMGB1-triggered inflammation IL-1β, Cox2 and c-Fos in the ischemic brains were examined by western blot analysis. (**C**)–(**E**) The relative expression levels of HMGB1, IL-1β, and Cox2, respectively, quantified and analyzed by using Gel-Pro analyzer software. Mean values ± SEM; * $p < 0.05$, ** $p < 0.01$ versus MCAO/R group; # $p < 0.05$, ## $p < 0.01$, versus sham group. Scale bar, 100 μm.

4. Discussion

Ischemic stroke remains one of the leading causes of death worldwide, which mainly caused by cerebral ischemia and reperfusion injury [1,3,4]. Numerous studies on stroke have been performed in recent decades, but the pathogenesis of ischemic stroke has not been fully elucidated, and few medicines are available [53,54]. Therefore, the development of novel therapeutic options and strategies is urgently needed to limit injury after cerebral infarction. In the current study, we initially proved that PNGL exerted neuroprotective effects against cerebral ischemia and reperfusion injury in middle cerebral artery occlusion/reperfusion (MCAO/R) model rats, and provided a novel mechanism by which PNGL may ameliorate cerebral I/R injury.

PNGL, as the total saponins of Panax notoginseng stem and leaf, has already been shown to exert potent neuroprotective and anti-apoptotic properties. Since the first beneficial effect of PNGL was detected on nervous diseases, several reports have not only revealed its diverse pharmacological properties but have also raised some speculative proposals concerning its mechanism of action. Moreover, currently there had been no clear evidence on whether PNGL has neuroprotective effects against cerebral I/R injury. Meanwhile, our research found that PNGL pretreatment improved the neurological functions, attenuated the brain swelling, and reduced the cortex infarct volume in MCAO/R rats (Figure 3). Additionally, PNGL may evidently alleviate BBB disruption (Figure 4), improve nervous density, and decreases neuronal apoptosis and neuron loss caused by cerebral I/R injury (Figure 5). All of these results proved neuroprotective effects of PNGL against cerebral I/R injury.

Immunity and inflammation are key elements that contribute to the pathobiology of stroke, and its caused-CI/RI and the secondary damage to brain tissues are closely associated with immunity and inflammation responses [5–8]. Previous research has shown that immunity and inflammation are integral parts of the pathogenesis of ischemic stroke [55–57]. Inflammatory signaling is activated and completed by blood-borne leukocytes that penetrate the brain during the ischemic phase [2]. Once ischemia/reperfusion occurs, HMGB1secretion, ROS production, glutamate toxicity, and Ca^{2+} overload promotes the activation of complements, platelets and endothelial cells, activates inflammatory transcription factors and the release inflammatory signals [57], and generates inflammatory cytokines and pro-inflammatory mediators including TNF-α, IL-1β, IL-6, ICAM-1, IFN-γ, IL-17, IL-23, MIP-1α, MIP-2, MMP-2, MMP-9, and anti-inflammatory IL-10 in ischemic brain [55–57]. In our research, compared with the sham group, the levels of the inflammatory mediators TNF-α, IL-1β, IL-6, ICAM-1, MMP-2, MMP-9, and HMGB1 significantly increased in the MCAO/R group (Figures 4 and 6). Interestingly, PNGL pretreatment markedly downregulated these concentrations of the inflammatory mediators indicating that the neuroprotective effects of PNGL may be related with inhibition of neurogenic inflammation caused by brain ischemia.

HMGB1 is a nuclear DNA-binding protein and an important DAMP, which activates TLR2/4 and RAGEs signaling following rapid translocation to the cytoplasm or release from dying cells after cerebral ischemia [9,10]. Additionally, cellular HMGB1 binds to pattern recognition receptors of microglia and subsequently leads to synthesis and release of pro-inflammatory mediators, aggravating neuronal injury and BBB disruption [20,58]. Subsequently, the activation of TLR4 signaling at the plasma membrane triggers NF-κB, MAPK, STAT3, and AP-1 signaling, which in turn increases innate and acquired immunity and further heightens the post-ischemic neuroinflammation response [10,59]. Accordingly, intercepting the HMGB1/TLR4 signaling pathway is a promising therapeutic strategy for alleviating cerebral stroke injury and limiting neuroinflammation. Our data indicated MCAO/R induced an obvious increase of the HMGB1 concentrations in serums and expressions in ischemic brains (Figures 4 and 9). Consequently highly released HMGB1 triggered post-ischemic neuroinflammation, and there was also a significant up-regulation of IL-6, TNF-α, IL-1β, ICAM-1, MMP-2 MMP-9 (Figure 6A, Figure 9A,B), and Cox2 accompanied by microglia activation (Figure 6), which was consistent with the previous existing reports [6,7]. However, PNGL (73, 146, 292 mg/kg) pretreatment markedly decreased HMGB1 expression in ischemic brains and concentrations in serums, inhibited the HMGB1-triggered inflammation, and downregulated the inflammatory cytokine levels (Figure 6A, Figure 9A,B).

Further research results suggested PNGL pretreatment dose-dependently inhibited the HMGB-1/TLR4 signaling-triggered downstream proteins including MAPKs, NF-κB, and cleaved caspase 3/8 [6–8], suggesting that the immunomodulatory effect of PNGL was associated with the inhibition of HMGB1-triggered inflammation, the NF-κB, and MAPK signaling pathways. Consistent with the current reports [6–8], there was a significant upregulation of p-P44/42, p-JNK1/2, and p-p38 MAPK in MCAO/R rats exposed to 2 h of MCAO and 24 h of reperfusion, and it also markedly caused the NF-κB activation and the p-NF-κB level increase. Interestingly, PNGL administration (146mg/kg) significantly downregulated the levels of p-P44/42, p-JNK1/2 and p-p38 MAPK (Figure 8), and also inhibited expressions of the total NF-κB and phosphorylated NF-κB in ischemic brains (Figure 7). No change in the expression of P44/42, JNK1/2, and P38 was observed. These studies indicated that the protective effects of PNGL against neuronal apoptosis could be associated with inhibiting HMGB1-triggered inflammation, suppressing the activation of MAPKs and NF-κB, and thus improved cerebral I/R-induced neuropathological changes. In additions, PNGL decreases neuronal apoptosis and loss caused by cerebral I/R injury.

These findings, together with our results, supported the neuroprotective effects of PNGL against cerebral I/R injury and neuronal apoptosis via decreasing the HMGB levels, inhibiting HMGB1-triggered inflammation, reduced the production of pro-inflammatory mediators, and suppressing the activation of MAPKs and NF-κB signaling pathways. However, neuroprotective effects of PNGL has not been convincingly confirmed by in vitro models of ischemic brain, and the mechanisms was not evidently sufficient to explain on how PNGL may regulate the subsequent immune and neuroinflammatory responses caused by the HMGB1/TLR2/4 pathway. Hence, further investigations are needed to elucidate the mechanisms more deeply and to investigate the clinical applications of PNGL.

Nevertheless, our results suggest that PNGL represents a potential treatment value for cerebral ischemic infarctions, and works through a mechanism of HMGB1-triggered inflammation inhibition through the MAPK and NF-κB pathway

5. Conclusions

In summary, this study supported the neuroprotective effects of PNGL on cerebral I/R injury, and the potential mechanisms may be largely associated with the inhibition of HMGB1-triggered inflammation, reduction of pro-inflammatory mediators including IL-6, TNF-α, IL-1 β, MMP-9, MMP-2, and ICAM-1, and attenuation of neuronal apoptosis and loss caused by ischemia via suppressing the activation of MAPKs and NF-κB signaling pathways. Although further studies are needed to elucidate the roles of MAPK signaling pathways in the cross talk between pro-inflammatory mediators and apoptosis, our findings may represent a novel mechanism of PNGL in focal cerebral I/R injury in rats, and provide new insights into therapeutic targets for ischemia stroke patients.

Supplementary Materials: The following are available online at http://www.mdpi.com/2218-273X/9/10/512/s1, Figure S1: The chromatograms and the chemical fingerprinting of PNGL established by the high performance liquid chromatography (HPLC). Figure S2: Effects of PNGL on the ICAM-1 concentration in serum, the JNK, P44/42, and P38 expression in MCAO/R rats.

Author Contributions: W.X., X.M., and P.Z. designed the research; W.X., X.D., and T.Z. performed the experimental work; W.X. and F.N. wrote the manuscript; W.X. and F.N. performed the statistical analysis; P.Z. and F.N. helped map the figures and revise the manuscript; G.S. and X.S. were responsible for the supervision and project administration. All authors discussed, edited, and approved the final version.

Funding: This work was supported by the National Natural Science Foundation of China (No. 81773938), the "Innovative Chinese Medicine *Qiye Tongmai Capsule* Clinical Research" Project (No. 2015ZX09101020), the "Study on the pharmacodynamic mechanism of the innovative Chinese medicine *Qiye Tongmai Capsule* III-clinical agent" Project (No. 20160307014YY), the Fundamental Research Funds for the Central Universities (No. 3332018152), and he National Natural Science Foundation of China (No. 81891012).

Conflicts of Interest: The authors declare no conflicts of interest.

References

1. Jamison, J.T. Mechanisms of persistent translation arrest following global brain ischemia and reperfusion. Dissertations Theses, Wayne State University, Detroit, MI, USA, January 2011.
2. Kamel, H.; Iadecola, C. Brain-Immune Interactions and Ischemic Stroke: Clinical Implications. *JAMA Neurol.* **2012**, *69*, 576–581.
3. Xie, W.; Zhou, P.; Sun, Y.; Meng, X.; Dai, Z.; Sun, G.; Sun, X. Protective Effects and Target Network Analysis of Ginsenoside Rg1 in Cerebral Ischemia and Reperfusion Injury: A Comprehensive Overview of Experimental Studies. *Cells* **2018**, *7*, 270. [CrossRef] [PubMed]
4. Antonino, T.; Riccardo, D.S.; Domenico, D.R.; Claudio, P.; Sergio, L.P.; Antonio, P.; Giuseppe, L. Effects of clinical and laboratory variables and of pretreatment with cardiovascular drugs in acute ischaemic stroke: A retrospective chart review from the GIFA study. *Int. J. Cardiol.* **2011**, *151*, 318–322.
5. Eltzschig, H.K.; Eckle, T. Ischemia and reperfusion—from mechanism to translation. *Nat. Med.* **2011**, *17*, 1391–1401. [CrossRef] [PubMed]
6. Jiang, M.; Li, J.; Peng, Q.; Liu, Y.; Liu, W.; Luo, C.; Peng, J.; Li, J.; Yung, K.K.L.; Mo, Z. Neuroprotective effects of bilobalide on cerebral ischemia and reperfusion injury are associated with inhibition of pro-inflammatory mediator production and down-regulation of JNK1/2 and p38 MAPK activation. *J. Neuroinflammation* **2014**, *11*, 167. [CrossRef] [PubMed]
7. Jianhua, Q.; Masaki, N.; Yumei, W.; Sims, J.R.; Sumei, Q.; Savitz, S.I.; Salvatore, S.; Moskowitz, M.A. Early release of HMGB-1 from neurons after the onset of brain ischemia. *J. Cereb. Blood Flow Metab.* **2008**, *28*, 927–938.
8. Tao, X.; Sun, X.; Yin, L.; Han, X.; Xu, L.; Qi, Y.; Xu, Y.; Li, H.; Lin, Y.; Liu, K.; et al. Dioscin ameliorates cerebral ischemia/reperfusion injury through the downregulation of TLR4 signaling via HMGB-1 inhibition. *Free. Radic. Boil. Med.* **2015**, *84*, 103–115. [CrossRef]
9. Yi, L.; Chang-Pei, G.; Shuang, Z.; Xi-Kun, Z.; Xue-Feng, L.; Yu-Quan, W.; Jin-Liang, Y.; Min, W. FIP200 is involved in murine pseudomonas infection by regulating HMGB1 intracellular translocation. *Cell. Physiol. Biochem. Pharmacol.* **2014**, *33*, 1733–1744.
10. Cheng, Y.; Wang, D.; Wang, B.; Li, H.; Xiong, J.; Xu, S.; Chen, Q.; Tao, K.; Yang, X.; Zhu, Y.; et al. HMGB1 translocation and release mediate cigarette smoke–induced pulmonary inflammation in mice through a TLR4/MyD88-dependent signaling pathway. *Mol. Boil. Cell* **2017**, *28*, 201–209. [CrossRef] [PubMed]
11. Lu, T.-H.; Hsieh, S.-Y.; Yen, C.-C.; Wu, H.-C.; Chen, K.-L.; Hung, D.-Z.; Chen, C.-H.; Wu, C.-C.; Su, Y.-C.; Chen, Y.-W.; et al. Involvement of oxidative stress-mediated ERK1/2 and p38 activation regulated mitochondria-dependent apoptotic signals in methylmercury-induced neuronal cell injury. *Toxicol. Lett.* **2011**, *204*, 71–80. [CrossRef]
12. Pietri, M.; Caprini, A.; Mouillet-Richard, S.; Pradines, E.; Ermonval, M.; Grassi, J.; Kellermann, O.; Schneider, B. Overstimulation of PrPCSignaling Pathways by Prion Peptide 106-126 Causes Oxidative Injury of Bioaminergic Neuronal Cells. *J. Boil. Chem.* **2006**, *281*, 28470–28479. [CrossRef] [PubMed]
13. Procaccio, V.; Bris, C.; De La Barca, J.C.; Oca, F.; Chevrollier, A.; Amati-Bonneau, P.; Bonneau, D.; Reynier, P. Perspectives of drug-based neuroprotection targeting mitochondria. *Rev. Neurol.* **2014**, *170*, 390–400. [CrossRef]
14. Sun, J.; Nan, G. The Mitogen-Activated Protein Kinase (MAPK) Signaling Pathway as a Discovery Target in Stroke. *J. Mol. Neurosci.* **2016**, *59*, 90–98. [CrossRef] [PubMed]
15. Yu, J.; Eto, M.; Kozaki, K.; Akishita, M.; Okabe, T.; Ouchi, Y. Raloxifene analogue LY117018 suppresses oxidative stress-induced endothelial cell apoptosis through activation of ERK1/2 signaling pathway. *Eur. J. Pharmacol.* **2008**, *589*, 32–36. [CrossRef] [PubMed]
16. Kovalská, M.; Kovalska, L.; Pavlíková, M.; Janickova, M.; Mikušková, K.; Adamkov, M.; Kaplan, P.; Tatarkova, Z.; Lehotský, J. Intracellular Signaling MAPK Pathway After Cerebral Ischemia–Reperfusion Injury. *Neurochem. Res.* **2012**, *37*, 1568–1577. [CrossRef] [PubMed]
17. Zhou, P.; Lu, S.; Luo, Y.; Wang, S.; Yang, K.; Zhai, Y.; Sun, G.; Sun, X. Attenuation of TNF-α-Induced Inflammatory Injury in Endothelial Cells by Ginsenoside Rb1 via Inhibiting NF-κB, JNK and p38 Signaling Pathways. *Front. Pharmacol.* **2017**, *8*. [CrossRef] [PubMed]

18. Sung-Chun, T.; Arumugam, T.V.; Xiangru, X.; Aiwu, C.; Mughal, M.R.; Gyu, J.D.; Lathia, J.D.; Siler, D.A.; Srinivasulu, C.; Xin, O. Pivotal role for neuronal Toll-like receptors in ischemic brain injury and functional deficits. *Proc. Natl. Acad. Sci USA* **2007**, *104*, 13798–13803.
19. Wang, X.; Wang, C.; Wang, J.; Zhao, S.; Zhang, K.; Wang, J.; Zhang, W.; Wu, C.; Yang, J. Pseudoginsenoside-F11 (PF11) exerts anti-neuroinflammatory effects on LPS-activated microglial cells by inhibiting TLR4-mediated TAK1/IKK/NF-κB, MAPKs and Akt signaling pathways. *Neuropharmacology* **2014**, *79*, 642–656. [CrossRef]
20. Liesz, A.; Dalpke, A.; Mracsko, E.; Antoine, D.J.; Roth, S.; Zhou, W.; Yang, H.; Na, S.-Y.; Akhisaroglu, M.; Fleming, T.; et al. DAMP Signaling is a Key Pathway Inducing Immune Modulation after Brain Injury. *J. Neurosci.* **2015**, *35*, 583–598. [CrossRef]
21. Eckert, B. Acute Stroke Therapy 1981–2009*. *Clin. Neuroradiol.* **2009**, *19*, 8. [CrossRef]
22. Yang, X.; Xiong, X.; Wang, H.; Wang, J. Protective Effects of Panax Notoginseng Saponins on Cardiovascular Diseases: A Comprehensive Overview of Experimental Studies. *Evidence-Based Complement. Altern. Med.* **2014**, *2014*, 1–13. [CrossRef] [PubMed]
23. Bao-Ying, H.; Xian-Jin, L.; Ren, Q.; Zheng-Lin, J.; Li-Hua, X.; Guo-Hua, W.; Xia, L.; Bin, P. Treatment with ginseng total saponins improves the neurorestoration of rat after traumatic brain injury. *J. Ethnopharmacol.* **2014**, *155*, 1243–1255.
24. Xie, W.; Meng, X.; Zhai, Y.; Zhou, P.; Ye, T.; Wang, Z.; Sun, G.; Sun, X. Panax Notoginseng Saponins: A Review of Its Mechanisms of Antidepressant or Anxiolytic Effects and Network Analysis on Phytochemistry and Pharmacology. *Molecules* **2018**, *23*, 940. [CrossRef] [PubMed]
25. Sun, K.; Fan, J.; Han, J. Ameliorating effects of traditional Chinese medicine preparation, Chinese materia medica and active compounds on ischemia/reperfusion-induced cerebral microcirculatory disturbances and neuron damage. *Acta Pharm. Sin. B* **2015**, *5*, 8–24. [CrossRef] [PubMed]
26. Qiang, H.; Zhang, C.; Shi, Z.-B.; Yang, H.-Q.; Wang, K.-Z. Protective effects and mechanism of Panax Notoginseng saponins on oxidative stress-induced damage and apoptosis of rabbit bone marrow stromal cells. *Chin. J. Integr. Med.* **2010**, *16*, 525–530. [CrossRef] [PubMed]
27. Zhou, P.; Xie, W.; He, S.; Sun, Y.; Meng, X.; Sun, G.; Sun, X. Ginsenoside Rb1 as an Anti-Diabetic Agent and Its Underlying Mechanism Analysis. *Cells* **2019**, *8*, 204. [CrossRef] [PubMed]
28. Zhou, P.; Xie, W.; Meng, X.; Zhai, Y.; Dong, X.; Zhang, X.; Sun, G.; Sun, X. Notoginsenoside R1 Ameliorates Diabetic Retinopathy through PINK1-Dependent Activation of Mitophagy. *Cells* **2019**, *8*, 213. [CrossRef]
29. Zhou, P.; Xie, W.; Sun, Y.; Dai, Z.; Li, G.; Sun, G.; Sun, X. Ginsenoside Rb1 and mitochondria: A short review of the literature. *Mol. Cell. Probes* **2019**, *43*, 1–5. [CrossRef] [PubMed]
30. Zhou, P.; Xie, W.; Luo, Y.; Lu, S.; Dai, Z.; Wang, R.; Zhang, X.; Li, G.; Sun, G.; Sun, X. Inhibitory Effects of Ginsenoside Rb1 on Early Atherosclerosis in ApoE-/- Mice via Inhibition of Apoptosis and Enhancing Autophagy. *Molecules* **2018**, *23*, 2912. [CrossRef]
31. Zhou, N.; Tang, Y.; Keep, R.F.; Ma, X.; Xiang, J. Antioxidative effects of Panax notoginseng saponins in brain cells. *Phytomedicine* **2014**, *21*, 1189–1195. [CrossRef]
32. Liu, X.-Y.; Wang, S.; Li, C.-J.; Ma, J.; Chen, F.-Y.; Peng, Y.; Wang, X.-L.; Zhang, D.-M. Dammarane-type saponins from the leaves of Panax notoginseng and their neuroprotective effects on damaged SH-SY5Y cells. *Phytochem.* **2018**, *145*, 10–17. [CrossRef] [PubMed]
33. Yao, C.-L.; Pan, H.-Q.; Wang, H.; Yao, S.; Yang, W.-Z.; Hou, J.-J.; Jin, Q.-H.; Wu, W.-Y.; Guo, D.-A. Global profiling combined with predicted metabolites screening for discovery of natural compounds: Characterization of ginsenosides in the leaves of Panax notoginseng as a case study. *J. Chromatogr. A* **2018**, *1538*, 34–44. [CrossRef] [PubMed]
34. Fu, J.H.; Li, X.Z.; Shang, X.H.; Liu, J.X. Protective effects of saponines of stem and leaf of Panax notoginseng on acute myocardial ischemia in anaesthetic dogs. *Chin. Mater. Med.* **2006**, *31*, 62–65. (In Chinese)
35. Chen, Z.H.; Wang, D.C.; Li, H.L.; Wei, J.X.; Wang, J.F.; Du, Y.C. Hemodynamic effects of san chi (Panax notoginseng) root, leaf, flower and saponins on anesthetized dogs. *Acta Pharm. Sin.* **1983**, *18*, 818–822. (In Chinese)
36. Meng, X.; Xie, W.; Xu, Q.; Liang, T.; Xu, X.; Sun, G.; Sun, X. Neuroprotective Effects of Radix Scrophulariae on Cerebral Ischemia and Reperfusion Injury via MAPK Pathways. *Molecules* **2018**, *23*, 2401. [CrossRef] [PubMed]
37. Oh, S.M.; Jung, B.J.; Lee, J.I.; Choi, S.K.; Kang, S.K. Middle Cerebral Artery Occlusion in Rats: Evaluation of the Model With or Without Craniectomy. *J. Korean Neurosurg Soc.* **1994**, *23*, 3–11.

38. Longa, E.Z.; Weinstein, P.R.; Carlson, S.; Cummins, R. Reversible middle cerebral artery occlusion without craniectomy in rats. *Stroke* **1989**, *20*, 84. [CrossRef] [PubMed]
39. Bederson, J.B.; Pitts, L.H.; Tsuji, M.; Nishimura, M.C.; Davis, R.L.; Bartkowski, H. Rat middle cerebral artery occlusion: evaluation of the model and development of a neurologic examination. *Stroke* **1986**, *17*, 472–476. [CrossRef] [PubMed]
40. Zhai, Y.; Meng, X.; Luo, Y.; Wu, Y.; Ye, T.; Zhou, P.; Ding, S.; Wang, M.; Lu, S.; Zhu, L. Notoginsenoside R1 ameliorates diabetic encephalopathy by activating the Nrf2 pathway and inhibiting NLRP3 inflammasome activation. *Oncotarget* **2018**, *9*, 9344–9363. [CrossRef] [PubMed]
41. Shu, Y.; Yang, Y.; Zhang, P. Neuroprotective effects of penehyclidine hydrochloride against cerebral ischemia/reperfusion injury in mice. *Brain Res. Bull.* **2016**, *121*, 115–123. [CrossRef] [PubMed]
42. Muir, K.W.; Pippa, T.; Naveed, S.; Elizabeth, W. Inflammation and ischaemic stroke. *Curr. Opin. Neurol.* **2007**, *20*, 334–342. [CrossRef] [PubMed]
43. Yang, X.; Feng, P.; Zhang, X.; Li, D.; Wang, R.; Ji, C.; Li, G.; Holscher, C. The diabetes drug semaglutide reduces infarct size, inflammation, and apoptosis, and normalizes neurogenesis in a rat model of stroke. *Neuropharmacology* **2019**, *158*, 107748. [CrossRef] [PubMed]
44. Ahmed, M.E.; Dong, Y.; Lu, Y.; Tucker, D.; Wang, R.; Zhang, Q. Beneficial Effects of a CaMKIIα Inhibitor TatCN21 Peptide in Global Cerebral Ischemia. *J. Mol. Neurosci.* **2017**, *61*, 42–51. [CrossRef] [PubMed]
45. Kim, Y.R.; Park, B.-K.; Kim, Y.H.; Shim, I.; Kang, I.-C.; Lee, M.Y. Antidepressant Effect of Fraxinus rhynchophylla Hance Extract in a Mouse Model of Chronic Stress-Induced Depression. *BioMed Res. Int.* **2018**, *2018*, 8249563. [CrossRef] [PubMed]
46. Zhou, P.; Xie, W.; Luo, Y.; Lu, S.; Dai, Z.; Wang, R.; Sun, G.; Sun, X. Protective Effects of Total Saponins of Aralia elata (Miq.) on Endothelial Cell Injury Induced by TNF-alpha via Modulation of the PI3K/Akt and NF-kappaB Signalling Pathways. *Int. J. Mol. Sci.* **2018**, *20*. [CrossRef]
47. Cheng, M.; Yang, L.; Dong, Z.; Wang, M.; Sun, Y.; Liu, H.; Wang, X.; Sai, N.; Huang, G.; Zhang, X. Folic acid deficiency enhanced microglial immune response via the Notch1/nuclear factor kappa B p65 pathway in hippocampus following rat brain I/R injury and BV2 cells. *J. Cell. Mol. Med.* **2019**, *23*, 4795–4807. [CrossRef] [PubMed]
48. Li, H.; Luo, X.B.; Xu, Y.; Hou, X.Y. A Brief Ischemic Postconditioning Protects Against Amyloid-beta Peptide Neurotoxicity by Downregulating MLK3-MKK3/6-P38MAPK Signal in Rat Hippocampus. *J. Alzheimer's Dis.* **2019**, 1–14.
49. Singh, R.; Kulikowicz, E.; Santos, P.T.; Koehler, R.C.; Martin, L.J.; Lee, J.K. Spatial T-maze identifies cognitive deficits in piglets 1 month after hypoxia-ischemia in a model of hippocampal pyramidal neuron loss and interneuron attrition. *Behav. Brain Res.* **2019**, *369*, 111921. [CrossRef]
50. Yin, H.Z.; Wang, H.L.; Ji, S.G.; Medvedeva, Y.V.; Tian, G.; Bazrafkan, A.K.; Maki, N.Z.; Akbari, Y.; Weiss, J.H. Rapid Intramitochondrial Zn^{2+} Accumulation in CA1 Hippocampal Pyramidal Neurons After Transient Global Ischemia: A Possible Contributor to Mitochondrial Disruption and Cell Death. *J. Neuropathol. Exp. Neurol.* **2019**, *78*, 655–664. [CrossRef]
51. Ramirez-Sanchez, J.; Pires, E.N.S.; Meneghetti, A.; Hansel, G.; Nunez-Figueredo, Y.; Pardo-Andreu, G.L.; Ochoa-Rodriguez, E.; Verdecia-Reyes, Y.; Delgado-Hernandez, R.; Salbego, C.; et al. JM-20 Treatment After MCAO Reduced Astrocyte Reactivity and Neuronal Death on Peri-infarct Regions of the Rat Brain. *Mol. Neurobiol.* **2019**, *56*, 502–512. [CrossRef]
52. Xiong, T.Q.; Chen, L.M.; Gui, Y.; Jiang, T.; Tan, B.H.; Li, S.L.; Li, Y.C. The effects of epothilone D on microtubule degradation and delayed neuronal death in the hippocampus following transient global ischemia. *J. Chem. Neuroanat.* **2019**, *98*, 17–26. [CrossRef] [PubMed]
53. Song, H.; Zhou, H.; Qu, Z.; Hou, J.; Chen, W.; Cai, W.; Cheng, Q.; Chuang, D.Y.; Chen, S.; Li, S.; et al. From Analysis of Ischemic Mouse Brain Proteome to Identification of Human Serum Clusterin as a Potential Biomarker for Severity of Acute Ischemic Stroke. *Transl. Stroke Res.* **2019**, *10*, 546–556. [CrossRef] [PubMed]
54. Chen, S.; Chen, Z.; Cui, J.; Mccrary, M.L.; Song, H.; Mobashery, S.; Chang, M.; Gu, Z. Early Abrogation of Gelatinase Activity Extends the Time Window for tPA Thrombolysis after Embolic Focal Cerebral Ischemia in Mice. *Eneuro* **2018**, *5*. [CrossRef] [PubMed]
55. Boehncke, W.H. Systemic Inflammation and Cardiovascular Comorbidity in Psoriasis Patients: Causes and Consequences. *Front. Immunol.* **2018**, *9*, 579. [CrossRef] [PubMed]

56. O'Connell, G.C.; Chantler, P.D.; Barr, T.L. Stroke-associated pattern of gene expression previously identified by machine-learning is diagnostically robust in an independent patient population. *Genom. Data* **2017**, *14*, 47–52. [CrossRef] [PubMed]
57. Xu, H.; Qin, W.; Hu, X.; Mu, S.; Zhu, J.; Lu, W.; Luo, Y. Lentivirus-mediated overexpression of OTULIN ameliorates microglia activation and neuroinflammation by depressing the activation of the NF-κB signaling pathway in cerebral ischemia/reperfusion rats. *J. Neuroinflammation* **2018**, *15*, 83. [CrossRef]
58. Laird, M.D.; Shields, J.S.; Sangeetha, S.R.; Kimbler, D.E.; R David, F.; Basheer, S.; Patrick, Y.; Nathan, Y.; Vender, J.R.; Dhandapani, K.M. High mobility group box protein-1 promotes cerebral edema after traumatic brain injury via activation of toll-like receptor 4. *Glia* **2013**, *62*, 26–38. [CrossRef] [PubMed]
59. Xiao-Juan, F.; Shu-Xia, L.; Chao, W.; Peng-Peng, K.; Qing-Juan, L.; Jun, H.; Hong-Bo, L.; Fan, L.; Yu-Jun, Z.; Xiao-Hui, F. The PTEN/PI3K/Akt signaling pathway mediates HMGB1-induced cell proliferation by regulating the NF-κB/cyclin D1 pathway in mouse mesangial cells. *Am. J. Physiology Cell Physiol.* **2014**, *306*, 1119–1128.

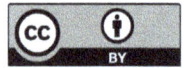

© 2019 by the authors. Licensee MDPI, Basel, Switzerland. This article is an open access article distributed under the terms and conditions of the Creative Commons Attribution (CC BY) license (http://creativecommons.org/licenses/by/4.0/).

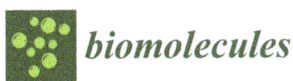

Article

Comparative Analysis of *Panax ginseng* Berries from Seven Cultivars Using UPLC-QTOF/MS and NMR-Based Metabolic Profiling

Dahye Yoon [1], Bo-Ram Choi [1,2], Young-Chang Kim [1], Seon Min Oh [1,2], Hyoung-Geun Kim [2], Jang-Uk Kim [1], Nam-In Baek [2], Suhkmann Kim [3] and Dae Young Lee [1,*]

[1] Department of Herbal Crop Research, National Institute of Horticultural and Herbal Science, RDA, Eumseong 27709, Korea
[2] Department of Oriental Medicine Biotechnology, Kyung Hee University, Yongin 17104, Korea
[3] Department of Chemistry, Center for Proteome Biophysics, and Chemistry Institute for Functional Materials, Pusan National University, Busan 46241, Korea
* Correspondence: dylee0809@gmail.com; Tel.: +82-43-871-5784

Received: 14 August 2019; Accepted: 27 August 2019; Published: 28 August 2019

Abstract: The commercial use of *Panax ginseng* berries is increasing as *P. ginseng* berries are known to contain large amounts of ginsenosides, and many pharmacological activities have been reported for the various ginsenosides. For the proper use of *P. ginseng* berries, it is necessary to study efficient and accurate quality control and the profiling of the overall composition of each cultivar. Ginseng berry samples from seven cultivars (Eumseung, Chung-buk Province, Republic of Korea) were analyzed using ultra-performance liquid chromatography-quadrupole-time-of-flight mass spectrometry (UPLC-QTOF/MS) for profiling of the ginsenosides, and high-resolution magic-angle-spinning nuclear magnetic resonance (HR-MAS NMR) spectroscopy for profiling of the primary metabolites. Comparing twenty-six ginsenoside profiles between the variant representatives and between the violet-stem variant, Kumpoong and Sunwon were classified. In the case of primary metabolites, the cultivars Kumpoong and Gopoong were classified. As a result of correlation analyses of the primary and secondary metabolites, in the Gopoong cultivar, the metabolism was found to lean toward energy metabolism rather than ginsenoside synthesis, and accumulation of osmolytes was low. The Gopoong cultivar had higher levels of most of the amino acids, such as arginine, phenylalanine, isoleucine, threonine, and valine, and it contained the highest level of choline and the lowest level of myo-inositol. Except for these, there were no significant differences of primary metabolites. In the Kumpoong cultivar, the protopanaxatriol (PPT)-type ginsenosides, ginsenoside Re and ginsenoside Rg2, were much lower than in the other cultivars, while the other PPT-type ginsenosides were inversely found in much higher amounts than in other cultivars. The Sunwon cultivar showed that variations of PPT-type ginsenosides were significantly different between samples. However, the median values of PPT-type ginsenosides of Sunwon showed similar levels to those of Kumpoong. The difference in primary metabolites used for metabolism for survival was found to be small in our results. Our data demonstrated the characteristics of each cultivar using profiling data of the primary and secondary metabolites, especially for Gopoong, Kumpoong, and Sunwon. These profiling data provided important information for further research and commercial use.

Keywords: Ginseng berries; UPLC-QTOF/MS; HR-MAS NMR spectroscopy; ginsenoside; primary metabolite

1. Introduction

Panax ginseng C.A. Mey. is one of the most important herbal products today, and its root has been widely used as a constituent of traditional medicine in Korea and other countries [1].

P. ginseng root contains diverse bioactive compounds, and ginsenosides are the major components. Previously, a number of studies have reported that ginsenosides show various pharmacological properties such as antitumor, antidiabetes, antifatigue, antistress, antioxidative, and antiaging effects, as well as enhancement of the immune system [2–5].

Due to their utility, the interest in the therapeutic potential of ginsenosides has increased. Ginsenosides are distributed in several parts of the *P. ginseng* plant, including not only the root but also the leaves and berries. Different parts of the plant contain distinct constituent compositions, and therefore may have different pharmacological activities [6–8].

Most of the previous reports on this topic have focused on the ginseng root as a reservoir of ginsenosides. Recent studies have also demonstrated that ginseng berries have a high content of ginsenosides, and their own various pharmacological properties [9–12].

Dey et al. compared the antihyperglycemic effect of both ginseng root and ginseng berries. They found that the berry exhibits more potent antihyperglycemic activity than the root, and only the berry shows marked antiobesity effects in mice [13].

Moreover, ginseng berry extract and compounds show potent antioxidative and antitumor activities [12,14,15].

In order to provide new insights for future study into *P. ginseng* berries, Lee et al. reviewed the chemical constituents and biological activities of the ginseng berry [16].

For the phytochemical study and quality control of ginseng berries, it is critical to assess the ginsenoside content in the berries. Analytical methods for assessing ginsenosides have been established by high-performance liquid chromatography (HPLC) coupled with a UV detector [6,17], or an evaporative light-scattering detector (ELSD) [18].

However, this method is limited to the simultaneous analysis of multiple target compounds. Additionally, such methods still lack the required sensitivity and selectivity to profile various ginsenosides. Recently, liquid chromatography (LC) coupled with mass spectrometry (MS) has emerged as a good tool for the sensitive and selective analysis of various ginsenosides. In particular, a quadrupole-time-of-flight (QTOF)/MS with ultra-performance liquid chromatography (UPLC) system is useful for the rapid and high-resolution separation of ginsenosides in ginseng [8,19,20].

The secondary metabolites of many plants have been studied extensively because they are characterized by the influence of plant characteristics and the environment. Although the primary metabolites are essential for growth and development, there is relatively less research focused on them compared to secondary metabolites. However, these secondary metabolites are produced from the primary metabolites. The study of primary metabolites, as well as secondary metabolites, is important in phytochemical research. For screening the major primary metabolites of a powdered sample, high-resolution magic-angle-spinning nuclear magnetic resonance (HR-MAS NMR) spectroscopy is a good tool without requiring extraction of the sample. The dipolar, chemical shift anisotropy and magnetic susceptibility interactions vanish when a powdered sample is spun with a magic angle (54.7°). Therefore, a reduced line width, which is similar to the resolution of the solution, can be observed by HR-MAS NMR spectroscopy [21].

Thus, in this study, UPLC-QTOF/MS was used to perform a comprehensive profiling of ginsenosides from extract of the ginseng berry and HR-MAS NMR spectroscopy was used to identify and quantify the major primary metabolites from a powder of the ginseng berry. The ginsenoside content and the major primary metabolites of ginseng berries may differ depending on the cultivars. The comprehensive profiling of various ginsenosides and the primary metabolites of the ginseng varieties that are currently grown by the National Institute of Horticultural and Herbal Science (NIHHS), Chunpoong, Chungsun, Kumpoong, Yunpoong, Gopoong, Sunwon, and Sunun, have not yet been fully reported. The metabolite profiling and classification of seven cultivars with this comparative method is applicable to the evaluation and control of the quality of ginseng berries.

2. Materials and Methods

2.1. Ginseng Berry Samples

Six-year-old ginseng berries were cultivated in the field of the Department of Herbal Crop Research (DHCR) located in Eumseung, Chung-buk Province (127°45′013.14″E, 36°56′36.63″N), Republic of Korea. This cultivation protocol was followed by the "ginseng GAP standard cultivation guideline" developed by the Rural Development Administration (RDA), Republic of Korea. On July 25, 2017, ginseng berries, randomly selected from those available on this date, were collected from the 10–15 samples of six-year-old ginseng of the seven cultivars (Figure 1). The seeds were removed from the ginseng berries, and the fruits were crushed and stored at –80 °C and freeze-dried by freeze dryer under reduced pressure (–30 °C, 100 mTorr) for 24 h. A voucher specimen (NIHHS-201707) was deposited at the Herbarium of DHCR, NIHHS, RDA, Republic of Korea.

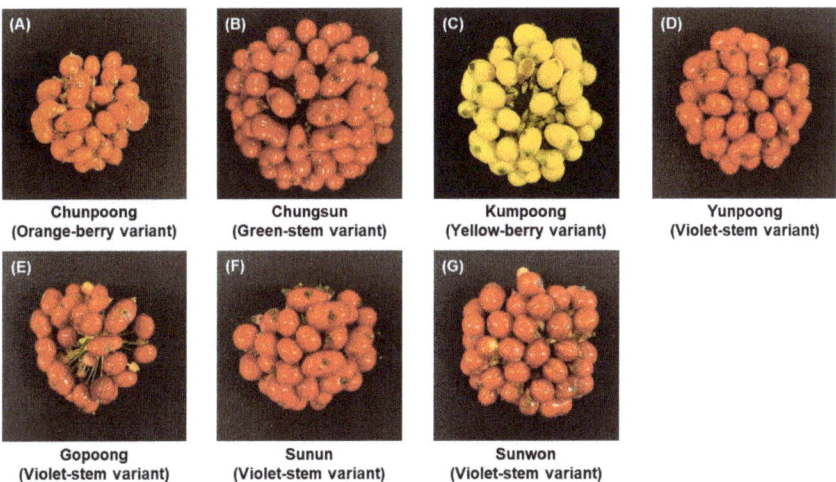

Figure 1. Characteristics of the fruit of varieties of ginseng. (**A**) Chunpoong. The color of the berries is orange. (**B**) Chungsun. The color of the berries is red. (**C**) Kumpoong. The color of the berries is yellow. (**D**) Yunpoong. The color of the berries is red. (**E**) Gopoong. The color of the berries is red. (**F**) Sunun. The color of the berries is red. (**G**) Sunwon. The color of the berries is red.

2.2. Standard Constituents and Reagents

HPLC-grade acetonitrile, methanol, and water were obtained from Merck (Darmstadt, Germany). Formic acid, deuterium oxide (D_2O), and 3-(trimethylsilyl) propionic-2,2,3,3-d_4 acid sodium salt (TSP-d_4) were purchased from Sigma-Aldrich (St. Louis, MO, USA). The ginsenosides were isolated and purified from *P. ginseng* roots by a series of chromatography procedures in our laboratory, and their structures were elucidated by comparison of spectroscopic data (MS, ^{1}H-NMR, and ^{13}C-NMR) with the literature data: ginsenoside Rb1, Ra2, Ra3, Rc, Ra1, Rb2, Rb3, Rd, F2, Rg3, Rh2, compound K, 20-O-glucoginsenoside Rf, ginsenoside Rg1, Rg2, Re, Rf, Rh1, notoginsenoside R2, ginsenoside F1, Rg6, Rk1, Ro, and Rk3, ginsenoside F4, Rh4, and Rg5 [8]. The purity of the isolated compounds was determined to be more than 98% by normalization of the peak areas detected by HPLC analysis.

2.3. Sample Preparation

Ginseng berries were lyophilized and ground (<0.5 mm) using a mixer (Hanil, Seoul, Korea) and thoroughly mixed, and subsamples were homogenized further using a Retsch MM400 mixer mill (Retsch GmbH, Haan, Germany) for later analyses.

For the UPLC-QTOF/MS analysis, fine powder was weighed (100 mg), suspended in 1 mL of 70% (v/v) methanol, and ultrasonically extracted for 1 h at 50 °C. After the centrifugation (13,500× g, 5 min at 4 °C), 900 µL of supernatant was transferred to a new Eppendorf tube. The solution was filtered through a syringe PTFE filter (0.2 µm) and diluted 20 times. Each sample was injected directly into the UPLC system.

For the HR-MAS NMR analysis, each powder sample was weighed to give 3 mg and transferred to the NMR nano tube (Agilent Technologies, Santa Clara, CA, USA). For the NMR analysis, 37 µL of D_2O containing 2 mM TSP-d_4 was added to each NMR nanotube before the NMR measurement.

2.4. UPLC-QTOF/MS Analysis

UPLC was carried out on a Waters ACQUITY H-Class UPLC (Waters Corp, Milford, MA, USA) Chromatographic separations were performed on a Thermo Hypersil Gold column (2.1 mm × 100 mm, 1.9 µm). The column oven was maintained at 40 °C and the mobile phases consisted of solvent A [Water + 0.1% formic acid (v/v)] and solvent B [Acetonitrile + 0.1% formic acid (v/v)]. The elution gradient was as follows: 0–0.5 min, B 15%; 0.5–1 min, B 15–20%; 1–6 min, B 20%; 6–13 min, B 20–30%; 13–23 min, B 30–35%; 23–24 min, B 35–38%; 24–27 min, B 38–60%; 27–31 min, B 60–90%; 31–32 min, B 90–15%; 32–34 min, B 15%. The injection volume was 2 µL and the flow rate was 500 µL/min for each run. Methanol was run after every sample as a blank. Next, MS analysis was conducted on a Waters Xevo G2-S QTOF MS (Waters Corp.) in the negative ion mode. The mass spectrometers performed the MS^E acquisition mode with alternative high- and low-energy scans. The operational parameters were set as follows: source temperature, 120 °C; desolvation temperature, 550 °C; cone voltage, 40 V; capillary, 3.0 kV; cone gas flow, 30 L/h; and desolvation gas flow, 800 L/h. Accurate mass measurements were achieved with the use of an automatic calibration delivery system, which contained the internal reference [Leucine-enkephalin, m/z 556.276 (ESI+), m/z 554.262 (ESI-)]. Data were collected from m/z 100 to 2000 [8].

2.5. HR-MAS NMR Analysis

All spectra were acquired with a 600.167 MHz Agilent NMR spectrometer equipped with a 4 mm gHX NanoProbe (Agilent technologies, Santa Clara, CA, USA). The spinning rate was 2000 Hz. A total of 128 transients were collected using CPMG (Carr–Purcell–Meiboom–Gill) with a PRESAT pulse sequence for the suppression of water and high molecular mass compounds [22]. The spectra were obtained using 1.704 s of acquisition time, 1 s of relaxation delay, and 128 transients. The TSP-d_4 peak at 0.00 ppm was used for the reference to calibrate the chemical shift [23]. All spectra were phased and the baselines corrected manually. Metabolite assignment and quantification for each sample were processed using Chenomx NMR Suite 7.1 Professional (Chenomx Inc., Canada) and the Chenomx 600 MHz library database. For the multivariate statistical analysis, each NMR spectrum was binned from 0.5 to 8.0 ppm, and the water peak was excluded. The binning size was 0.001 ppm and normalization was conducted with total area. The binned spectra were aligned using the icoshift algorithm of MATLAB R2013b (The MathWorks, Natick, MA, USA). After the alignment, multivariate statistical analyses were conducted using SIMCA-P+ 12.0 software (Umetrics, Umeå, Sweden). The principal component analysis (PCA), partial least squares discriminant analysis (PLS-DA), and orthogonal partial least squares discriminant analysis (OPLS-DA) were processed.

3. Results

3.1. Construction of LC-MS Conditions to Profile Various Ginsenosides

For a comprehensive profiling of various ginsenosides from the *P. ginseng* berry, an analytical method based on UPLC-QTOF/MS was constructed. Extracts of natural products generally have complex metabolites, including known and unknown compounds. To identify the metabolites in a mixture, it is critical to measure the exact mass values of target metabolites. QTOF/MS, which provides a full mass scan at high resolution, is an effective way to analyze ginsenosides in a complex mixture. Among the various ginsenosides, there are several isomers that have the same mass values but different molecular structures. To determine the isomers, chromatographic separation is also required. A UPLC system with a small particle size column provides the rapid and effective separation of various compounds, including isomers. Thus, we used UPLC-QTOF/MS to profile various ginsenosides from the ginseng berry.

First, 37 standard samples of ginsenosides were used to optimize the LC-MS conditions. In the negative mode of electrospray ionization (ESI), the 37 ginsenosides were mainly detected as $[M - H]^-$ and $[M + COOH]^-$ ions. Under a flow rate of 500 µL/min using a Thermo Hypersil Gold column (2.1 mm × 100 mm, 1.9 µm particle size), various ginsenoside standards were separated well and eluted in 34 min. Although several compounds were eluted at almost the same times, the exact mass values could differentiate the ginsenosides. For a reliable and high-throughput analysis of various ginsenosides from many ginseng berry samples, it is required to construct an in-house library for the ginsenosides. The molecular formula and retention time (RT) of 37 ginsenosides were listed in the library. The m/z of ions from the ginsenoside profile data was automatically matched to the library compounds.

To construct the in-house library for the 37 ginsenosides, the molecular formula of each compound was added into the UNIFI software (v1.8, Waters Corp., Milford, MA, USA).

Next, we optimized the protocols to extract the ginsenosides from the ginseng berries. For effective extraction, it is critical to select a suitable solvent. Previously, several solvents such as water, ethanol (EtOH), and methanol (MeOH) have been widely used to extract ginsenosides from ginseng berries. First, we tried to compare the extraction efficiency of both EtOH and MeOH. A cultivar of ginseng berry, called Kumpoong, was used in this experiment. The EtOH or MeOH extracts of the ginseng berry were subjected to UPLC-QTOF/MS analysis. There was no significant difference between these two solvents, and we selected MeOH.

3.2. Profiling of Various Ginsenosides from Seven Different Cultivars of Ginseng Berries

The UPLC-QTOF/MS-based metabolomics approach was applied to identify the ginsenosides. Total ion chromatograms were obtained from seven different cultivars of ginseng berries using optimized conditions for UPLC-QTOF/MS (Figure 2).

After metabolite profiling of individual samples by UPLC-QTOF/MS, each set of data was processed using the UNIFI software. Progenesis QI v2.3 (Nonlinear Dynamics, Newcastle, UK) was used for data processing, including peak picking, alignment, and univariate analysis for filtering the peaks as follows: fold change >2, and p-value < 0.05. In total, 5655 peaks were filtered, and then the peaks were matched with the ginsenoside library. Therefore, 26 ginsenosides were identified. Heatmap analysis was conducted with these ginsenoside profiles of representative cultivars in each variant (Figure 3A). Kumpoong in the yellow-berry variant showed a different pattern to the other cultivars, and Chunpoong in the orange-berry variant and Yunpoong in the violet-stem variant, which are native cultivars, had similar patterns to each other. On the other hand, in the results of heatmap analysis with four cultivars of the violet-stem variant, Sunwon showed patterns different from the other cultivars (Figure 3B).

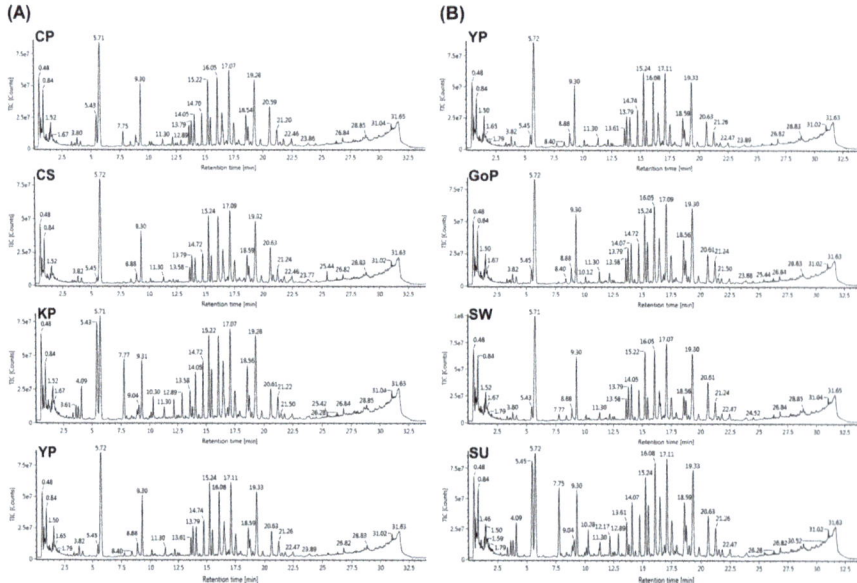

Figure 2. Representative ultra-performance liquid chromatography-quadrupole-time-of-flight mass spectrometry (UPLC–QTOF/MS) total ion chromatograms (TIC) of ginseng berry extracts. (**A**) Comparison of representative cultivars in each variant (CP, Chunpoong; CS, Chungsun; KP, Kumpoong; YP, Yunpoong). (**B**) Comparison of cultivars in the violet-stem variant (YP, Yunpoong; GoP, Gopoong; SW, Sunwon; SU, Sunun). See retention time in Table 1.

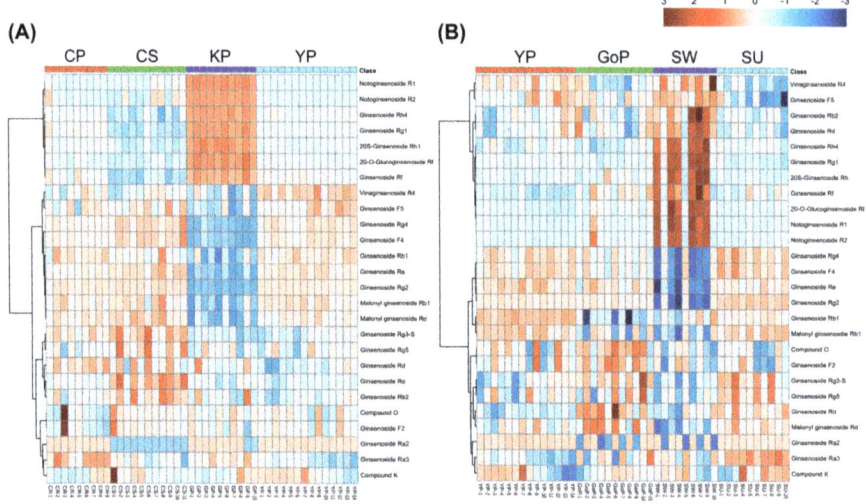

Figure 3. Heatmap of ginsenoside profiles from different cultivars. (**A**) Comparison of representative cultivars in each variant (CP, Chunpoong; CS, Chungsun; KP, Kumpoong; YP, Yunpoong). (**B**) Comparison of cultivars in the violet-stem variant (YP, Yunpoong; GoP, Gopoong; SW, Sunwon; SU, Sunun).

Table 1. Relative percentages of ginsenosides in each cultivar (%).

No.	Expected RT (min)	Component Name	Formula	Observed m/z	Observed RT (min)	Adducts	Average of Relative Percentage (%)						
							CP	CS	KP	YP	GoP	SW	SU
1	3.6	20-O-Glucoginsenoside Rf	C48H82O19	1007.5265	3.62	+HCOO, -H	0.0732	0.0563	0.2943	0.0764	0.0899	0.2539	0.0787
2	4.07	Notoginsenoside R1	C47H80O18	977.5161	4.09	+HCOO, -H	0.0478	0.0570	0.7476	0.0409	0.0511	0.4965	0.0406
3	5.35	Ginsenoside Rg1	C42H72O14	845.4773	5.45	+HCOO, -H	0.8297	0.2613	3.4380	0.5507	0.5116	2.4831	0.4419
4	5.66	Ginsenoside Re	C48H82O18	991.5347	5.71	+HCOO, -H	6.7781	7.3395	4.5799	7.3372	6.7865	5.3904	6.7817
5	11.2	vinaginsenoside R4	C48H82O19	1007.5265	11.30	+HCOO, -H	0.2449	0.2195	0.2489	0.2805	0.2415	0.3290	0.2317
6	12.11	Ginsenoside Rf	C42H72O14	845.4770	12.17	+HCOO, -H	0.1992	0.1142	0.4025	0.1991	0.2414	0.3307	0.2202
7	12.81	Notoginsenoside R2	C41H70O13	815.4644	12.89	+HCOO, -H	0.0368	0.0528	0.5008	0.0193	0.0384	0.2823	0.0203
8	13.43	Ginsenoside F5	C41H70O13	815.4669	13.58	+HCOO, -H	0.4852	0.4637	0.4576	0.5050	0.4842	0.5796	0.4123
9	13.56	20(S)-Ginsenoside Rh1	C36H62O9	683.4246	13.66	+HCOO	0.0128	0.0090	0.0354	0.0114	0.0119	0.0258	0.0107
10	13.7	Ginsenoside Rg2	C42H72O13	829.4824	13.79	+HCOO, -H	0.9250	0.9064	0.2598	0.9042	0.8504	0.4588	1.0673
11	14.51	Ginsenoside Ra3	C59H100O27	1285.6185	14.27	+HCOO, -H	0.0033	0.0023	0.0032	0.0022	0.0026	0.0027	0.0031
12	14.35	Ginsenoside Ra2	C58H98O26	1255.6049	14.52	+HCOO, -H	0.0054	0	0.0057	0.0051	0.0031	0.0027	0.0038
13	14.53	Ginsenoside Rb1	C54H92O23	1153.5806	14.72	+HCOO, -H	0.5071	0.4411	0.4727	0.4999	0.3281	0.4326	0.4280
14	15.12	Malonyl ginsenoside Rb1	C57H94O26	1193.5794	15.24	-H	3.0830	2.9241	2.6016	3.1462	2.5714	2.5060	3.1080
15	15.69	Ginsenoside Ro	C48H76O19	955.4726	15.73	-H	0.0486	0.0705	0.0530	0.0437	0.0621	0.0506	0.0563
16	16.3	Ginsenoside Rb2	C53H90O22	1123.5710	16.48	+HCOO, -H	0.9968	1.0124	1.1320	0.9467	0.9372	1.1441	0.9034
17	18.34	Ginsenoside Rd	C48H82O18	991.5318	18.58	+HCOO, -H	1.6839	1.4716	1.7702	1.4030	1.4115	1.7513	1.3188
18	19.11	Malonyl ginsenoside Rd	C51H84O21	1031.5279	19.32	-H	5.0173	4.8832	4.3847	4.8414	5.1380	4.6440	4.9302
19	23.46	Ginsenoside Rg4	C42H70O12	811.4684	23.75	+HCOO, -H	0.0430	0.0489	0.0249	0.0459	0.0397	0.0310	0.0488
20	23.5	Compound O	C47H80O17	961.5136	23.77	+HCOO, -H	0.0930	0.0498	0.0527	0.0439	0.0610	0.0338	0.0317
21	24.28	Ginsenoside F4	C42H70O12	811.4695	24.52	+HCOO, -H	0.0964	0.1100	0.0566	0.1013	0.0864	0.0678	0.1077
22	24.68	Ginsenoside Rh4	C36H60O8	665.4140	24.90	+HCOO	0.0003	0.0001	0.0024	0.0003	0.0002	0.0016	0.0003
23	25.19	Ginsenoside F2	C42H72O13	829.4626	25.44	+HCOO, -H	0.0655	0.0346	0.0276	0.0238	0.0333	0.0201	0.0185
24	26.01	Ginsenoside Rg3-S	C42H72O13	829.4784	26.19	+HCOO, -H	0.0240	0.0252	0.0219	0.0198	0.0224	0.0199	0.0223
25	27.35	Compound K	C36H62O8	667.4320	27.54	+HCOO	0.0028	0.0060	0.0038	0.0039	0.0034	0.0038	0.0043
26	27.55	Ginsenoside Rg5	C42H70O12	811.4685	27.75	-H	0.0135	0.0153	0.0157	0.0135	0.0140	0.0134	0.0148

3.3. Profiling of Primary Metabolites from Different Cultivars of Ginseng Berries Using HR-MAS NMR

The primary metabolites from seven different cultivars of ginseng berry were analyzed using HR-MAS NMR spectroscopy (Figures S1 and S2). The representative ^{1}H-NMR spectrum is shown in Figure 4.

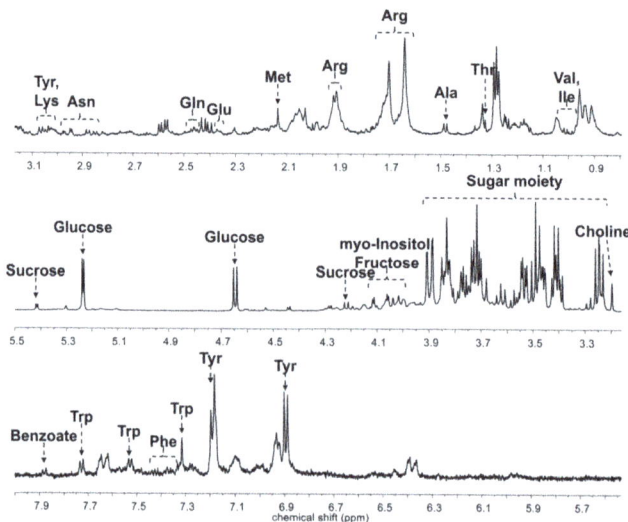

Figure 4. Representative ^{1}H-nuclear magnetic resonance (NMR) spectrum with metabolite annotation. Ala, alanine; Arg, arginine; Asn, asparagine; Gln, glutamine; Glu, glutamate; Ile, isoleucine; Lys, lysine; Met, methionine; Phe, phenylalanine; Thr, threonine; Trp, tryptophan; Tyr, tyrosine; Val, valine.

Twenty-four primary metabolites were identified and quantified, and a one-way analysis of variance (ANOVA) was conducted using MetaboAnalyst 4.0 (https://www.metaboanalyst.ca). In the results of the one-way ANOVAs on all cultivars, alanine, arginine, benzoate, choline, glucose, glutamate, lysine, methionine, phenylalanine, sucrose, tyrosine, valine, and myo-inositol were found to be the significant metabolites (p-value <0.05). In the comparison of the representative cultivars in each variant, glutamate, methionine, choline, glucose, asparagine, phenylalanine, and lysine were significant, and in the comparison of the four cultivars in the violet-stem variant, myo-inositol, alanine, sucrose, arginine, methionine, choline, valine, tyrosine, phenylalanine, glutamate, tryptophan, sn-glycero-3-phosphocholine, lysine, and fructose were significant.

Multivariate statistical analyses of the NMR spectra were conducted for a spectral pattern comparison of cultivars. Multivariate statistical analyses were performed on the Pareto-scaled NMR spectra of all samples. PCA, PLS-DA, and OPLS-DA were performed, but the clustering pattern was not good in the PCA models. PLS-DA and OPLS-DA showed the same clustering pattern, and OPLS-DA showed a clearer classification. Therefore, we presented the OPLS-DA score plots (Figure 5). The OPLS-DA score plot of representative cultivars in each variant showed the clustering of Chunpoong with Chungsun. Kumpoong was clearly differentiated. In the comparison of cultivars in the violet-stem variant, the score plot showed similar patterns for Sunun and Yunpoong.

However, Gopoong showed a clear classification. These clustering patterns were different from the results of UPLC-QTOF/MS. From this, it was predicted that the perturbation patterns of primary and secondary metabolites differed according to the cultivars.

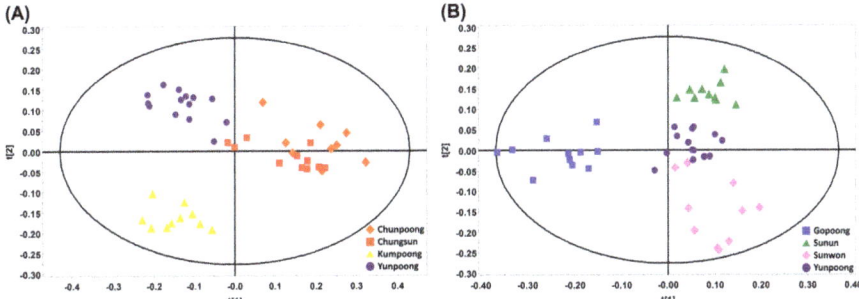

Figure 5. Multivariate statistical analyses of NMR spectra from different cultivars. (**A**) Comparison of representative cultivars in each variant (♦, Chunpoong; ■, Chungsun; ▲, Kumpoong; ●, Yunpoong). (**B**) Comparison of cultivars in violet-stem variant (■, Gopoong; ▲, Sunun; ♦, Sunwon; ●, Yunpoong).

3.4. Pearson Correlation Analysis of Metabolites

The results of clustering showed differences in the primary and secondary metabolites of different cultivars. These results suggest that the degree of metabolic pathway activation among cultivars may be different. Therefore, a Pearson correlation analysis was performed using MetaboAnalyst 4.0 (Xia Lab, McGill University, Montréal, Quebec, Canada) to confirm the correlation between the primary metabolites and the secondary metabolites, and to interrelate this with the metabolic pathway (Figure 6). Samples were normalized by a pooled sample from the Yunpoong cultivar, which is one of the native species. Log transformation was used to obtain a normal distribution. Data were scaled with Pareto scaling.

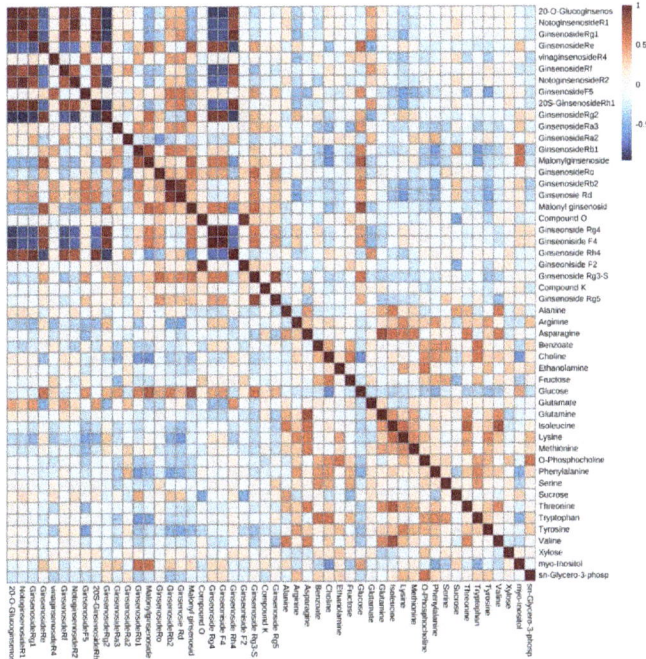

Figure 6. Correlation matrix of primary metabolites and ginsenosides. The scale bar shows the correlation coefficient from −1 to +1.

The range of the correlation coefficient (r) is from −1 to +1. In the case of a value less than 0, it is considered a negative correlation, and a value over 0 is considered a positive correlation [24]. The r value can be divided by the degree of correlation: 0.40–0.69, moderate correlation; 0.70–0.89, strong correlation; 0.90–1.00, very strong correlation [25].

4. Discussion

The purpose of this study was to investigate the metabolite profiles of various ginseng berry cultivars and to investigate the differences among the cultivars by profiling the primary metabolites, which are required for survival, and the ginsenosides, which are functional metabolites. From the analysis results, it was confirmed that the primary metabolites and ginsenosides were different among cultivars, and correlation analysis was performed to confirm the relationship between them. The r value obtained from the correlation analysis indicates the degree of correlation, and the interval is divided into specific standards. However, these standards are controversial, and researchers use different standards in various ways. In our results, the data was cut off based on the r value of 0.4. Most of the amino acids which had r values > 0.4 with ginsenosides showed negative correlations. Conversely, glucose had positive correlations with the ginsenosides, with an r value > 0.4. These metabolites are all on the energy metabolic pathway, and the cultivars that had abundant glucose had also abundant ginsenosides (Re, Rb1, Rb2, and Rg3(S)). The synthesis of ginsenosides requires acetyl-CoA which is formatted through glycolysis from glucose, therefore abundant glucose can make more ginsenosides. On the other hand, when acetyl-CoA is utilized in the synthesis of ginsenosides, amino acids should supplement the acetyl-CoA and TCA intermediates for normal energy metabolism. Therefore, ginsenosides have negative correlations with amino acids (Figure 7) [26].

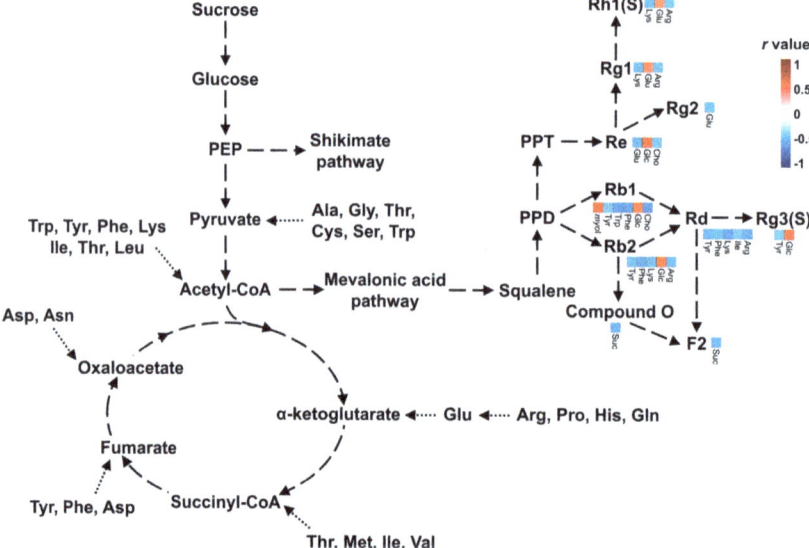

Figure 7. Pathway of energy metabolism and ginsenoside synthesis. Selected correlation matrix plots of primary metabolites with $r > 0.4$ are shown for each ginsenoside.

Sucrose synthesized from leaves is transported to nonphotosynthetic organs to supply energy and carbon skeletons [27]. Glucose is obtained from sucrose and used for synthesis of ginsenosides. Therefore, sucrose and ginsenosides showed negative correlations in our results. Choline is the precursor of glycinebetaine, which has the role of protecting plants from stress through the structural stabilization of complex proteins and membranes [28]. Myo-inositol is an osmolyte that plays an important role in phosphate storage, cell wall biosynthesis, stress-related molecular production, intercellular communication, and plant hormone transport [29]. From these results, choline and myo-inositol showed the opposite pattern of concentrations. Choline had a negative correlation with ginsenoside Rb1 and malonyl ginsenoside Rb1. On the other hand, myo-inositol had a positive correlation with them. These results were combined to link the more active metabolic pathway to the cultivars. The most specific cultivar was Gopoong. Most of the amino acids (arginine, phenylalanine, isoleucine, threonine, and valine) were present at higher levels in this cultivar, and most of the ginsenosides showed lower or similar levels than in the other cultivars. This seems to be due to normal energy metabolism rather than ginsenoside synthesis being prioritized in Gopoong. Gopoong contained the highest amount of choline among the cultivars, and the lowest amount of myo-inositol. It is thought to undergo less osmotic stress than the other cultivars. The other cultivars showed no significant differences in primary metabolites (Figure S3), and although the ginsenosides showed differences, they were not characteristic in the protopanaxadiol (PPD)-type (Figure S4). However, Kumpoong and Sunwon showed characteristic patterns in protopanaxatriol (PPT)-type ginsenosides (Figure 8). Notoginsenoside R1, R2, ginsenoside Rg1, Rh4, Rf, Rh1(S), and 20-O-glucoginsenoside Rf were present in higher levels in Kumpoong than in the other cultivars, while Re and Rg2 existed in much smaller amounts. In PPT-type ginsenosides, Sunwon showed a larger variation among samples than the other cultivars, however, the median values of these ginsenosides had levels similar to those of Kumpoong. Ginsenoside Rg4 and F4 were also weak, but showed patterns similar to Re and Rg2. Since there are few differences in the primary metabolites between cultivars, which are essential for general survival, there is little difference in the basic metabolism among the cultivars. However, the ginsenoside contents were different in each cultivar because of the different pathways and degree of response to the external environment in each cultivar.

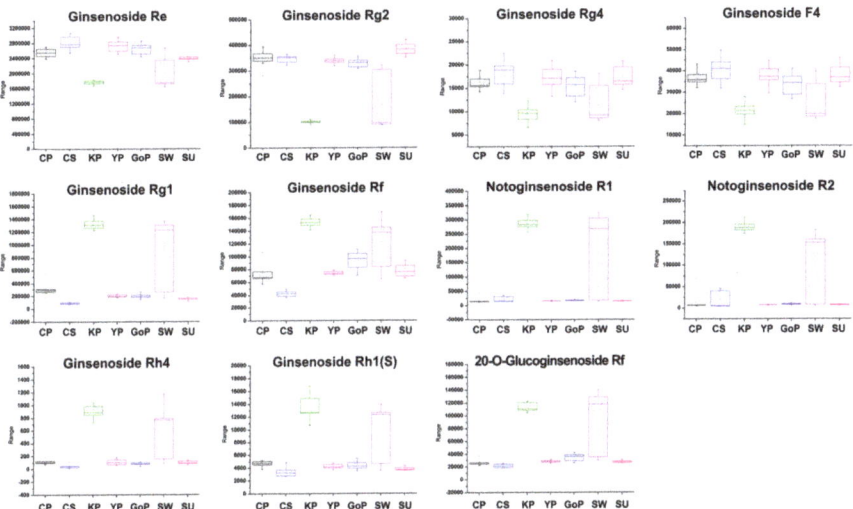

Figure 8. Box plots of protopanaxatriol (PPT)-type ginsenosides which showed characteristic patterns in the Kumpoong (KP) and Sunwon (SW) cultivars.

These results can provide information on the cultivars that is useful for the production of pharmaceuticals, cosmetics, and so forth containing specific bioactivity. It is advantageous to use Chunpoong, Chungsun, Yunpoong, Gopoong, and Sunun for producing antidiabetic agents, based on the biological activity of ginsenoside Re [2,30–32]. On the other hand, the use of notoginsenoside R1, R2, ginsenoside Rg1, Rf, and Rh1-rich Kumpoong and Sunwon will be of benefit in the production of pharmaceuticals with neuroprotective effects [33–40] and cardioprotective effects [41–45].

5. Conclusions

This study was conducted to profile the overall metabolites of ginseng berries with pharmacological activities for commercial enhancement and quality control. There are various cultivars of ginseng berry, and representative cultivars of them were analyzed by UPLC-QTOF/MS and HR-MAS NMR spectroscopy for profiling of the primary and secondary metabolites. As a result, primary and secondary metabolites showed different patterns among cultivars. Therefore, the correlations between primary and secondary metabolites were analyzed. A characteristic metabolic pattern in Gopoong and the differential content of PPT-type ginsenosides in Kumpoong and Sunwon were confirmed. It was a new approach to the analysis of the correlation between primary and secondary metabolites in the ginseng berries. Through this study, it was possible to confirm the overall constituents by profiling the primary and secondary metabolites of the ginseng berry, and the characteristics of each variant were compared by confirming their differences.

Supplementary Materials: The following are available online at http://www.mdpi.com/2218-273X/9/9/424/s1, Figure S1: Representative ^{1}H-NMR spectra of representative cultivars in each variant, Figure S2: Representative ^{1}H-NMR spectra of cultivars in the violet-stem variant, Figure S3: Box plots of quantified primary metabolites, Figure S4: Box plots of quantified ginsenosides.

Author Contributions: Conceptualization, N.-I.B. and D.Y.L.; Data curation, D.Y.; Formal analysis, B.-R.C., S.M.O., H.-G.K. and S.K.; Investigation, D.Y.; Resources, Y.-C.K. and J.-U.K.; Writing – original draft, D.Y. and D.Y.L.; Writing – review & editing, D.Y.L.

Funding: This research was funded by the "Cooperative Research Program for Agriculture Science & Technology Development" (Project No. PJ01420402) of the Rural Development Administration, Republic of Korea.

Conflicts of Interest: The authors declare no conflicts of interest. The founding sponsors had no role in the design of the study; collection, analyses, or interpretation of the data; writing of the manuscript; or decision to publish the results.

Abbreviations

ANOVA	analysis of variance
ELSD	evaporative light-scattering detector
ESI	electrospray ionization
HPLC	high-performance liquid chromatography
HR-MAS	high-resolution magic angle spinning
HR-MAS	high-resolution magic angle spinning
LODs	limits of detection
MS	mass spectrometry
NMR	nuclear magnetic resonance
OPLS-DA	orthogonal partial least squares discriminant analysis
PCA	principal component analysis
PLS-DA	partial least squares discriminant analysis
PPD	protopanaxadiol
PPT	protopanaxatriol
QTOF	quadrupole time of flight
RT	retention time

References

1. Wang, Y.; Pan, J.Y.; Xiao, X.Y.; Lin, R.C.; Cheng, Y.Y. Simultaneous determination of ginsenosides in *Panax ginseng* with different growth ages using high-performance liquid chromatography–mass spectrometry. *Phytochem. Anal.* **2006**, *17*, 424–430. [CrossRef]
2. Xie, J.-T.; Mehendale, S.R.; Li, X.; Quigg, R.; Wang, X.; Wang, C.-Z.; Wu, J.A.; Aung, H.H.; Rue, P.A.; Bell, G.I. Anti-diabetic effect of ginsenoside Re in ob/ob mice. *BBA-Mol. Basis Dis.* **2005**, *1740*, 319–325. [CrossRef] [PubMed]

3. Kenarova, B.; Neychev, H.; Hadjiivanova, C.; Petkov, V.D. Immunomodulating activity of ginsenoside Rg1 from *Panax ginseng*. *Jpn. J. Pharmacol.* **1990**, *54*, 447–454. [CrossRef] [PubMed]
4. Yue, P.Y.K.; Mak, N.K.; Cheng, Y.K.; Leung, K.W.; Ng, T.B.; Fan, D.T.P.; Yeung, H.W.; Wong, R.N.S. Pharmacogenomics and the Yin/Yang actions of ginseng: Anti-tumor, angiomodulating and steroid-like activities of ginsenosides. *Chin. Med.-UK* **2007**, *2*, 6. [CrossRef] [PubMed]
5. Tang, W.; Zhang, Y.; Gao, J.; Ding, X.; Gao, S. The anti-fatigue effect of 20 (R)-ginsenoside Rg3 in mice by intranasally administration. *Biol. Pharm. Bull.* **2008**, *31*, 2024–2027. [CrossRef] [PubMed]
6. Kang, O.-J.; Kim, J.-S. Comparison of Ginsenoside Contents in Different Parts of Korean Ginseng (*Panax ginseng* C.A. Meyer). *Prev. Nutr. Food Sci.* **2016**, *21*, 389–392. [CrossRef] [PubMed]
7. Shi, W.; Wang, Y.T.; Li, J.; Zhang, H.Q.; Ding, L. Investigation of ginsenosides in different parts and ages of *Panax ginseng*. *Food Chem.* **2007**, *102*, 664–668. [CrossRef]
8. Lee, J.W.; Choi, B.-R.; Kim, Y.-C.; Choi, D.J.; Lee, Y.-S.; Kim, G.-S.; Baek, N.-I.; Kim, S.-Y.; Lee, D.Y. Comprehensive Profiling and Quantification of Ginsenosides in the Root, Stem, Leaf, and Berry of *Panax ginseng* by UPLC-QTOF/MS. *Molecules* **2017**, *22*, 2147. [CrossRef]
9. Attele, A.S.; Zhou, Y.P.; Xie, J.T.; Wu, J.A.; Zhang, L.; Dey, L.; Pugh, W.; Rue, P.A.; Polonsky, K.S.; Yuan, C.S. Antidiabetic effects of *Panax ginseng* berry extract and the identification of an effective component. *Diabetes* **2002**, *51*, 1851–1858. [CrossRef] [PubMed]
10. Jang, H.J.; Han, I.H.; Kim, Y.J.; Yamabe, N.; Lee, D.; Hwang, G.S.; Oh, M.; Choi, K.C.; Kim, S.N.; Ham, J.; et al. Anticarcinogenic Effects of Products of Heat-Processed Ginsenoside Re, a Major Constituent of Ginseng Berry, on Human Gastric Cancer Cells. *J. Agric. Food Chem.* **2014**, *62*, 2830–2836. [CrossRef]
11. Mehendale, S.; Aung, H.; Wang, A.; Yin, J.-J.; Wang, C.-Z.; Xie, J.-T.; Yuan, C.-S. American ginseng berry extract and ginsenoside Re attenuate cisplatin-induced kaolin intake in rats. *Cancer Chemother. Pharmacol.* **2005**, *56*, 63–69. [CrossRef] [PubMed]
12. Xie, J.-T.; Shao, Z.-H.; Vanden Hoek, T.L.; Chang, W.-T.; Li, J.; Mehendale, S.; Wang, C.-Z.; Hsu, C.-W.; Becker, L.B.; Yin, J.-J.; et al. Antioxidant effects of ginsenoside Re in cardiomyocytes. *Eur. J. Pharmacol.* **2006**, *532*, 201–207. [CrossRef] [PubMed]
13. Dey, L.; Xie, J.T.; Wang, A.; Wu, J.; Maleckar, S.A.; Yuan, C.-S. Anti-hyperglycemic effects of ginseng: Comparison between root and berry. *Phytomedicine* **2003**, *10*, 600–605. [CrossRef] [PubMed]
14. Xie, J.-T.; Du, G.-J.; McEntee, E.; Aung, H.H.; He, H.; Mehendale, S.R.; Wang, C.-Z.; Yuan, C.-S. Effects of Triterpenoid Glycosides from Fresh Ginseng Berry on SW480 Human Colorectal Cancer Cell Line. *Cancer Res. Treat.* **2011**, *43*, 49–55. [CrossRef] [PubMed]
15. Shao, Z.-H.; Xie, J.-T.; Vanden Hoek, T.L.; Mehendale, S.; Aung, H.; Li, C.-Q.; Qin, Y.; Schumacker, P.T.; Becker, L.B.; Yuan, C.-S. Antioxidant effects of American ginseng berry extract in cardiomyocytes exposed to acute oxidant stress. *BBA-Gen. Subj.* **2004**, *1670*, 165–171. [CrossRef] [PubMed]
16. Lee, S.Y.; Kim, Y.K.; Park, N.I.; Kim, C.S.; Lee, C.Y.; Park, S.U. Chemical constituents and biological activities of the berry of *Panax ginseng*. *J. Med. Plants Res.* **2010**, *4*, 349–353.
17. Wang, C.-Z.; Wu, J.A.; MCENTEE, E.; Yuan, C.-S. Saponins Composition in American Ginseng Leaf and Berry Assayed by High-Performance Liquid Chromatography. *J. Agric. Food Chem.* **2006**, *54*, 2261–2266. [CrossRef]
18. Kim, S.N.; Ha, Y.W.; Shin, H.; Son, S.H.; Wu, S.J.; Kim, Y.S. Simultaneous quantification of 14 ginsenosides in *Panax ginseng* CA Meyer (Korean red ginseng) by HPLC-ELSD and its application to quality control. *J. Pharm. Biomed.* **2007**, *45*, 164–170. [CrossRef]
19. Mao, Q.; Bai, M.; Xu, J.-D.; Kong, M.; Zhu, L.-Y.; Zhu, H.; Wang, Q.; Li, S.-L. Discrimination of leaves of *Panax ginseng* and *P. quinquefolius* by ultra-high performance liquid chromatography quadrupole/time-of-flight mass spectrometry based metabolomics approach. *J. Pharm. Biomed. Anal.* **2014**, *97*, 129–140. [CrossRef]
20. Xie, G.X.; Ni, Y.; Su, M.M.; Zhang, Y.Y.; Zhao, A.H.; Gao, X.F.; Liu, Z.; Xiao, P.G.; Jia, W. Application of ultra-performance LC-TOF MS metabolite profiling techniques to the analysis of medicinal *Panax* herbs. *Metabolomics* **2008**, *4*, 248–260. [CrossRef]
21. Alam, T.M.; Jenkins, J.E. HR-MAS NMR spectroscopy in material science. In *Advanced Aspects of Spectroscopy*; IntechOpen: London, UK, 2012; pp. 279–306.
22. Mun, J.-H.; Lee, H.; Yoon, D.; Kim, B.-S.; Kim, M.-B.; Kim, S. Discrimination of Basal Cell Carcinoma from Normal Skin Tissue Using High-Resolution Magic Angle Spinning ^{1}H NMR Spectroscopy. *PLoS ONE* **2016**, *11*, e0150328. [CrossRef] [PubMed]

23. Raja, G.; Kim, S.; Yoon, D.; Yoon, C.; Kim, S. ^{1}H-NMR-based Metabolomics Studies of the Toxicity of Mesoporous Carbon Nanoparticles in Zebrafish (*Danio rerio*). *Bull. Korean. Chem. Soc.* **2017**, *38*, 271–277. [CrossRef]
24. Sedgwick, P. Pearson's correlation coefficient. *BMJ* **2012**, *345*, e4483. [CrossRef]
25. Schober, P.; Boer, C.; Schwarte, L.A. Correlation coefficients: Appropriate use and interpretation. *Anesth. Analg.* **2018**, *126*, 1763–1768. [CrossRef] [PubMed]
26. Vickers, C.E.; Williams, T.C.; Peng, B.; Cherry, J. Recent advances in synthetic biology for engineering isoprenoid production in yeast. *Curr. Opin. Chem. Biol.* **2017**, *40*, 47–56. [CrossRef]
27. Ward, J.M.; Kühn, C.; Tegeder, M.; Frommer, W.B. Sucrose transport in higher plants. *Int. Rev. Cytol.* **1997**, *178*, 41–71.
28. Falasca, A.; Melck, D.; Paris, D.; Saviano, G.; Motta, A.; Iorizzi, M. Seasonal changes in the metabolic fingerprint of *Juniperus communis* L. berry extracts by ^{1}H NMR-based metabolomics. *Metabolomics* **2014**, *10*, 165–174. [CrossRef]
29. Loewus, F.A.; Murthy, P.P. myo-Inositol metabolism in plants. *Plant Sci.* **2000**, *150*, 1–19. [CrossRef]
30. Cho, W.C.; Chung, W.S.; Lee, S.K.; Leung, A.W.; Cheng, C.H.; Yue, K.K. Ginsenoside Re of Panax ginseng possesses significant antioxidant and antihyperlipidemic efficacies in streptozotocin-induced diabetic rats. *Eur. J. Pharmacol.* **2006**, *550*, 173–179. [CrossRef]
31. Liu, Y.W.; Zhu, X.; Li, W.; Lu, Q.; Wang, J.Y.; Wei, Y.Q.; Yin, X.X. Ginsenoside Re attenuates diabetes-associated cognitive deficits in rats. *Pharmacol. Biochem. Behav.* **2012**, *101*, 93–98. [CrossRef]
32. Zhang, Z.; Li, X.; Lv, W.; Yang, Y.; Gao, H.; Yang, J.; Gao, H.; Yang, J.; Shen, Y.; Ning, G. Ginsenoside Re reduces insulin resistance through inhibition of c-Jun NH2-terminal kinase and nuclear factor-κB. *Mol. Endocrinol.* **2008**, *22*, 186–195. [CrossRef] [PubMed]
33. Meng, X.; Wang, M.; Wang, X.; Sun, G.; Ye, J.; Xu, H.; Sun, X. Suppression of NADPH oxidase-and mitochondrion-derived superoxide by Notoginsenoside R1 protects against cerebral ischemia?reperfusion injury through estrogen receptor-dependent activation of Akt/Nrf2 pathways. *Free Radic. Res.* **2014**, *48*, 823–838. [CrossRef] [PubMed]
34. Meng, X.; Sun, G.; Ye, J.; Xu, H.; Wang, H.; Sun, X. Notoginsenoside R1-mediated neuroprotection involves estrogen receptor-dependent crosstalk between Akt and ERK1/2 pathways: A novel mechanism of Nrf2/ARE signaling activation. *Free Radic. Res.* **2014**, *48*, 445–460. [CrossRef] [PubMed]
35. Zhai, Y.; Meng, X.; Luo, Y.; Wu, Y.; Ye, T.; Zhou, P.; Ding, S.; Wang, M.; Lu, S.; Zhu, L.; et al. Notoginsenoside R1 ameliorates diabetic encephalopathy by activating the Nrf2 pathway and inhibiting NLRP3 inflammasome activation. *Oncotarget* **2018**, *9*, 9344. [CrossRef] [PubMed]
36. Meng, X.B.; Sun, G.B.; Wang, M.; Sun, J.; Qin, M.; Sun, X.B. P90RSK and Nrf2 activation via MEK1/2-ERK1/2 pathways mediated by notoginsenoside R2 to prevent 6-hydroxydopamine-induced apoptotic death in SH-SY5Y cells. *Evid. Based Complement. Altern.* **2013**, *2013*, 1–15. [CrossRef] [PubMed]
37. Chen, X.C.; Zhu, Y.G.; Zhu, L.A.; Huang, C.; Chen, Y.; Chen, L.M.; Fang, F.; Zhou, Y.C.; Zhao, C.H. Ginsenoside Rg1 attenuates dopamine-induced apoptosis in PC12 cells by suppressing oxidative stress. *Eur. J. Pharmacol.* **2003**, *473*, 1–7. [CrossRef]
38. Chen, X.C.; Zhou, Y.C.; Chen, Y.; Zhu, Y.G.; Fang, F.; Chen, L.M. Ginsenoside Rg1 reduces MPTP-induced substantia nigra neuron loss by suppressing oxidative stress 1. *Acta Pharmacol. Sin.* **2005**, *26*, 56–62. [CrossRef] [PubMed]
39. Jung, J.S.; Ahn, J.H.; Le, T.K.; Kim, D.H.; Kim, H.S. Protopanaxatriol ginsenoside Rh1 inhibits the expression of matrix metalloproteinases and the in vitro invasion/migration of human astroglioma cells. *Neurochem. Int.* **2013**, *63*, 80–86. [CrossRef] [PubMed]
40. Jung, J.S.; Kim, D.H.; Kim, H.S. Ginsenoside Rh1 suppresses inducible nitric oxide synthase gene expression in IFN-γ-stimulated microglia via modulation of JAK/STAT and ERK signaling pathways. *Biochem. Biophys. Res. Commun.* **2010**, *397*, 323–328. [CrossRef] [PubMed]
41. Gai, Y.; Ma, Z.; Yu, X.; Qu, S.; Sui, D. Effect of ginsenoside Rh1 on myocardial injury and heart function in isoproterenol-induced cardiotoxicity in rats. *Toxicol. Mech. Method* **2012**, *22*, 584–591. [CrossRef] [PubMed]
42. Yu, Y.; Sun, G.; Luo, Y.; Wang, M.; Chen, R.; Zhang, J.; Ai, Q.; Xing, N.; Sun, X. Cardioprotective effects of Notoginsenoside R1 against ischemia/reperfusion injuries by regulating oxidative stress-and endoplasmic reticulum stress-related signaling pathways. *Sci. Rep.-UK* **2016**, *6*, 21730. [CrossRef] [PubMed]

43. Zhong, L.; Zhou, X.L.; Liu, Y.S.; Wang, Y.M.; Ma, F.; Guo, B.L.; Yan, Z.Q.; Zhang, Q.Y. Estrogen receptor α mediates the effects of notoginsenoside R1 on endotoxin-induced inflammatory and apoptotic responses in H9c2 cardiomyocytes. *Mol. Med. Rep.* **2015**, *12*, 119–126. [CrossRef] [PubMed]
44. Ge, Z.R.; Xu, M.C.; Huang, Y.U.; Zhang, C.J.; Lin, J.E.; Ruan, C.W. Cardioprotective effect of notoginsenoside R1 in a rabbit lung remote ischemic postconditioning model via activation of the TGF? β1/TAK1 signaling pathway. *Exp. Ther. Med.* **2016**, *11*, 2341–2348. [CrossRef] [PubMed]
45. Lee, H.; Gonzalez, F.J.; Yoon, M. Ginsenoside Rf, a component of ginseng, regulates lipoprotein metabolism through peroxisome proliferator-activated receptor α. *Biochem. Biophys. Res. Commun.* **2006**, *339*, 196–203. [CrossRef] [PubMed]

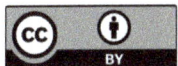

© 2019 by the authors. Licensee MDPI, Basel, Switzerland. This article is an open access article distributed under the terms and conditions of the Creative Commons Attribution (CC BY) license (http://creativecommons.org/licenses/by/4.0/).

MDPI
St. Alban-Anlage 66
4052 Basel
Switzerland
Tel. +41 61 683 77 34
Fax +41 61 302 89 18
www.mdpi.com

Biomolecules Editorial Office
E-mail: biomolecules@mdpi.com
www.mdpi.com/journal/biomolecules

www.ingramcontent.com/pod-product-compliance
Lightning Source LLC
LaVergne TN
LVHW070456100526
838202LV00014B/1734